Health Economics of Well-being and Well-becoming across the Life-course

Health Economics of Well-being and Well-becoming across the Life-course

Edited By

Rhiannon T. Edwards

Professor of Health Economics, Centre for Health Economics
and Medicines Evaluation (CHEME), School of Health
Sciences, Bangor University, UK

Catherine L. Lawrence

Research Officer, Centre for Health Economics and Medicines
Evaluation (CHEME), School of Health Sciences, Bangor
University, UK

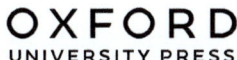

OXFORD
UNIVERSITY PRESS

OXFORD
UNIVERSITY PRESS

Great Clarendon Street, Oxford, OX2 6DP,
United Kingdom

Oxford University Press is a department of the University of Oxford.
It furthers the University's objective of excellence in research, scholarship,
and education by publishing worldwide. Oxford is a registered trade mark of
Oxford University Press in the UK and in certain other countries

Published in the United States of America by Oxford University Press
198 Madison Avenue, New York, NY 10016, United States of America

British Library Cataloguing in Publication Data
Data available

Library of Congress Control Number 2024938219

ISBN 9780192896964

DOI: 10.1093/9780191919336.001.0001

Printed and bound by
CPI Group (UK) Ltd, Croydon, CR0 4YY

Oxford University Press makes no representation, express or implied,
that the drug dosages in this book are correct. Readers must therefore always check
the product information and clinical procedures with the most up-to-date
published product information and data sheets provided by the manufacturers
and the most recent codes of conduct and safety regulations. The authors and
the publishers do not accept responsibility or legal liability for any errors in the
text or for the misuse or misapplication of material in this work. Except where
otherwise stated, drug dosages and recommendations are for the non-pregnant
adult who is not breast-feeding

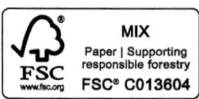

'With stout hearts may we see in every calamity an opportunity, and not give way to the pessimism that sees in every opportunity a calamity.'

Peter Marshall
(Lived 1902–1949; Chaplain of the United States Senate)

Contents

Preface

To write a book entitled *Health Economics of Well-being and Well-becoming across the Life-course* at a time in the United Kingdom (UK) when life-expectancy is falling and many are facing unprecedented economic and health challenges may seem strange. It is a book written with hope. This is not perhaps the most traditional of academic books. It is wide-ranging and, by definition, a normative venture. Having completed it, I still believe the idea of the book to be very important and the way we should shape future health economics research and approach wider evidence-based public policy with respect to the prevention of avoidable ill-health, disability, and premature death.

This book was written during 2020 to 2023. These were extraordinary years for all living through the experience of the coronavirus disease 2019 (COVID-19) pandemic. As the original sole editor, I had planned the book and agreed its content with Oxford University Press prior to the COVID-19 pandemic. However, watching our society grapple with the ethical and economic challenges of the pandemic noticeably sharpened my reasons for editing and writing this book with colleagues, and I found that the content of the book needed to reference early lessons from the pandemic. The pandemic has widened the gulf between the wealthy and the poor, often along ethnicity lines, made stark by the Black Lives Matter movement. The pandemic has made clear what is 'good work' and 'bad work' for people and made stark the unequal division of labour in the home that still prevails. The pandemic has shown us the need for a gender lens in the analysis of data in medical and health services research. What is interesting to consider is what we mean by 'health' and what we mean by 'well-being', and the way many people through the pandemic have re-evaluated what is really important in their lives.

Increasingly we hear reference to the term 'well-being', but we do not often talk about 'well-becoming', that is, how we create opportunities for the individual and groups in society to grow and flourish in later stages of life. Fifty per cent of mental health problems, such as depression, anxiety, eating disorders, substance abuse disorders, and psychosis, emerge before the age of fourteen years and 75 per cent by age twenty-four (Blakemore, 2019; Kessler et al., 2005). Likewise, the lifestyle choices we make in our fifties determine how we age and whether we age well (Cavendish, 2019).

As health economists will be aware, the National Institute for Health and Care Excellence (NICE) has a threshold of £20,000 to £30,000 per quality-adjusted life year (QALY). This threshold is based on a now questioned view on what society should and should not be prepared to spend to produce an additional statistical healthy year of life. Having worked with this reference point as a professor of health economics, I stood incredulous as all budget boundaries evaporated in front of our eyes in meeting and dealing with the wider health costs and costs to the economy of the COVID-19 pandemic. If we were to spend one-tenth of what we spent on the pandemic in a concerted effort to improve general health and well-being across the life-course, what could we achieve and what pressure could we potentially take off the UK National Health Service (NHS) and social care services? In hindsight, we are now far more able to judge and evaluate the relative costs and benefits to our society and the economy of the path taken, mandatory lockdowns, and ceasing all planned health care, leaving capacity to meet the new and poorly understood demands of the pandemic. More people will have died from not receiving necessary care than from COVID-19. People's lives are being affected by the long NHS waiting lists, partly a result of the COVID-19 pandemic, but also a decade of austerity and Brexit. These budget boundaries are now back with a vengeance as we face a cost of living crisis, unprecedented heating and fuel costs, in part a result of the war in Ukraine. We are learning to live alongside new variants of COVID-19. We will need more than ever evidence of 'value for money' in terms of public, private, and voluntary sector spending, promoting health and well-being and managing demand on overstretched NHS and social care systems. Sadly, a need to re-pay government borrowing accrued during the pandemic may make policy horizons very short, cure taking priority over prevention. Prior to the pandemic, only 5 per cent of the NHS budget was spent on prevention (Office for National Statistics, 2020, 2021; Faculty of Public Health, 2019). Prevention involves 'co-production' between us as individuals and health and other services, and many opportunities for prevention of ill-health and disability in society lie in government policy, the hands of local planners, employers, schools, and those custodians of our natural environment. We need to make available more comparative evidence of the cost-effectiveness or value for money of spending on prevention to redress the cure-prevention imbalance. To this end, this book is a call to arms to fellow health economists to pick up this admittedly normative challenge, improve the way we undertake economic evaluation of preventative interventions, and get the evidence out there on both health and well-being and on well-becoming.

Coming to the end of editing this book, and reading other books that have been published in this area, I realize that 'context is everything'. I am undoubtably one of Paul Dolan's 'middle class folk', as he points out in his book *Happy ever after*, and am aware that many people face life circumstances that make co-production of better health extremely challenging (Dolan, 2019). I also am acutely aware of the challenge or potential accusation of 'confirmation bias', that is, presenting evidence that bolsters our view of the world, about what is, and what should be. However, I think it is worth risking a bit of confirmation bias to move health economists towards the 'well-being' end of the 'health and well-being' spectrum.

This book unapologetically blurs boundaries between conventional academic health economics, educational economics, and labour economics. I think advances in behavioural economics hold huge promise in the design of future effective and cost-effective public health and preventative interventions to promote health and well-being. The examples of cost-effectiveness studies drawn from these four fields, amongst others, are exactly that: illustrative examples. It would not be possible to apply systematic reviewing methodology across the breadth of the life-course approach we have taken. We have made the most use we can of published systematic reviews pertaining to each chapter of the book. As first editor, I find myself very much aligned with the precautionary principle agenda that combines gold standard evidence from randomized controlled trials (RCTs) with evidence from prior beliefs, based on theory, observation, and experience, for example, natural experiments (Skivington et al., 2021; Deidda et al., 2019; Edwards & McIntosh, 2019; Fischer & Ghelardi, 2016). This basic set of beliefs is updated as new evidence becomes available. This is indeed what we have all lived with in terms of how the UK Government and governments internationally have responded to the COVID-19 pandemic. At the same time, there is a need to be conscious of heuristics that guide our thinking and expectations. As health economists working in the field of public health we appreciate the importance of robust, unbiased evidence, but also an openness to learn from natural experiments, international case studies, and expert patient or public opinion, to support policy and funding decisions about the use of scarce resources. Sometimes in public health the questions at a population level have to be:

- If this is a low-cost public health intervention, universal or targeted with reach (e.g. giving out toothbrushes and toothpaste to all children through primary schools to combat dental caries in young children and the associated avoidable costs to the NHS of extraction), is this likely to do any harm?
- Is this good value for money at a population level?
- How does the effectiveness and cost-effectiveness of these interventions vary from context to context, or geographical or socioeconomic setting to setting?

- What is the opportunity cost of using these resources to meet this need?
- Could we use them to better effect in another way to achieve our objective?
- Beyond the immediate life-course stage, what is the potential for the intervention to have a knock-on effect into subsequent life-course stages?

We offer examples of evidence at each life-course stage, not to be prescriptive, but to show in some way the magnitude of benefits that might be generated by investing in programmes to improve well-being and well-becoming in future life-course stages where this evidence exists, and how health economists and health services researchers more widely are attempting to capture relative costs and benefits and understand the processes involved. We also try to highlight the costs of 'not acting', the huge social costs that are, at least in theory, preventable through early intervention. By organizing the book in this way, I hope we will encourage the reader to apply a 'life-course lens' when, traditionally, NHS budgets and the way we evaluate cost-effectiveness of different health technologies in no way encourages us to do this (i.e. think across the life-course).

This book was planned around life-course stages: from birth and the early years, through to adolescence, through to working-age (which is also largely a parenting and caring stage of life), through to early or late retirement and later life, and death. This was akin to the 'Ages of man' monologue of the character Jaques in Shakespeare's play *As you like it*. We are all different and our life paths are all different, but thinking in this way may help the UK Government and those who are in a position to fund and commission services, large or small, national or local, to tip the balance between prevention and treatment across the life-course, and in this way, over time, improve the well-being and well-becoming chances of us all. I have always wondered why the NHS budgets are defined by clinical departments and services rather than thinking about how much of the budget is spent on different age groups through the life-course with a view to moving from cure to prevention in an overstretched service. This is why I was so taken by the Office for Budget Responsibility (OBR; 2022) graph of public spending on education, health, adult social care, tax, and welfare (see Figure 1.7 in Chapter 1). Internationally, we currently spend between 13 per cent and 25 per cent of lifetime spend on health care during the last year of life (Dolan, 2021). In this sense we need to 'shift the curve' of public spending from the end of life to the early years on efficiency and equity grounds, as is explored in this book and illustrated in our infographic (see Figure 3.3 in Chapter 3).

In terms of a readership, I hope, as first editor, that this book is first and foremost of interest to fellow health economists working in the evaluation of public health interventions and thinking about health, well-being, and well-becoming. It may be that this book is also a useful textbook for postgraduate students on public health, health economics, population health or prevention science courses. It is hoped that this book will be of interest to a wider readership from public health practitioners, policymakers, through to those on the ground working in the NHS, social care, and voluntary sector, to improve well-being and well-becoming in society. It should also be on the reading list of every undergraduate medical course.

The final chapter of this book opens up an agenda for diversifying health economics as a discipline in order to meet the need for evidence to support public policy. Diversification means more attention on both the Global South as well as the Global North. Diversification means further interdisciplinary working across subdisciplines of economics along with other relevant fields. The overarching direction of research needs to be within the context of sustainability and climate change.

I want to thank all the contributors to the chapters of this book, many of whom are my colleagues at the Centre for Health Economics and Medicines Evaluation (CHEME) at Bangor University, some of whom were my PhD students and postdoctoral researchers, and are going on to achieve great things. I want to thank my co-editor, Dr Catherine Lawrence, who has brought her psychology and coaching background and experience to the development of this book. I want to thank the Welsh Government through Health and Care Research Wales for infrastructure funding that made some of the time spent on this book possible. I want to thank Public Health Wales for giving permission for the three reports we produced for them to be updated and incorporated into this book (Edwards et al., 2016, 2018, 2019). I want to thank my husband, Paul Gash, for his unwavering support to me. I would also like to thank my mother, Eleri, and children, William and Non. Finally, Bailey, my German Shepherd guide dog should get a mention.

Rhiannon T. Edwards

References

Blakemore, S. J. (2019). Adolescence and mental health. *The Lancet*, **393**(10185), 2030–2031. https://doi.org/10.1016/S0140-6736(19)31013-X

Cavendish, C. (2019). *Extra time: 10 lessons for an ageing world*. Harper Collins.

Deidda, M., Geue, C., Kreif, N., Dundas, R., & McIntosh, E. (2019). A framework for conducting economic evaluations alongside natural experiments. *Social Science & Medicine*, **220**, 353–361. https://doi.org/10.1016/j.socscimed.2018.11.032

Dolan, P. (2019). *Happy ever after: A radical new approach to living well*. Penguin Random House UK.

Dolan, P. (2021). *Policymakers should focus healthcare more on achieving wellbeing over whole lifetimes*. The London School of Economics and Political Science. https://blogs.lse.ac.uk/politicsandpolicy/healthcare-wellbeing/

Edwards, R. T., Bryning, L., & Lloyd-Williams, H. (2016). *Transforming young lives across Wales: The economic argument for investing in early years.* Centre for Health Economics and Medicines Evaluation, Bangor University. https://cheme.bangor.ac.uk/documents/transforming-young-lives/CHEME%20transforming%20Young%20Lives%20Full%20Report%20Eng%20WEB%202.pdf

Edwards, R. T., & McIntosh, E. (Eds.). (2019). *Applied health economics for public health practice and research.* Oxford University Press.

Edwards, R. T., Spencer, L. H., Anthony, B. F., & Bryning, L. (2019). *Wellness in work: The economic arguments for investing in the health and wellbeing of the workforce in Wales.* Centre for Health Economics and Medicines Evaluation, Bangor University. https://cheme.bangor.ac.uk/documents/Wellness-in-Work-Report.pdf

Edwards, R. T., Spencer, L. H., Bryning, L., & Anthony, B. F. (2018). *Living well for longer: The economic argument for investing in the health and wellbeing of older people in Wales.* Centre for Health Economics and Medicines Evaluation, Bangor University. https://cheme.bangor.ac.uk/documents/livingwell2018.pdf

Faculty of Public Health. (2019). *What the NHS thinks about prevention.* https://www.fph.org.uk/media/2515/fph-what-the-nhs-thinks-about-prevention-final.pdf

Fischer, A. J., & Ghelardi, G. (2016). The precautionary principle, evidence-based medicine, and decision theory in public health evaluation. *Frontiers in Public Health, 7*(4), 107. https://doi.org/10.3389/fpubh.2016.00107

Kessler, R. C., Berglund, P., Demler, O., Jin, R., Merikangas, K. R., & Walters, E. E. (2005). Lifetime prevalence and age-of-onset distributions of DSM-IV disorders in the National Comorbidity Survey Replication. *Archives of General Psychiatry, 62*(6), 593–602. https://doi.org/10.1001/archpsyc.62.6.593

Office for Budget Responsibility. (2022, July). *Fiscal risks and sustainability.* CP702. UK Government. https://obr.uk/docs/dlm_uploads/Fiscal_risks_and_sustainability_2022-1.pdf

Office for National Statistics. (2020). *Healthcare expenditure, UK Health Accounts: 2018.* https://www.ons.gov.uk/peoplepopulationandcommunity/healthandsocialcare/healthcaresystem/bulletins/ukhealthaccounts/2018

Office for National Statistics. (2021). *Healthcare expenditure, UK Health Accounts: 2019.* https://www.ons.gov.uk/peoplepopulationandcommunity/healthandsocialcare/healthcaresystem/bulletins/ukhealthaccounts/2019

Skivington, K., Matthews, L., Simpson, S. A., Craig, P., Baird, J., Blazeby, J. M., Boyd, K. A., Craig, N., French, D. P., McIntosh, E., Petticrew, M., Rycroft-Malone, J., White, M., & Moore, L. (2021). A new framework for developing and evaluating complex interventions: Update of Medical Research Council guidance. *BMJ, 374*(2061), 1–11. http://dx.doi.org/10.1136/bmj.n2061

List of Contributors

Bethany F. Anthony, PhD is Research Officer, Centre for Health Economics and Medicines Evaluation, Bangor University, Bangor, United Kingdom. https://orcid.org/0000-0002-2593-1069

Nathan Bray, PhD is Senior Lecturer, Academy for Health Equity, Prevention and Wellbeing, Bangor University, Bangor, United Kingdom. https://orcid.org/0000-0001-7646-5435

Lucy Bryning, PhD is Lecturer in Health Sciences, Bangor University, Bangor, United Kingdom. https://orcid.org/0000-0002-9076-4682

Joanna Charles, PhD is Research Fellow in Health Economics, Centre for Health Economics and Medicines Evaluation, Bangor University, Bangor, United Kingdom. https://orcid.org/0000-0002-5306-3887

Rhiannon T. Edwards, DPhil is Professor of Health Economics and Co-director of the Centre for Health Economics and Medicines Evaluation, Bangor University, Bangor, United Kingdom. https://orcid.org/0000-0003-4748-5730

Victory Ezeofor, PhD is Mathematical/Statistical Modeller in Health Economics, Centre for Health Economics and Medicines Evaluation, Bangor University, Bangor, United Kingdom. https://orcid.org/0000-0002-4211-8942

Ned Hartfiel, PhD is Research Fellow in Public Health and Prevention Economics, School of Health Sciences, Bangor University, Bangor, United Kingdom. https://orcid.org/0000-0001-9976-4294

Catherine L. Lawrence, PhD is Research Officer, Centre for Health Economics and Medicines Evaluation, Bangor University, Bangor, United Kingdom. https://orcid.org/0000-0002-6453-4912

Huw Lloyd-Williams, PhD is Senior Consultant, Wavehill Limited, Aberaeron, United Kingdom.

Mary Lynch, PhD is Executive Vice Dean for Research, Faculty of Nursing and Midwifery, Royal College of Surgeons, Dublin, Ireland. https://orcid.org/0000-0001-6887-3447

Abraham Makanjuola, MscRes is Research Assistant, Faculty of Life Sciences and Education, University of South Wales, United Kingdom. https://orcid.org/0000-0002-9577-0424

Kalpa Pisavadia, MA is Research Project Support Officer, Centre for Health Economics and Medicines Evaluation, Bangor University, Bangor, United Kingdom. https://orcid.org/0000-0003-1435-163X

Llinos H. Spencer, PhD is Research Officer, Centre for Health Economics and Medicines Evaluation, Bangor University, Bangor, United Kingdom. https://orcid.org/0000-0002-7075-8015

Carys Stringer, PhD is Lecturer, School of Health Sciences, Bangor University, Bangor, United Kingdom. https://orcid.org/0000-0001-6159-1842

Alexander Torbuck, MSc is PhD candidate, University of Rochester, Rochester, United States.

Lorna Tuersley, PhD is Research Officer (retired), Centre for Health Economics and Medicines Evaluation, Bangor University, Bangor, United Kingdom. https://orcid.org/0000-0003-1780-258X

Eira Winrow, PhD is Lecturer, School of Health Sciences, Bangor University, Bangor, United Kingdom. https://orcid.org/0000-0002-1399-0651

Chapter 1

Introduction

Rhiannon T. Edwards, Catherine L. Lawrence,
Bethany F. Anthony, and Lucy Bryning

Health Economics—The Starting Point

Health economics is the study of how we use health and social care resources to meet our health care needs, or at least that is what it used to be about (Drummond et al., 2015; Edwards, 2001; Edwards & McIntosh, 2019; Morris et al., 2007). When we are now increasingly recognizing that so much of our health and well-being is determined by factors other than access to health care, and by policy and budget decisions beyond the health sector, there is an opportunity for some of us to re-appraise the task now facing health economists over the next two decades. Advances in behavioural economics and psychology, as well as systems thinking in economics more broadly, probably, as we stand today, have more to offer the agenda of improving population health and well-being than the traditional toolbox of economic evaluation. At a minimum, we need to re-appraise this toolbox, add to it and be ready to work in an interdisciplinary way with the above protagonists. On the one hand, we are meant to be 'dispassionate analysts' (Cookson & Claxton, 2012) and on the other, particularly those in the 'extra-welfarist' camp, take the normative view that greater health gain is preferable to less health gain for the population. The operationalization by health economists of this societal goal is potentially legitimized by research undertaken by the London School of Economics. A survey of nearly 13,000 people from the United Kingdom (UK) and United States (US) found that people preferred affective happiness (feeling good) over evaluative (life satisfaction) and eudaimonic (worthwhile-ness) components. They also found that individuals were willing to trade off levels of happiness by sacrificing income, physical health, family status, career success, and education. More respondents would prefer to be healthy than to be 'happy' (Adler et al., 2017). We think many health economists would also embrace the central tenet of public health, that is, that we should, as a society, be increasing the health of the worst off, or to put it another way, reducing

Rhiannon T. Edwards, Catherine L. Lawrence, Bethany F. Anthony, and Lucy Bryning, *Introduction* In: *Health Economics of Well-being and Well-becoming across the Life-course*. Edited by: Rhiannon T. Edwards and Catherine L. Lawrence, Oxford University Press. © Oxford University Press 2024. DOI: 10.1093/9780191919336.003.0001

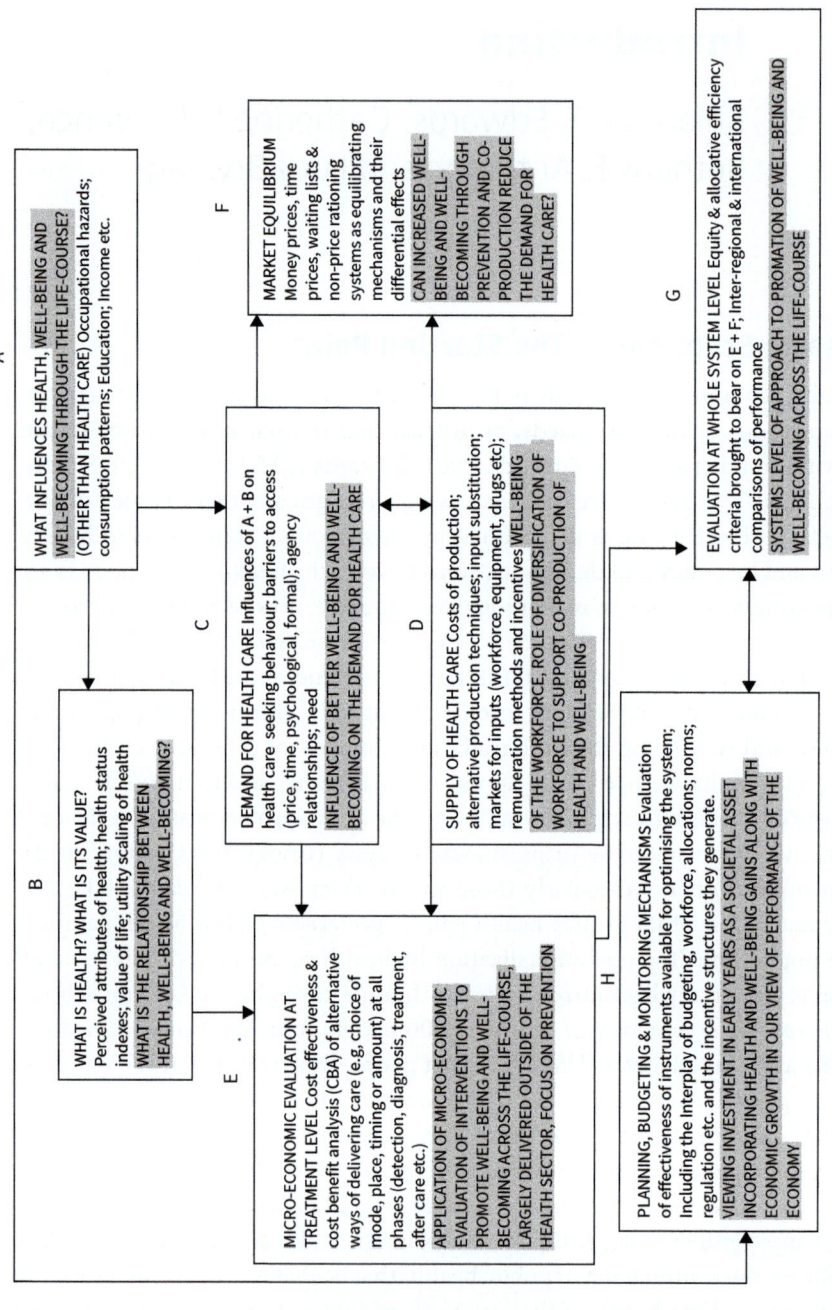

Figure 1.1 Incorporating well-being and well-becoming into health economics: The adapted plumbing diagram

Adapted from: Williams, A. (1987) *Health and economics. Proceedings of section F (economics) of the British Association for the Advancement of Science, Bristol, 1986.* Palgrave Macmillan. Reproduced with permission of Springer Nature Customer Service Center.

A

WHAT INFLUENCES HEALTH, WELL-BEING AND WELL-BECOMING THROUGH THE LIFE-COURSE? (OTHER THAN HEALTH CARE) Occupational hazards; consumption patterns; Education; Income etc.

B

WHAT IS HEALTH? WHAT IS ITS VALUE? Perceived attributes of health; health status indexes; value of life; utility scaling of health WHAT IS THE RELATIONSHIP BETWEEN HEALTH, WELL-BEING AND WELL-BECOMING?

C

DEMAND FOR HEALTH CARE Influences of A + B on health care seeking behaviour; barriers to access (price, time, psychological, formal); agency relationships; need INFLUENCE OF BETTER WELL-BEING AND WELL-BECOMING ON THE DEMAND FOR HEALTH CARE

D

SUPPLY OF HEALTH CARE Costs of production; alternative production techniques; input substitution; markets for inputs (workforce, equipment, drugs etc); remuneration methods and incentives WELL-BEING OF THE WORKFORCE, ROLE OF DIVERSIFICATION OF WORKFORCE TO SUPPORT CO-PRODUCTION OF HEALTH AND WELL-BEING

E

MICRO-ECONOMIC EVALUATION AT TREATMENT LEVEL Cost effectiveness & cost benefit analysis (CBA) of alternative ways of delivering care (e.g. choice of mode, place, timing or amount) at all phases (detection, diagnosis, treatment, after care etc.). APPLICATION OF MICRO-ECONOMIC EVALUATION OF INTERVENTIONS TO PROMOTE WELL-BEING AND WELL-BECOMING ACROSS THE LIFE-COURSE, LARGELY DELIVERED OUTSIDE OF THE HEALTH SECTOR, FOCUS ON PREVENTION

F

MARKET EQUILIBRIUM Money prices, time prices, waiting lists & non-price rationing systems as equilibrating mechanisms and their differential effects CAN INCREASED WELL-BEING AND WELL-BECOMING THROUGH PREVENTION AND CO-PRODUCTION REDUCE THE DEMAND FOR HEALTH CARE?

G

EVALUATION AT WHOLE SYSTEM LEVEL Equity & allocative efficiency criteria brought to bear on E + F; Inter-regional & international comparisons of performance SYSTEMS LEVEL OF APPROACH TO PROMATION OF WELL-BEING AND WELL-BECOMING ACROSS THE LIFE-COURSE

H

PLANNING, BUDGETING & MONITORING MECHANISMS Evaluation of effectiveness of instruments available for optimising the system; Including the interplay of budgeting, workforce, allocations; norms; regulation etc. and the incentive structures they generate. VIEWING INVESTMENT IN EARLY YEARS AS A SOCIETAL ASSET INCORPORATING HEALTH AND WELL-BEING GAINS ALONG WITH ECONOMIC GROWTH IN OUR VIEW OF PERFORMANCE OF THE ECONOMY inequalities in health. But this probably involves an 'efficiency-equity trade-off' (Cookson et al., 2020).

Alan Williams, influential health economist and one of the chapter co-author's PhD supervisors (Rhiannon T. Edwards), distinguished between health economics as a topic and health economics as a discipline (Mason & Towse, 2008; Williams, 1987). His famous plumbing diagram is reproduced in Figure 1.1 with added text showing where greater consideration of well-being and well-becoming through the life-course could fit into this schematic (see shaded text) (Williams, 1987).

Why This Book Is Extra Welfarist in Nature

Von Neumann and Morgenstern have a lot to answer for. Our whole approach to modern economics is built on the theory of what 'rational economic man' values, how his utility is 'individually judged', and that collective good is measured by adding up the utility of individuals. In all this, there is no verbalized concept of 'common good' or 'shared well-being or well-becoming', which evidence throughout this book points to being so important for societal happiness. On re-reading Anthony Culyer's (1989) seminal paper, *The normative economics of health care finance and provision*, it becomes clear that our book is essentially embedded in principles of extra-welfarism. Culyer defined extra-welfarism as transcending traditional welfare economics, specifically stating that 'it does not exclude individual welfare from the judgement about the social state, but it does supplement them with other aspects of individuals (including even the quality of the relationships between individuals, groups, and social classes)' (Culyer, 1989, p. 36). He supported the idea of adjusting the theoretical scheme to accommodate 'merit goods', for example, which we could identify today as health care, education, access to legal aid as of normative importance in a social welfare function. We would like to explicitly add to this list the societal prevention of avoidable ill-health, disability, and premature mortality (Culyer, 1989, p. 36).

Culyer raised the uncomfortable need to overrule individual judgements of value and raised the question of the weights to be attached to individual utilities in a social welfare function and of who should be assigning those weights. He asked, 'should the values of some members of society count for more than those of others?' (Culyer, 1989, p. 36). A similarly paternalistic (admittedly benevolent in intention) approach can be seen in Layard and Wards' book, *Can we be happier?: Evidence and ethics* (Layard & Ward, 2020; Seymour, 2020). Culyer acknowledged the cost-benefit analysis (CBA) based decision-making approach put forward by Sugden and Williams (1978), which challenged the Paretian optimality approach of welfare economics. This decision-making approach acknowledges that government and other decision-makers may have other objectives, which today we might view as collective societal value creation, well-being, or happiness. Culyer argued that a justification for an extra-welfarist approach in health economics is that, 'If the characteristics of people are a way of describing deprivation, desired states, or significant changes in people's characteristics, then commodities and characteristics of commodities are what is often needed to remove the deprivation or to move towards the desired state, or to help people cope with change' (Culyer, 1989, p. 50). He goes on to say, 'Since health services are needed only for what they enable to be accomplished, in a world of scarcity, judgements must be made about the value of what might be accomplished . . . . One of the first lessons of 'needology' is the lesson of the ethical acceptability of unmet need' (Culyer, 1989, p. 51).

Marmot: Ten Years On

'If health has stopped improving it is a sign that society has stopped improving'. (Marmot et al., 2020a, p. 5)

Health is determined by many factors including our genetic make-up. It is shaped by the multifaceted conditions in which we are born, grow, live, work, and age. These factors are influenced by broad social and economic circumstances known as the 'social determinants of health', which are predominantly accountable for health inequalities between and within countries (Marmot & Wilkinson, 2005). These health inequalities are not caused by chance; our health follows a social or class gradient whereby those living in a less advantaged situation have worse health and shorter lives than those living in a more advantaged situation in society (Buck & Maguire, 2015; Dolan, 2019; Marmot et al., 2010, 2020a). This phenomenon has been expressed as the 'Marmot curve', which plots healthy life expectancy against neighbourhood by income deprivation, showing that place or geographical region is overridingly important in determining this gradient (see Figure 1.2). This figure shows how health outcomes vary across different social gradients (Marmot et al., 2020a). While poverty negatively impacts health, the gradient highlights that health inequalities are more significant and far reaching. People living in poorer communities not only die sooner, but they also live more of their lives with chronic disease and disability.

The Marmot curve arose from the landmark 2010 Marmot review into health inequalities which proposed evidence-based strategies to address the social determinants of health in England (Marmot et al., 2010). The review estimated

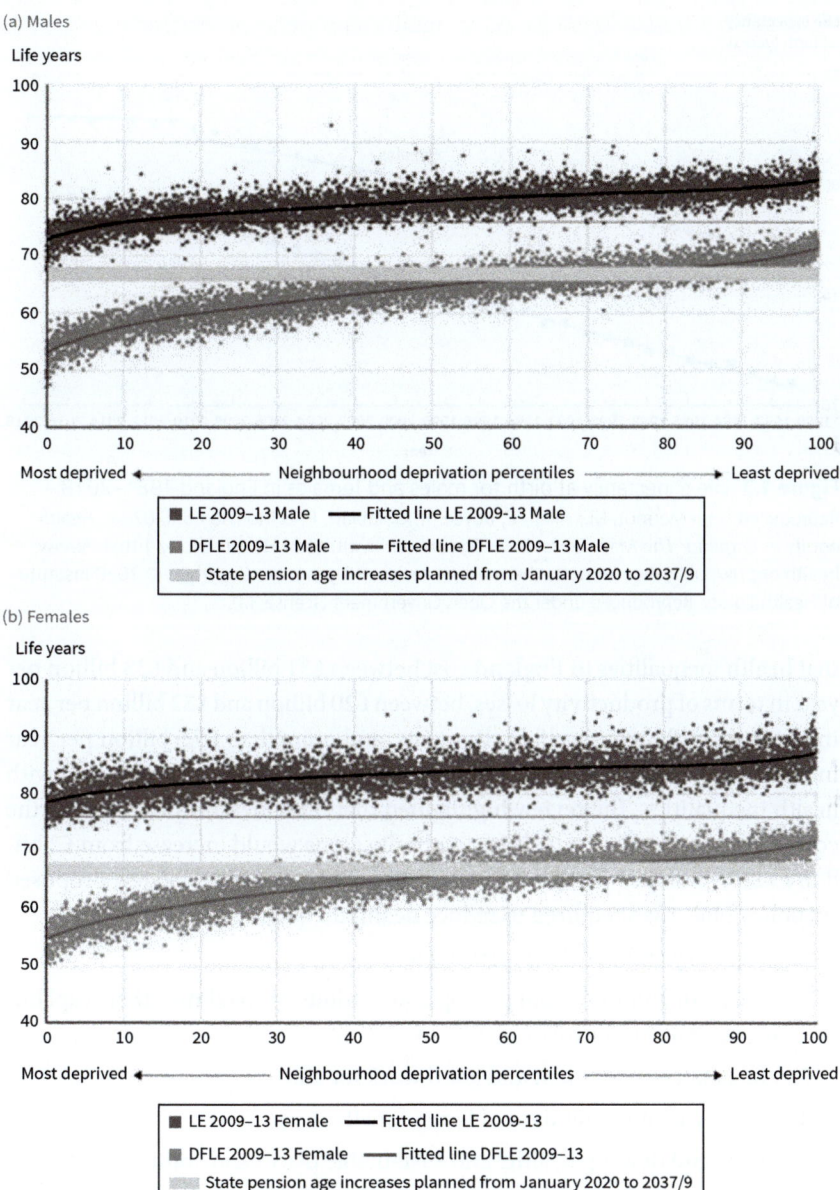

Note: Each dot represents life expectancy (LE) or disability-free life expectancy (DFLE) of a neighbourhood (middle level super output area)

Figure 1.2 The 'Marmot curve': Life expectancy and disability-free life expectancy at birth by neighbourhood deprivation percentiles in England 2009–2013

Reproduced from Marmot, M., Allen, J., Boyce, T., Goldblatt, P., & Morrison, J. (2020a). *Health equity in England: The Marmot review 10 years on*. Institute of Health Equity. https://www.hea lth.org.uk/publications/reports/the-marmot-review-10-years-on. Copyright © 2020 Institute of Health Equity. Reproduced under the Open Government License 3.0.

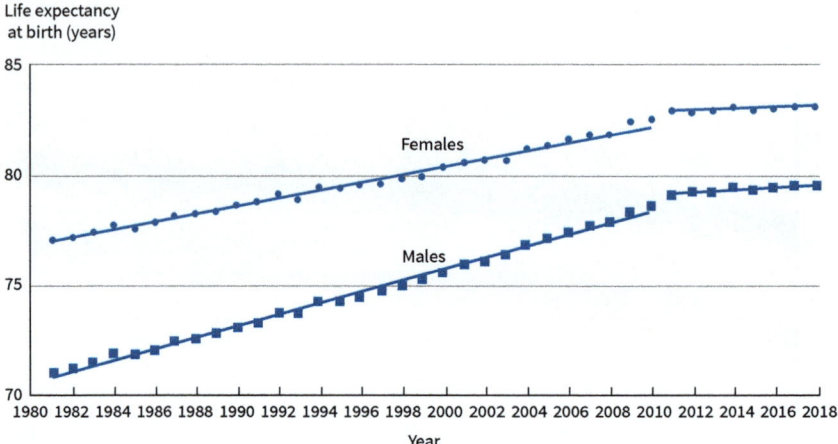

Figure 1.3 Life expectancy at birth for males and females in England 1981–2018
Reproduced from Marmot, M., Allen, J., Boyce, T., Goldblatt, P., & Morrison, J. (2020a). *Health equity in England: The Marmot review 10 years on*. Institute of Health Equity. https://www.health.org.uk/publications/reports/the-marmot-review-10-years-on. Copyright © 2020 Institute of Health Equity. Reproduced under the Open Government License 3.0.

that health inequalities in England cost between £31 billion and £33 billion per year in terms of productivity losses, between £20 billion and £32 billion per year in lost taxes and higher welfare payments, and more than £5.5 billion per year in additional National Health Service (NHS) health care costs associated with health inequalities. The review highlighted that if no measures were taken, the cost of treating health inequalities in obesity alone would increase from £2 billion to £5 billion per year by 2025 (Marmot et al., 2010). The review proposed six policy objectives required to reduce health inequalities:

1. give every child the best start in life;
2. enable all children, young people and adults to maximise their capabilities and have control over their lives;
3. create fair employment and good work for all;
4. ensure a healthy standard of living for all;
5. create and develop healthy and sustainable places and communities; and
6. strengthen the role and impact of ill-health prevention.

(Marmot et al., 2010, p. 15)

We have kept these policy objectives close in our minds in writing this book and in thinking about a future role of some health economists in providing evidence to enable the UK to achieve these policy goals.

In 2020, Marmot and colleagues published the report 'Health equity in England: The Marmot review 10 years on', which argued that after a decade of austerity, life expectancy has stopped increasing and ground down almost to a halt from 2011 (Marmot et al., 2020a). This is shown in Figure 1.3. Put into context, this compares with life expectancy having increased over the last ninety years in England by approximately one year every four years (Marmot et al., 2020a). More recent statistics suggest cohort life expectancy at birth in the UK is projected to increase by 2.8 years to reach 90.1 years for boys and by 2.4 years to 92.6 years for girls born in 2045. It is estimated that 13.6 per cent of boys and 19.0 per cent of girls born in 2020 will live to be at least one hundred years old. This percentage is expected to rise to 20.9 per cent for boys and 27.0 per cent for girls born in 2045 (Office for National Statistic (ONS), 2022).

The 2019 Coronavirus (COVID-19) Pandemic

This book was conceived prior to the COVID-19 pandemic in 2020. It was in recognition that we have historically spent far more on treating the outcome of poor health and disability than preventing it across the life-course. A virus that has claimed over 220,000 lives in the UK (UK Government, 2023), with deaths and long-COVID symptoms falling disproportionately heavily on poorer communities, people from ethnic minority backgrounds, and key workers has brought into stark relief the existing inequalities in society before the pandemic. School closures that were part of measures to stem the spread of COVID-19 have had a disproportionately catastrophic impact on the well-being of poor children and those living in homes affected by domestic violence. These experiences will have a lasting impact on this generation, with school exams cancelled, unequal access to online learning opportunities determined by access to computers and the internet, and whether there was any parental support.

The longer-term psychosocial consequences of the COVID-19 pandemic may be particularly prevalent in families with adverse childhood experiences (ACEs) (Roubinov et al., 2020). Highlighting the scientific evidence on the effectiveness and cost-effectiveness of early childhood interventions can aid in developing and implementing evidence-based practices that reduce risk and promote resilience within vulnerable families through the life-course and across generations. The trauma and unpredictability of the pandemic has likely added to the types, intensity, and duration of ACEs in the short term with life-long consequences (Roubinov et al., 2020). Known risk factors of ACEs, including parental unemployment, substance use, marital strain, and parent-child conflict (Cicchetti & Toth, 2005) were intensified during the pandemic and the series of lockdowns in the UK, the true impact of which is only beginning to emerge. Through the pandemic, children and parents with pre-existing mental health conditions did not have access to their usual treatments or support, and the availability of protective family routines may have been disrupted

(Roubinov et al., 2020). In contrast, there is some evidence that during times of crisis, some families can develop resilience, drawing on social support, religious or spiritual beliefs, and other coping strategies to maintain (or even increase) well-being (Masten, 2018). However, as time goes on, we are seeing the cracks in society that undoubtably widened through the pandemic.

Social and community networks play an important role in maintaining our health and well-being. Table 1.1 summarizes some of the key impacts of the COVID-19 pandemic on the social determinants of health and well-being (Health and Equity in Recovery Plans Working Group, 2020).

In 2019/2020, the UK Government borrowed £57 billion and was forecast to borrow £55 billion in 2020/2021. However, as a result of the COVID-19 pandemic, the actual amount borrowed in 2020/2021 was significantly higher at £313 billion. Money was spent on public services (such as the NHS), support for businesses, support for individuals, and schemes such as the Coronavirus Job Retention Scheme (the furlough scheme) and NHS Test and Trace (Brien & Keep, 2023). It felt as if traditional budget limits became limitless. Going forward, the cost-effectiveness of mediating policies and programmes will need to be assessed as we come out of these pandemic years, closely followed by a cost of living crisis that has hit the worst off in society hardest. It is difficult to see how, with a struggling NHS system and social care system, there can be the necessary emphasis in government spending on prevention rather than treatment and cure in future. Will there be more emphasis on well-being and well-becoming rather than treatment and cure? This remains to be seen and looks more and more doubtful with the cost of living crisis in the UK and many other countries, in part a result of the war in Ukraine. A report by the Organisation for Economic Co-operation and Development (OECD) called for an increased proportion internationally of gross domestic product (GDP) of around 1.4 per cent to be directed to funding prevention over and above treatment in health systems (Morgan & James, 2022). This is as a precaution of readiness in the event of another pandemic and in recognition of 80 per cent of chronic health problems, such as premature heart disease, stroke, and diabetes, being preventable (World Health Organization (WHO), 2005).

There has been an opportunity to view the COVID-19 pandemic as a natural experiment. Interventions deemed effective and cost-effective during the pandemic may or may not be effective and cost-effective in future years under normal circumstances. Whilst research in the fields of paediatrics, neuroscience, epigenetics, psychology, and public health can be used to understand the consequences of this pandemic, health economists can help provide evidence for interventions that are likely to be cost-effective to promote well-being and well-becoming in future. Online delivery of mental health support is a good example of innovations that have arisen or expanded during the pandemic which may be cost-effective in

Table 1.1 Summary of the key impacts of the COVID-19 pandemic on the social determinants of health and well-being

Impact	Type of impact	Likelihood of impact	Findings	Direction of cost savings or added costs to the public sector
Civic participation	Positive	Definite	Thousands of new volunteer groups established (Stansfield et al., 2020). Voluntary sector infrastructure reported receiving many offers of help.	⬇
Social cohesion	Positive	Possible	Majority of adults believe that the country will be more united and kinder once we have recovered from the pandemic (ONS, 2020a; All Party Parliamentary Group on Social Integration, 2020).	Unknown
Social isolation and loneliness	Negative	Probable	Well-being has been affected by the lockdown measures (ONS, 2020b). Young adults, women, people with lower education or income, the economically inactive, people living alone, and urban residents are most at risk of being lonely (Bu et al., 2020). Adults with disabilities are also identified as a group at particular risk of loneliness (ONS, 2020c, 2020d).	⬆
Family violence and abuse	Negative	Probable	Domestic and family violence increases following disasters (COVID-19 Critical Intelligence Unit, 2020; Peterman et al., 2020). Calls to domestic abuse helplines have increased during lockdown (Home Affairs Select Committee, 2020).	⬆
Social disorder	Unclear	Unclear	Robbery and serious assaults lower than in the same period in 2019 (Swann & Shaw, 2020). However, risk of criminal gangs recruiting young people out of school possibly increased (Children's Commissioner, 2020).	⬆

(continued)

Table 1.1 Continued

Impact	Type of impact	Likelihood of impact	Findings	Direction of cost savings or added costs to the public sector
Hidden safeguarding issues	Negative	Probable	Access to the safety net of support and supervision of professionals is reduced (Isba et al., 2020). Vulnerable children and families are likely to be missing out on vital support (Early Intervention Foundation, 2020; Local Government Association, 2020; Wilson & Waddell, 2020).	⬆

Adapted from the table in Health and Equity in Recovery Plans Working Group. (2020). *Direct and indirect impacts of COVID-19 on health and wellbeing.* https://www.ljmu.ac.uk/~/media/phi-reports/2020-07-direct-and-indirect-impacts-of-covid19-on-health-and-wellbeing.pdf

the long term (Richards et al., 2020). A systematic review of the evidence of the cost-effectiveness of mental health prevention and promotion interventions prior to the pandemic identified a significant growth in the economic evaluations on the prevention of mental disorders or promotion of mental health and well-being over the previous ten years (Le et al., 2021). Of the sixty-five included papers, twenty-three targeted children and adolescents, thirty-five targeted adults, and the remaining seven targeted older adults. There are undoubtably lessons to be learnt from the pandemic and we revisit the theme of mental health and well-being through subsequent chapters in this book.

The Dangers of an Austerity Policy

At the beginning of 2021, Angus Deaton, Nobel Prize winning economist, warned that austerity as a public policy instrument had been shown to fail. He warned that it should not be used in future as a means of repaying the enormous national debt that has built up due to the COVID-19 pandemic (Rajan, 2021). From 2008, a decade of austerity in the UK had a shattering impact on equality and health, which could have been avoided (Marmot et al., 2020a). In response to the global financial crisis in 2008, the UK Government rolled out an austerity programme that involved reductions in public spending and tax increases, which were implemented in the hope of controlling the government budget deficit. These measures have had devastating consequences and have prevented those who are most in need of help from receiving it (Roy, 2019). Although annual government borrowing decreased from £158.3 billion in 2009/2010 to

£38.4 billion in 2018/2019, the economy has now been temporarily hit once more by the COVID-19 pandemic (Eaton, 2020). The UK Government's gross debt was £2,516 billion at the end of 2022, equivalent to 101 per cent of GDP (ONS, 2023). In their updated report, Marmot and colleagues (2020a) stated that the social gradient and inequalities in life expectancy have increased. They appealed to the UK Government to deliver its assurance to reduce health inequalities for individuals living in the more deprived areas of the country in a bid to reverse the harm created during the ten years of austerity, compounded since then by the pandemic. Marmot and colleagues called for action to be taken to improve the lives of those who are relatively disadvantaged and for policies to 'level up' so that everyone can enjoy good health and well-being experienced by those at the top of the social hierarchy (Marmot et al., 2020a).

'Build Back Better' was the UK Government's strategy to recover from the damage caused by the COVID-19 pandemic by rethinking ways to support growth through investments in infrastructure, skills, and innovation, in order to pursue more inclusive, resilient, and environmentally friendly outcomes (HM Treasury, 2021a). Marmot and colleagues warned that our nation will not fully recover from the pandemic or adequately prepare for any future outbreaks unless the interaction between the biological and social determinants of COVID-19 are fully understood and represented (Marmot et al., 2020b). As outlined in the report 'Health equity in England: The Marmot review 10 years on', health inequalities in the UK were already a major cause for concern, but have now been exacerbated by the pandemic and have contributed to the high and unequal death toll from COVID-19 (Marmot et al., 2020a, 2020b). People from ethnic minority backgrounds and people living in areas of deprivation had a greater risk of serious health outcomes and death (Bibby et al., 2020). In their report entitled 'Build back fairer: The COVID-19 Marmot review', Marmot and colleagues advocated the need for an inequalities strategy to be at the centre of the UK Government's recovery plan to reduce the widening socioeconomic inequalities and worsening health outcomes in our society (Marmot et al., 2020b). Increased investment in public health and efforts to prioritize the damaging impacts caused by the pandemic on education, employment, and income were some of the key recommendations outlined in the report. Jennifer Dixon, chief executive of The Health Foundation, stated: 'Putting the health and welfare of the next generation at the heart of the UK's recovery plans will be critical in the years ahead. It should concern us all that the pandemic has hit young people so hard, affecting their education, their work and income' (The Health Foundation, 2020a). Standing out amongst the four nations of the UK, the Welsh Government (2015) has demonstrated this vision through the Well-being of Future Generations (Wales) Act 2015 (see Box 1.1).

Box 1.1 Well-being of Future Generations (Wales) Act

In 2015, Wales passed the Well-being of Future Generations (Wales) Act to make long-lasting improvements to the social, economic, environmental, and cultural well-being of Wales (Welsh Government, 2015). The Act gives a legally-binding common purpose—the seven well-being goals—for national government, local government, local health boards, and other specified public bodies to not only consider current well-being, but also the well-being of future generations (see Figure 1.4). The Act requires these public bodies in Wales to consider the long-term impact of decisions to

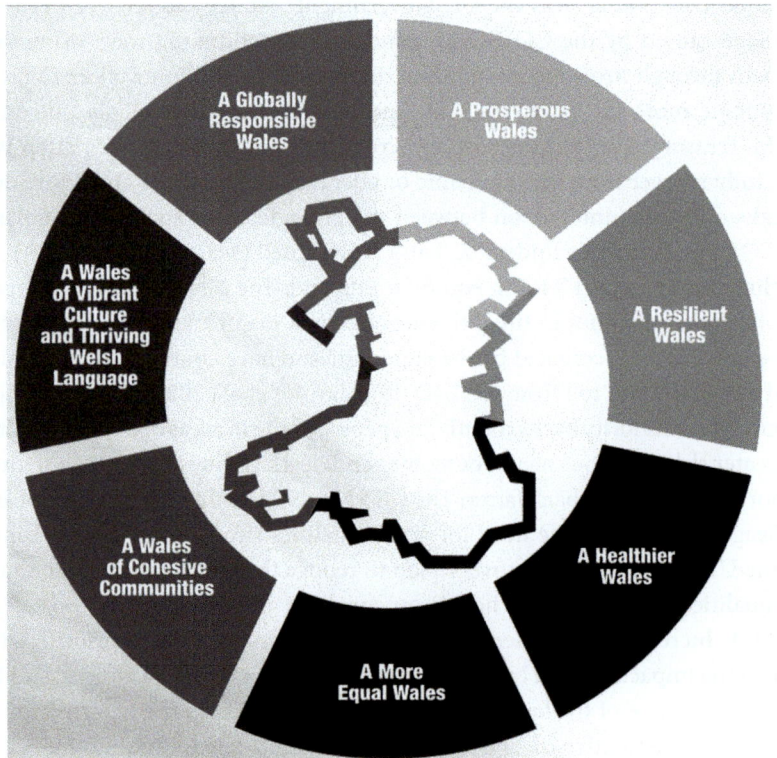

Figure 1.4 Well-being goals related to the Well-being of Future Generations (Wales) Act

Reproduced from Welsh Government. (2015). *Well-being of Future Generations (Wales) Act 2015*. https://gov.wales/sites/default/files/publications/2021-10/well-being-future-generations-wales-act-2015-the-essentials-2021.pdf. Crown copyright © 2021 Welsh Government. Reproduced under the Open Government License 3.0.

proactively address ongoing challenges such as poverty, health inequalities, and climate change. The legislation outlines a vision for a healthier Wales as, 'a society in which people's physical and mental wellbeing is maximised and in which choices and behaviours that benefit future health are understood'.

In the 'Welsh Government's Well-being of Future Generations continuous learning and improvement plan for 2023 to 2025' report, fifty-two specific actions were outlined that will be undertaken between 2023 to 2025 to further strengthen the integration of sustainable development principles within the government. It plans to do this through six themes:

1. Welsh ministers—maximize the government's contribution to the well-being goals by establishing and delivering well-being objectives.

2. Welsh Government civil services—improve the support and guidance to Welsh ministers by incorporating the five ways of working into all aspects of their operations.

3. Enabling others—facilitate, lead, and influence others to contribute to achieving the well-being goals.

4. Understanding Wales—gain a deeper understanding of both the current state of Wales and its future trajectory to formulate more sustainable decisions and policies.

5. Culture change—strive to integrate sustainable practices into actions.

6. Making it happen—continually driving the improvements in aligning with the sustainable development principle, backed by the support and oversight of a wide range of officials.

(Welsh Government, 2023)

Widening Inequalities as a Result of the COVID-19 Pandemic

The COVID-19 pandemic has highlighted inequality in society with the virus and lockdown disproportionally affecting the most disadvantaged groups and the poorest communities across the UK particularly impacted. In order to prevent the virus from spreading, the UK Government shut down entire sections of the economy, such as hospitality and retail (excluding food and pharmaceuticals), schools and nurseries, and arts and leisure services. Working from home became the new norm for many. However, the economic impact of these changes has not been experienced equally across the population, exacerbating existing inequalities (Blundell et al., 2020). There have been higher death rates among certain occupations, ethnic minority groups, and poorer localities.

The COVID-19 pandemic has also widened the gender divide. For example, the pandemic has had a greater effect on men medically as they are more likely to experience serious illness or death from the virus, whereas women are disproportionately affected societally. During lockdowns across the UK, schools closed, forcing many people to work from home and make alternative childcare arrangements. Real-time survey evidence suggests that in the US and the UK women were significantly more likely than men to lose their jobs, while people with a university degree were significantly less likely to do so than those without a degree (Adams-Prassl et al., 2020). Findings from the survey also showed that women spent more time home-schooling and caring for children than men (Adams-Prassl et al., 2020). In another study, 61 per cent of women found it more challenging to stay positive on a daily basis compared with 47 per cent of men (Ipsos MORI and The Fawcett Society, 2020). There is now a new norm, and we are unlikely to return to a work environment identical to pre-COVID-19 pandemic times. This provides the opportunity to create a new work environment that addresses gender inequalities and factors around flexible or blended working (see Chapter 5).

The COVID-19 pandemic has made stark the socioeconomic inequalities and inequalities in healthy life expectancy that we have lived with but have not talked about enough for many years. Figure 1.5 takes a life-course perspective to tease out factors impacting on mental health related to the COVID-19 pandemic (Local Government Association, 2023). Increase in life expectancy has slowed down to almost a halt and has actually declined for women in the poorest 10 per cent of neighbourhoods (Marmot et al., 2020a). The health inequality gap has widened between wealthy and deprived areas. There are marked differences in life expectancy depending on the region in which you live. A person from a deprived area in the North East has a life expectancy of almost five years less than a person from a comparable deprived area in London. Socioeconomic gradients in preventable mortality rates are evident. Poorer neighbourhoods have the highest preventable mortality rates, whereas the wealthiest areas have the lowest (Marmot et al., 2020a).

The Office for Budget Responsibility (OBR) forecasted that as a result of Brexit, over a five-year horizon, UK productivity will be 4 per cent lower, exports and imports will be around 15 per cent lower in the long run, and new trade deals with non-European Union (non-EU) countries will not have a material impact (OBR, 2023). This has also contributed to growing inequality. The impact on household earnings is forecast to be unequal, with middle earners disproportionally disadvantaged (Levell et al., 2020).

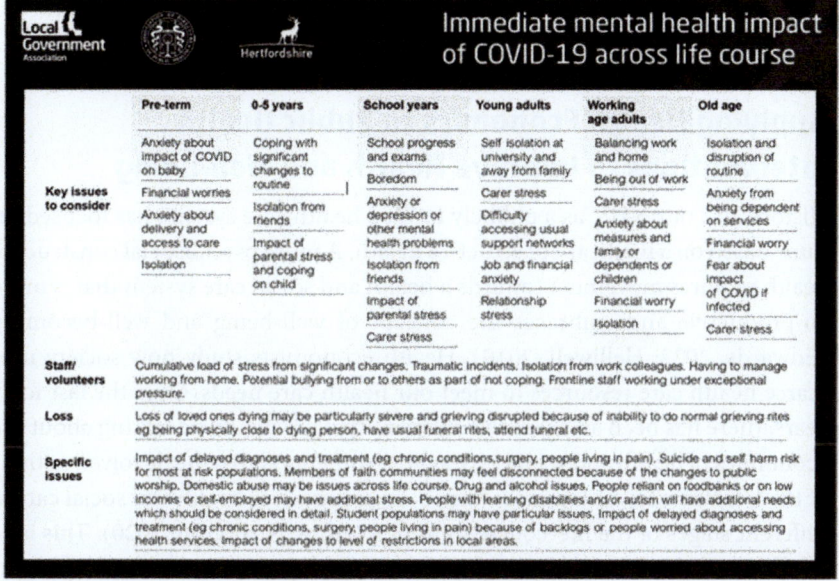

Figure 1.5 Mental health impact of the COVID-19 pandemic across the life-course
Reproduced with permission from Local Government Association. (2023). *Public mental health and wellbeing and COVID-19*. https://www.local.gov.uk/public-mental-health-and-wellbe ing-and-covid-19

An Emerging Framework for Well-being Economics

Whilst neoclassical economics is the study of how society uses scarce resources to meet our wants, an alternative paradigm of well-being economics has been put forward, described recently by Dalziel and colleagues (2018) in their book *Wellbeing economics: The capabilities approach to prosperity*. The premise of this framework is that economics should be the study of how to improve human well-being through guiding private and public sector efforts to expand the cap-abilities of persons to enable them to lead lives they value and have reason to value. The well-being economics framework focuses on seven types of capital investment (i.e. human, cultural, social, economic, natural, knowledge, and diplomatic) at seven levels of human choice (i.e. persons, households and fam-ilies, civil society, market participation, local government, nation state, and global community; for more information, see Dalziel et al., 2018, Table 1.1). This framework draws heavily on the work of Amartya Sen (1999), Nobel Prize winning economist, and aligns with capability-based outcome measurement developed by health economists, as described later in this chapter. We return full circle to this line of argument in Chapter 8 where we set out priorities for fu-ture research in health economics within a more diverse health and well-being paradigm, acknowledging the overarching challenges of sustainability and climate change.

Applying Health Economics to Public Health Interventions to Improve Health and Well-being

Historically, our NHS, as a publicly funded health care system, has focused on 'cure' based on a medical 'construct' of health. A more psychosocial construct of health requires movement towards a health and social care system that is more co-productive and embraces the concept of well-being and well-becoming (Edwards, 2022; Helliwell, 2019). Health economists study how society uses scarce health care resources to meet our health care needs. Over the last forty years, there has been an acknowledgement that we should be talking about the economics of health and social care as governments across the devolved nations of the UK strive towards a more joined-up approach to health and social care at different stages of the life-course (Shuttleworth & Nicholson, 2020). This is as much in recognition of the need for demand management with an ageing population and a recognition that the cause and solution to many challenges in life are more about social support than medical care. Growing interest in what can be called 'public health economics', or the economic evaluation of public health interventions with the potential to change health and well-being at a population level, raises all sorts of additional questions beyond those that we have had some success in tackling in an increasingly standardized manner. The focus has been on applying these increasingly standardized methods to health technology assessment, for example, new medicines and hospital-based care (Morris et al., 2007). Weatherly and colleagues (2009) set out four key methodological challenges to assess the cost-effectiveness of public health interventions:

1. attribution of effects;
2. measuring and valuing outcomes;
3. identifying intersectoral costs and consequences; and
4. incorporating equity considerations.

We explore many of these challenges through the rest of this book with reference to examples of evidence on the relative cost-effectiveness of public health and prevention interventions across the life-course.

What Do We Mean by Well-being and Well-becoming?

We saw how a wider consideration of well-being and well-becoming alongside health could fit into William's plumbing diagram in Figure 1.1. The WHO's 'Constitution of the World Health Organization' (1995) has promoted the concept of well-being since 1948. However, there is still little consensus as to how it should be measured across many academic disciplines, including health economics. It can be thought of as 'the balance point between an individual's resource pool and the challenges faced' (Dodge et al., 2012, p. 230). Research approaches have diverged into two different interpretations of what is meant by well-being: 'hedonic well-being' and 'eudaimonic well-being' (Ryan & Deci, 2001). The hedonic viewpoint is based on the notion that increased pleasure and avoidance of pain leads to happiness (Kahneman et al., 1999). The eudaimonic viewpoint is defined more broadly to incorporate dynamic processes such as self-actualization and the degree to which a person is fully functioning in society (Martela & Sheldon, 2019; Ryff & Singer, 1998). Well-being is often made up of multiple components, is normative or subjective, and is used synonymously with the terms 'quality of life' and 'happiness'. Attempts are made to measure some components objectively, such as health-related quality of life in health economics using the EuroQol-5 Dimensions (EQ-5D) questionnaire, and more recently, the EuroQol-Health and Wellbeing (EQ-HWB) questionnaire (EuroQol Research Foundation, 2018, Brazier et al., 2022). Objective measures are useful for comparing and monitoring trends over time in self-reported population well-being or cross-sectionally in comparing groups within the population or across countries internationally. At a national policy level, having an umbrella definition and measure of subjective well-being makes it possible to track and acknowledge its importance and compare across place and time. Concepts of well-being are being included in alternative measures of economic growth to traditional measures of GDP (see Table 1.3 later in this chapter).

Table 1.2 illustrates four survey questions that the ONS (2018a) uses to measure national personal well-being. Respondents are asked to choose a response to each measure on a scale from 0 to 10 where 0 refers to 'not at all' and 10 refers to 'completely'. These measures provide a harmonized standard for assessing personal well-being.

Table 1.2 Four measures of personal well-being

Measure	Question
Life satisfaction	Overall, how satisfied are you with your life nowadays?
Worthwhile	Overall, to what extent do you feel that the things you do in your life are worthwhile?
Happiness	Overall, how happy did you feel yesterday?
Anxiety	Overall, how anxious did you feel yesterday?

Reproduced from Office for National Statistics. (2018a, 26 September). *Surveys using our four personal well-being questions*. https://www.ons.gov.uk/peoplepopulationandcommunity/wellbeing/methodolog ies/surveysusingthe4officefornationalstatisticspersonalwellbeingquestions.Copyright © 2018 Office National Statistics. Reproduced under the Open Government License 3.0.

The importance of 'social context' is key to understanding subjective well-being at a population and individual level. The 'World happiness report' identified six determinants of happiness/life evaluation: GDP per capita, social support, healthy life expectancy, freedom, generosity, and absence of corruption (Helliwell et al., 2020). These determinants explained 75 per cent of variation across 150 countries, where over 1,000 people in each country had been interviewed through the Gallup World Poll (Helliwell et al., 2020).

Paul Dolan's books, *Happy ever after: A radical new approach to living well* and *Happiness by design: Finding pleasure and purpose in everyday life*, address aspects of happiness through ideas relating to wealth, success, education, marriage, children, altruism, health, and volition (Dolan, 2019, 2014). It is genetics compounded by the class system that seems to be perpetuating inequalities in society and, similarly, inequalities in our happiness. Dolan questions accepted social narratives about what makes us happy using UK and international data, and challenges us to keep thinking about context. This is a theme taken up by the co-editors of this book in relation to the use of CBA and social return on investment (SROI) analysis in health economics (Edwards & Lawrence, 2021).

'Well-becoming' can be thought of as 'our multitude of life-journeys towards meaning and purposefulness, not some steady-state of managed contentment' (Kane, 2007). The term well-becoming is not new, but it is not a term we routinely use in our everyday language or in research. Where it has appeared, it has predominantly been in early years research (Cassidy, 2017; Nsamenang, 2010). In the field of health economics, the only place we have found reference to the term well-becoming is in the sense of 'capability well-being' at different life-course stages. This has been a programme of research to develop capability measures at distinct stages of the life-course (Coast, 2019; Coast et al., 2015; Helter et al., 2020; Mitchell et al., 2021).

The financial benefits of investing in well-becoming are found in the work of James Heckman, the Chicago Nobel Prize winning economist (Heckman, 2008, 2012). Heckman demonstrated the lifetime benefits of investing in high-quality preschool care and the mitigating influence this can have on those with the worst start in life. Heckman has revised downwards some of his original estimates, but his arguments are still very powerful (see Chapter 3 in this book).

Well-becoming is based on the concept of assets-based public health (Morgan & Ziglio, 2007). Relevant to this assets-approach is user-based innovation theory—the idea that the public contribute to the design of interventions that boost local assets such as social cohesion (von Hippel, 2018). There is no doubt that the COVID-19 pandemic saw examples of increased social cohesion out of necessity, for example, charitable giving, including food banks. The pandemic, with associated national lockdowns, can be seen as a natural experiment in social inclusion. Taylor-Gooby and colleagues (2021) tracked charitable appeals, donations, cases of COVID-19 per 100 per week, deaths per 100 per week, and number of people in households claiming universal credit per 10,000. They showed how policy discourse that stresses common humanity in the face of a collective challenge, rather than social divisions, can help build social cohesion.

A Life-course Approach to Well-being and Well-becoming

ACEs are defined as stressful events that occur in childhood which have life-long impacts on health, well-being, and health-related behaviours (Hughes et al., 2017). Examples of ACEs include: domestic violence; physical, sexual, or verbal abuse; physical or emotional neglect; or a family member who has a mental health issue or who is experiencing substance misuse. The antithesis of society investing in well-becoming in children has been a growing recognition of the long-term detrimental impact of ACEs, reflecting a deficit model (Treanor, 2019). In health economics, the dominant paradigm in our discussion of cost-effectiveness relates to that of the cost per quality-adjusted life year (QALY), an extra-welfarist paradigm underpinning recommendations by the National Institute for Health and Care Excellence (NICE). Importantly, this paradigm takes a life horizon approach, but the reality is that most published cost-effectiveness analyses (CEAs) conducted alongside, for example, randomized controlled trials (RCTs), report findings after a few years of within trial follow-up and do not consider or hypothesize longer-term impacts. This is due largely to the high costs of running and recruiting to large RCTs, with very few funded to run more than five years.

There are substantial methodological challenges facing, for example, those undertaking economic evaluations (particularly CBA and return on investment (ROI) analysis) of early child development programmes. For example, a long follow-up period, the need to discount costs and outcomes at an appropriate discount rate, and differing methods for monetizing benefits with no market price (Karoly & Bigelow, 2005). The evaluation of some early childhood development programmes has been particularly challenging as a result of having several components and goals, which we would now define as 'complex interventions within complex systems' (Skivington et al., 2021; Craig et al., 2008; Karoly & Bigelow, 2005; Rutter et al., 2017; Shiell et al., 2008).

Well-becoming is not just about the early years of childhood. In her book, *Extra time: 10 Lessons for an ageing world,* Camilla Cavendish (2019) writes about the recent changes in our life-course, in that we can expect a far longer 'old age', and that well-becoming in the middle years can set up for physical and mental well-being in very old age. We address these issues in Chapters 5 and 6 in this book. Specific to the health and well-being of women, Mishra and colleagues (2023) present a life-course approach to women's health spanning reproductive health; health, ageing, and disease; biological and behavioural pathways; and social issues impacting women's health.

It Is Time for Prevention

Eighty per cent of chronic health problems, such as premature heart disease, stroke, and diabetes, are preventable (WHO, 2005). Back in 2012, 50 per cent of general practitioner (GP) appointments, 64 per cent of outpatient appointments, and 70 per cent of inpatient bed stays were for preventable conditions (Department of Health, 2012). Prior to the COVID-19 pandemic, it was estimated that a 24 per cent reduction in funding to local government was having a knock-on effect on the provision of public health interventions funded through local government, with the potential to prevent ill-health and chronic disease (The Health Foundation, 2023). This is counter-intuitive when cost per QALY calculations reveal that public health expenditure, at about £3,800 per QALY, appears to be about three to four times more productive at the margin than health care expenditure (which costs about £13,500 per QALY; Martin et al., 2019). In 2015, McDaid and colleagues published a book entitled *Promoting health, preventing disease: The economic case*. They provided an economic perspective on health promotion and chronic disease prevention, and gave a rationale for assessing the economic case for action. They focused on specific health-harming issues such as smoking, alcohol, road accidents, and the potential benefits of improving nutrition, promoting physical exercise and supporting mental health (McDaid et al., 2015).

It is interesting to consider how much money could be saved if we focused our efforts on prevention. Taking diabetes as an example, the NHS spends around £10 billion a year on treating diabetes (NHS England, 2022). In 2020/2021, there were 57.9 million drugs used in treating diabetes prescribed in England at a cost of £1.19 billion, 12.5 per cent of the total spend on all prescription items prescribed in England (NHS Business Services Authority, 2021). There are currently 3.8 million people in the UK living with diabetes, 90 per cent of whom have type 2 diabetes. There are 12.3 million people at risk of developing type 2 diabetes. Many cases of type 2 diabetes could be prevented through lifestyle choices, such as healthy eating, being more active, and losing weight (if overweight) (Diabetes UK, 2019). By focusing on prevention, the NHS could save billions of pounds in avoidable treatment costs. Evidence from large studies on the preventative health benefits of exercise are becoming available. A meta-analysis of 196 large prospective studies found that walking just eleven minutes a day could prevent 10 per cent of premature deaths (Garcia et al., 2023). These researchers highlighted that such a moderate increase in exercise was inversely associated with the prevalence of chronic disease in inactive adults. Here it is worth pausing to reconsider concerns that individuals actually have less autonomy and options to co-produce better health for themselves than theory might suggest (Dolan, 2019). It may be that changing contexts and environments where we live and work, and how we travel, may reduce the need for such co-production (Rutter, 2018), but the argument still stands that in the long run, achievable prevention is a necessary way forward for an over-stretched NHS and social care system.

The prediction of the NHS plan for England in 2014, that failure to 'get real' about prevention would lead to a flattening in increased life expectancy, widening inequalities, and a crowding-out of new medical interventions due to the need to care for people living with preventable chronic disease, has in part been borne out, even before the as yet unclear overall impact of the COVID-19 pandemic (Marmot et al., 2020b; NHS England, 2014). When local authorities and NHS organizations are under pressure within annual funding cycles to cut costs within reduced budgets, making a case for investment of any kind, even in prevention, can be difficult. Although we do not know across the whole economy what is spent on prevention (i.e. sectors such as housing, education, local government, and central government), the figure of 5 per cent is often quoted for what is spent as a proportion of the NHS budget (ONS, 2020e). Internationally, this figure is in the range of 5 per cent to 12 per cent (Xu et al., 2018). Several commentators have argued that what is needed is a 'system-wide shift' towards prevention (Edwards & McIntosh, 2019; Ferguson, 2016). This was illustrated in the case of obesity prevention in the UK 'Government foresight report', which emphasized the complex nature of obesity and argued for it to be addressed using systems approaches (Butland et al., 2007; Rutter, 2018).

Taking a long-term view, health economists in the field of public health have argued that prevention is cost-effective, may save the health service money in the short and long term, and the benefits of prevention reach far beyond the health care system (Edwards & McIntosh, 2019; Ferguson, 2016). To this, we would add that prevention in early life can have benefits far beyond that stage in life and help shape lifetime health experience, and with this, well-being and well-becoming through subsequent stages of the life-course with associated potential savings to health and social care systems.

Half of all mental health problems begin by age fifteen, rising to three-quarters by early adulthood (Kessler et al., 2005). Ten per cent of children in secondary schools require some mental health support (Rethink Mental Illness,

2020). The prevalence of depression in children and young people is increasing (Pitchforth et al., 2018). Depression in adolescence often goes undetected (and untreated) until adulthood, with symptoms often attributed to more typical teenage emotions and behaviours (Thapar et al., 2012). The life trajectory of children who experience poor mental health is similar to that of children raised in poverty, with a higher likelihood of poor outcomes into adulthood, with lower academic attainment, reduced rates of employment, poorer career progression opportunities, and a higher likelihood of contacts with social justice and welfare systems (Khan, 2016). All of these consequences have high economic and social costs. There are high rates of returns from investment in the earliest years of life. There continues to be an interesting debate between the evidence that this rate of return declines with age, known as the 'Heckman Curve' (Heckman, 2008), and more recent evidence, predominantly from the Washington State Institute for Public Policy. Rea and Burton (2020) argued that early intervention can be cost-effective, but in addition, later treatment and amelioration ('second chance') using evidence-based programmes can also succeed. If prevention is so important going forward, then there needs to be a shift in the balance of spending in research and development between what we spend on research into prevention and what we spend globally on cure, particularly via the pharmaceutical industry. An example of the enormous global spend on research and development (R&D) by the pharmaceutical industry is provided by Bayer's plans to spend $1 billion on drug R&D in the US to double its sales in the US by 2030 (Erman & Wingrove, 2023).

Investing in well-being and well-becoming

Putting a monetary value on non-market goods, such as well-being and well-becoming, can be challenging. However, it is important to acknowledge that market prices themselves are subjective, variable, and inexact as they are often a result of negotiating power rather than being reflective of the real incurred costs (Vardakoulias, 2013). This challenge is explored further on in this introductory chapter and also in later chapters in this book in the presentation of the use of CBA and SROI, which aim to capture and monetize wider social value creation where there are no traditional markets such as in health care, preventative interventions, and social policies aiming to improve health and well-being.

Maintaining well-being and well-becoming through the life-course

Like many other countries, the UK's population is ageing due to people living longer (ONS, 2019). While living longer may be a cause for celebration, what does this impact of longevity have on the economy, services, and society? As life expectancy increases, so does the amount of time spent in poor health (ONS, 2018b). But what happens if we shift our focus from reactively 'curing' ill-health and invest more in proactively 'preventing' ill-health by maintaining well-being and well-becoming throughout the life-course, starting from preconception? This is the focus of our book.

All too often, discussions about spending on health and social care fall into budget silos, determined by disease or cause of premature death, cancer, heart disease, and mental ill-health. We rarely think about spending on health and social care along the lines of a life-course model. It seems obvious that the start that children and young people have in their lives will impact their later life and old age. As health economists, what we do in this book is to collate and present examples of evidence on the relative cost-effectiveness and/or financial ROI or SROI of spending public money through different phases of the life-course, from preconception right through to death. What we have learnt is that different decision-makers at national and local level gravitate towards different kinds of evidence, which broadly fall into the NICE (2022) reference case paradigm and alternatively the HM Treasury (2022) social CBA, ROI, and SROI paradigm. This is very much the case in the economic evaluation of public health interventions delivered across multiple sectors (Hill, 2019). This book has arisen out of our previous three reports series prepared for Public Health Wales, which focused on some of these aspects specifically in the context of Wales (Edwards et al., 2016, 2018, 2019). We believe these issues to be of far wider interest, so this book presents such evidence at a UK level with some international examples.

Understandably, current post-pandemic pressure on the UK NHS and on social care services means that we continue to prioritize 'cure' today over the prevention of future chronic disease, disability, and premature death. As we noted earlier, though many public health interventions provide relatively convincing value for money compared to the NICE threshold of £20,000 per QALY, we have historically only spent 5 per cent of the NHS budget on preventative health care (ONS, 2020e). Public health interventions, unlike surgical or pharmacological clinical interventions, are charged with 'saving money today' for the health and social care system. This seems illogical when we do not expect high-cost cancer drugs, for example, to 'save money'.

In his book, *Thinking, fast and slow*, Daniel Kahneman, Nobel Prize winning psychologist and economist, warns researchers to be aware of the potential for bias in our everyday use of evidence and statistics to build a story or explain a phenomenon in a way that seems rational to us. He describes this bias as 'what you see is all there is' and uses the acronym WYSIATI (Kahneman, 2012). Writing any book, this is probably exactly what we are doing: building a narrative and referring to evidence. With this in mind, and as health economists brought up in the paradigm of evidence-based medicine and the gold standard of the RCT, we approach evidence referenced in this book as follows. We acknowledge that NICE (2012) recommends the use of CBA and other methods beyond QALYs to evaluate public health interventions because the benefits and costs fall across many sectors in the economy. This includes methods such as social CBA (HM Treasury, 2022), ROI (Public Health England, 2021), and SROI (New Economics Foundation (NEF) Consulting, 2023; Nicholls et al., 2009). The reality is that it is very expensive to conduct large-scale trials in public health, requiring a large sample size and long follow-up period. Using the 'precautionary principle', the reality is that there is a need to use different types of evidence, such as from historical cohort studies and natural experiments (e.g. changes in policy such as the introduction of the ban on smoking in public places and the introduction of minimum alcohol pricing), and these are not all RCT gold standard (Deidda et al., 2019; Fischer & Ghelardi, 2016).

A life-course approach to health

A 'life-course' approach to health is the idea that experiences in earlier life shape adult health, valuing the health and well-being of both current and future generations. It emphasizes a temporal and social perspective of health and ageing by assessing life experiences across generations to help explain current patterns of health and disease (WHO, 2005). There are numerous protective factors and risk factors that interplay in health and well-being over the life-course. The main outcome of this approach is to maintain good functioning ability, which can be influenced by health policies, societal norms, economic factors, and environmental factors. Protective factors include good educational attainment, living in good quality housing, and having a healthy, balanced diet. Risk factors include ACEs, smoking, and poor mental health (Public Health England, 2019). The life-course approach emphasizes primary interventions in addition to cure or palliation (WHO, 2005).

In Figure 1.6, functional ability and intrinsic capacity are shown diagrammatically as idealized curves across the life-course. Intrinsic capacity refers to the physical and mental attributes a person was born with, and can be enhanced by supportive environments and social factors throughout the life-course, thereby contributing to a person's functional ability (Kuruvilla et al., 2018). For example, the availability of affordable healthy food to support a healthy diet and glasses to correct poor vision supports functional ability, whereas a lack of a safe space to play might have a negative impact on mobility and functional ability. Adopting a life-course approach involves identifying opportunities for minimizing risk factors and enhancing protective factors through evidence-based

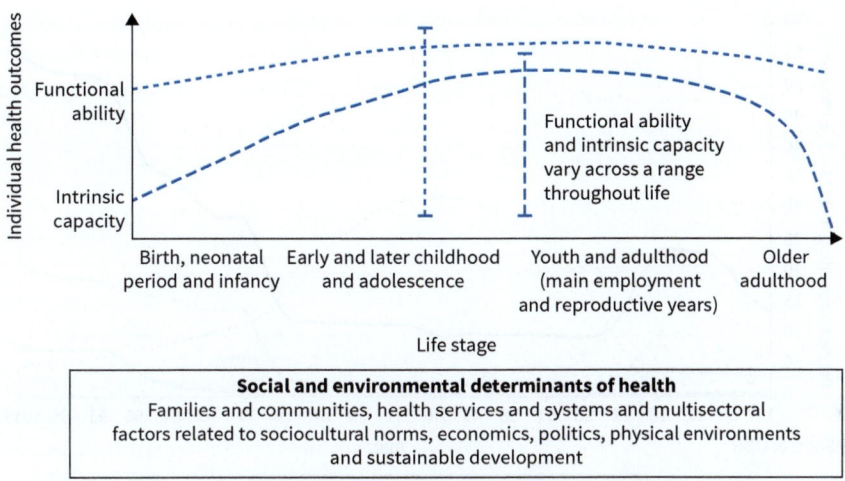

Figure 1.6 Conceptual framework for a life-course approach to health

Reproduced from Kuruvilla, S., Sadana, R., Montesinos, E. V., Beard, J., Vasdeki, J. F., de Carvalho, I. A., Thomas, R. B., Drisse, M.-N. B., Daelmans, B., Goodman, T., Koller, T., Officer, A., Vogel, J., Valentine, N., Wootton, E., Banerjee, A., Magar, V., Neira, M., Bele., J. M. O., . . . Bustreo, F. (2018). A life-course approach to health: synergy with sustainable development goals. *Bulletin of the World Health Organization*, 96(1), 42–50. https://doi.org/10.2471/BLT.17.198358. Licence: Creative Commons BY 3.0 IGO.

interventions at important life stages (Public Health England, 2019). Spending on health and social care across the life-course is disproportionally high towards the end of life. There are potentially opportunities to shift the curve to spend more in early life to prevent poor health and disability in later life with associated cost savings to society.

Figure 1.7 shows the representative tax, public services, and welfare spending profiles by age that form the basis of the projections for 2026 to 2027 by the OBR (2022). This graph plots total spending, education, health, adult social care, tax, and welfare across the life-course. What is clear from this figure is that the majority of spending will continue to be in the latter part of the life-course.

NICE and the cost-effectiveness of preventative interventions

Growing evidence of the cost-effectiveness of public health preventative interventions across the life-course is not sinking into the UK Government consciousness at scale. In a review of economic evaluations of public health interventions assessed by NICE between 2005 and 2018, Owen and Fischer

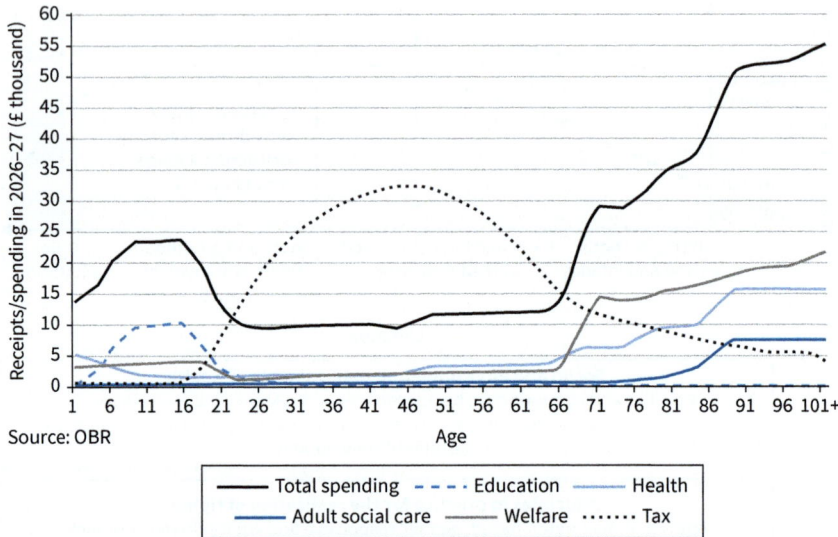

Figure 1.7 UK public spending across the life-course

Reproduced from Office for Budget Responsibility. (2022). *Fiscal risks and sustainability.* HM Government. https://obr.uk/docs/dlm_uploads/Fiscal_risks_and_sustainability_2022-1.pdf. Copyright © 2022 Office for Budget Responsibility. Reproduced under the Open Government License 3.0.

(2019) found that 75 per cent of interventions were cost-effective at a threshold of £20,000 per QALY when disregarding clustering, and 68 per cent were cost-effective when clusters were represented by a single incremental cost-effectiveness ratio (ICER). They found that the median cost per QALY ICER for the 380 estimates was £1,986. Twenty-one per cent of these were cost-saving, 54 per cent ranged from £1 to £20,000, 3 per cent were between £20,001 and £30,000, 16 per cent were above £30,000 per QALY, and 5 per cent were dominated. Taking into account clustering of interventions made relatively little difference to these findings. Owen and Fischer (2019) found that reducing the threshold from £20,000 per QALY to £15,000 per QALY would result in 2 per cent of ICERs moving across the threshold. Overall, they concluded that 75 per cent of public health interventions assessed were cost-effective.

Saying this, NICE and some health economists have recognized the narrow nature of the cost per QALY model underpinning estimates of the cost-effectiveness of health technology assessment and its limited relevance to the evaluation of public health interventions (Edwards & McIntosh, 2019; NICE, 2011, 2012). It is, however, useful to keep going back to cost per QALY estimates for preventative, often public health, interventions and compare them with the cost per QALY of new high-cost medicines—just to check in on the prevention-cure paradigm. There has been some movement to increase the use of CBA and develop the use of SROI (showing a broader measure of social and economic benefit right across society and the economy) in the evaluation of public health interventions. However, much of this remains in the grey literature. A review of published SROI studies across the life-course between 1996 and 2019 identified forty articles, of which thirty-seven were in the grey literature (Ashton et al., 2020). Methods of CBA and SROI analysis are less standardized than methods of CEA and cost-utility analysis (CUA; Edwards & McIntosh, 2019; Fujiwara, 2014, 2015).

An Increased Focus by Health Economists on Inequalities

Health economists have traditionally focused on the concept of efficiency (both allocative efficiency and technical efficiency). More recently, there has been growing interest in distributional analysis in the process of CEA. This aims to help health care and public health organizations make fairer decisions with better outcomes. Whereas standard CEA provides information about total mean costs and effects, distributional CEA provides added information about fairness in the distribution of costs and effects across the population. Attention is focused on who gains, who loses, by how much, and whether there are opportunities for compensation. Distributional analysis can also provide information about the trade-offs that sometimes occur between efficiency objectives, such as improving the total health of the population, and equity objectives, such as reducing unfair inequality in health (Cookson et al., 2020). This is relevant to the application of economic evaluation methods to the evaluation of public health interventions given that one of the central tenets of public health is the goal of increasing the health of the worst-off (Elwell-Sutton et al., 2019).

The COVID-19 pandemic, the Black Lives Matter movement, and the need for greater consideration of sex, gender, and ethnicity in research

The recent experience of deaths from COVID-19 and the increased awareness of the Black Lives Matter movement have raised social and research community consciousness of the role of age and ethnicity, and the need for representativeness in health economics, health services, and population health research. Lindsay et al. (2020) reviewed a purposive sample of 200 RCTs of peri-operative care and found that only 2 per cent of trials published data on the race or ethnicity of participants. In ninety-two of the RCTs, the proportion of each sex in the study sample was more than 25 per cent different from the proportion in the registry population (Lindsay et al., 2020). In 2017, a systematic review of international literature on the representation of people from ethnic minority backgrounds in patient and public involvement (PPI) in health and social care research found that published papers on this topic mainly came from the US (Dawson et al., 2018). These researchers also found that the involvement of people from ethnic minority backgrounds was limited to particular phases of research, such as the research design phase (Dawson et al., 2018). The National Institute for Health and Care Research (NIHR) has strengthened its commitment to ensuring that participants from ethnic minority backgrounds have the opportunity to take part in COVID-19 research studies (Khunti & Farooqi, 2020). This has been a response to the fact that people from ethnic minority backgrounds were disproportionately affected by the COVID-19 pandemic. Despite reporting poorer health outcomes, people from ethnic minority backgrounds are under-represented in health and social care research. Inclusion of people from ethnic minority backgrounds in research is necessary to avoid inequalities and increase the representativeness of a health and social care evidence base (Osuafor et al., 2021). This should be a basis for improving the representativeness of all health services research in future, including economic evaluation alongside RCTs and other study designs.

Caroline Criado Perez has documented a systemic lack of consideration of gender differences in trials of new medicines. She highlights how early research into the treatment of cardiovascular disease focused on men, and that women have continued to be under-represented, with women making up only 25 per cent of participants across thirty-one landmark trials for congestive heart failure between 1987 and 2012 (Perez, 2019). The same argument can be made for how we approach subgroup analysis in CEA where gender is relevant.

Economic Growth and Alternative Ideas for the Measurement of Economic Well-being

The conventional metric of the well-being of an economy has been growth in gross national product (GNP) or GDP. The GDP of an economy is a measure of total production. More precisely, it is the monetary value of all goods and services produced within a country or region within a given time period. Critics have questioned the continued use of GDP as a measure of public well-being and quality of life as it focuses on income and material wealth and disregards the fact that the economy profits from natural, social, and human capital (Giannetti et al., 2015). In this book, we present examples of evaluations of

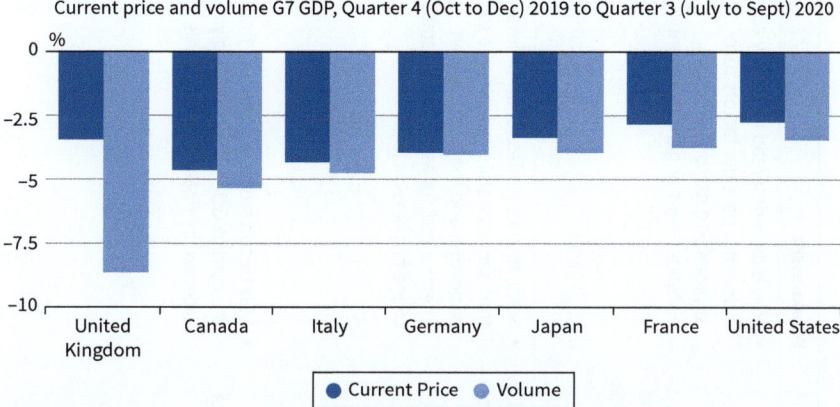

Figure 1.8 International comparisons of GDP highlight how the UK was hit relatively worse than other advanced economies during 2019 and 2020
Reproduced from Office for National Statistics. (2021,1 February). *International comparisons of GDP during the coronavirus (COVID-19) pandemic*. https://www.ons.gov.uk/economy/grossdom esticproductgdp/articles/internationalcomparisonsofgdpduringthecoronaviruscovid19pande mic/2021-02-01. Copyright © 2021 Office for National Statistics. Reproduced under the Open Government License 3.0.

the cost-effectiveness of interventions across the life-course aimed to promote well-being and well-becoming. However, revisiting these estimates is against the backdrop of the COVID-19 pandemic and a fall in the UK economy's GDP during 2019 and 2020, greater than any other Group of Seven (G7) country (see Figure 1.8; ONS, 2021). At a macro-level, there are concerns that GDP and GNP do not tell the whole story or adequately represent what we value in terms of a wider sense of economic growth, or what we should, in future, value. A number of alternative measures to GDP and GNP are described in Table 1.3.

Middle and low-income countries have been exploring well-being measurement. For example, in 2018 the Indian Government launched the Ease of Living Index to assess the development of cities and improve the well-being and living standards of residents. The framework provides information across three pillars of quality of life, economic ability, and sustainability, fourteen categories (education; health; housing and shelter; water supply to household and solid waste management; mobility; safety and security; recreation; level of economic development; economic opportunities; Gini coefficient (an inequality index based on consumption expenditure); environment; green spaces and buildings; energy consumption; and city resilience) and fifty indicators (Ministry of Housing and Urban Affairs, 2019).

Table 1.3 Methods for measuring the well-being of a country

Measure	Origin	Strengths	Weaknesses
Human Development Index (HDI)	• Developed by the United Nations (UN) Development Programme (2020) • A geometric means of normalized indices across three dimensions: life expectancy, average years of schooling, and gross national income per capita • Recognizes people and their capabilities in assessing a country's development	• Provides a broader picture of an economy that includes social development • Demonstrates that, while there is a correlation between economic and social development, the former does not guarantee the latter	• May hide widespread inequality as it does not consider factors such as protecting personal freedom, pollution levels or gender disparity
Genuine Progress Indicator (GPI)	• American metric • Incorporates social and environmental factors not measured by GDP, such as the cost of ozone depletion, crime, or poverty on a nation's economic health • Nets the positive and negative results to decide whether economic growth has benefited the population overall, for example, balancing GDP spending against external costs	• Shifts the value basis of a product by adding its social and environmental impacts to the equation • Assigns values to non-financial human contributions, such as volunteering	• Some finance professionals believe that non-economic variables are too subjective, and that GPI is not an effective tool for assessing the state of the business cycle
Thriving Places Index (TPI)	• Developed by the Centre for Thriving Places, UK • Provides a breakdown of holistic elements that help support thriving communities and economies • Includes a wide variety of factors: mental and physical health, education and learning, work and local economy, and 'green' infrastructure	• Supports a move away from defining success purely in terms of consumption • Looks at factors such as land use, recycling, and income disparity to help planners understand how to better support communities	• May be too radical a departure from the current GDP paradigm widely accepted by finance professionals

Green GDP	• China's Green GDP measures the cost of environmental damage as the result of economic growth by subtracting factors such as resource depletion and environmental degradation from the GDP, with local governments accountable for ecological conservation	• Local governments that do not want their economic growth statistics affected by environmental factors have been resistant to adopting this as a GDP alternative
	• Embraces broader accounting of economic development that considers the effects of pollution and resource depletion	
Better Life Index (BLI)	• Allows for a comparison of well-being across thirty-five countries, based on eleven topics identified by the OECD	• For finance professionals, the information in the index may not contain enough economic indicators to provide a satisfactory GDP alternative
	• Topics include: housing, income, community, education, environment, civic engagement, and health	• Some of the assessment criteria may be too vague
	• Includes eighty indicators of well-being that provide a comprehensive picture of natural, human, economic and social capital	
	• Allows a comparison of gender differences	
Inclusive Wealth Index (IWI)	• Developed by the UN	• The IWI needs to be part of broader macroeconomic planning, alongside other indicators, if economic progress is to be evaluated based on a balanced assessment of capital
	• Measures the wealth of a nation using a comprehensive analysis of a country's productive base, including the assets from which human well-being is derived—manufactured and human and natural capital	
	• By injecting 'green' accounting into the assessment of capital assets, and assessing changes in natural capital, such as forests or waterways, the IWI could help drive climate change policies and action	
Genuine Savings Indicator (GSI)	• The World Bank's savings analysis argues that factors such as public investments of resource revenues and the social costs of pollution emissions are equally relevant in determining the overall level of saving	• Until tools have been developed to measure this reliably, it is a fundamentally flawed way of measuring economic health
	• Encourages discussion around natural resources in a language familiar to finance policymakers	

(continued)

Table 1.3 Continued

Measure	Origin	Strengths	Weaknesses
Happy Planet Index (HPI)	• Developed by the UK's New Economics Foundation • Combines four elements: life expectancy, well-being, ecological footprint, and inequality • Shows how efficiently people in different countries are using environmental resources to lead long, happy lives	• A nicely rounded, composite measure considering the social and environmental aspects of life to measure economic health	• Ecological footprint is a contentious measure of economic development • Fails to account for some key 'happiness killers', such as human rights violations and modern slavery
Index of Economic Well-being	• Developed by Osberg (1985) and Osberg and Sharpe (2001) • Comprises four domains of economic well-being: effective per capita consumption flows, net societal accumulation of stocks of productive resources, income distribution, and economic security	• Indicates the 'command over resources' of people living in a country and includes genuine savings rate, inequality and insecurity	• Measures the risk of catastrophe • Measures the dollar values of the levels of resources and emissions costs, without reference to optimal or sustainable levels
National Well-being Index	• Developed by Vemuri and Constanza (2006) • Combines data on national levels of subjective well-being (measured by life satisfaction) with data on objective measures of built, human, social, and natural capital	• Focuses on land use and access to green space as part of the measurement of well-being	• There are a number of national well-being indexes used in different countries with this name

Source: Hawkes, H. (2021, 6 September). *8 ways of measuring economic health.* In The Black. https://www.intheblack.com/articles/2021/06/8-ways-of-measuring-economic-health. Copyright © 2023 CPA Australia Ltd.

A study by Kubiszewski and colleagues (2013) reported that estimates of genuine progress indicator (GPI) per capita between 1950 and 2003 for seventeen nations showed that global GPI per capita peaked in 1978. At the same time, the global ecological footprint (a measure of humanity's demand on nature) exceeded global biocapacity (a measure of the biologically productive land available for producing resource materials and absorbing waste). In this study, life satisfaction in most countries had also not significantly improved since 1975 (Kubiszewski et al., 2013).

The Wellbeing Economy Alliance has argued that we must shift how we understand and build societal health and prosperity, looking beyond economic growth to collective well-being and environmental sustainability (Chrysopoulou, 2020). In particular, a well-being economy should strive for a congruent relationship between society and nature, where individuals enjoy a fair distribution of resources, living in healthy and resilient communities (Chrysopoulou, 2020). Aligned with this but springing from the business sector has been what is referred to as the 'kindness economy', led by Mary Portas. The kindness economy moves away from the tenets of capitalism that 'more equals better' and instead focuses on adding social value. The triple bottom line is: people, planet, and profit (Portas, 2020).

Happiness Economics

The economics of happiness has three basic principles: 1) the state of a nation should be measured by the happiness of the individuals living there, particularly the happiness of the least happy individuals; 2) focus should be on trying to produce the largest amount of happiness in the world possible through how individuals live their lives; and 3) governments should aim to produce the greatest happiness in individuals and prevent misery (Layard & Ward, 2020). The field has grown substantially since the late twentieth century, for example, with the development of methods, surveys, and indices to measure happiness (Wiking, 2019). We recall from earlier in the chapter the conceptualization of happiness as experience and purpose. Dolan (2014) argues that happiness is a combination of experiences of both pleasure and purpose over time, and depends on how we allocate our attention to the various stimuli vying for it.

Denmark consistently scores top in international comparisons of societal happiness. This is largely down to having a large welfare state, with most Danes paying 45 per cent tax on their income. With societal shared values of common good, Danes are happy to do this knowing that they have free health care, free university tuition with a stipend of over €600 per month, and generous maternity and paternity leave. This combined with five weeks of paid holiday per year, family-friendly working hours, and a city infrastructure that makes it possible for 45 per cent of Danes to commute to and from work, school, and other activities by bicycle. Many Nordic countries with centrist socialist democratic governments share these characteristics of society and again score highly on international comparisons of societal well-being or happiness. Governments of the past decade in both the UK and US place us at what may feel a considerable distance from such consensus about shifting from a GDP and growth model of economic progress to a well-being model of what constitutes progress in terms of well-being and happiness. This has been disastrously played out under the brief Truss Government of October 2022, where an almost messianic preoccupation with economic growth damaged the UK economy with widespread impact on, for example, mortgage payments of households, pension plans, and government borrowing, which households are still feeling today.

Well-being-adjusted Life Years (WELLBYs) and the Well-being Manifesto

Proponents of well-being measurement at societal level have argued that the main aim of the government should be to improve well-being and reduce suffering by as much as possible in those whose suffering matters the most to society (Dolan et al., 2021). It has been proposed that subjective measurement of life satisfaction could be used to weight years of life gained measured in terms of well-being-adjusted life years (WELLBYs), in the same way as in health economics we have used QALYs (Dolan et al., 2021). A single metric allows for the value of all possible uses of scarce resources to be estimated in terms of their relative cost per WELLBY. Proponents do not specify how it should be measured but that ideally the measure should allow for the duration of different levels of subjective well-being to be properly accounted for in a well-becoming sense across the life-course (Dolan & Kahneman, 2008). This approach accounts for well-being across the life-course as a 'concept of flow'. Akin to the fair innings argument put forward by Alan Williams (1987) is the idea that a person is entitled to some 'normal' span of life in terms of WELLBYs and that their right to more WELLBYs diminishes as they get older. Though this is controversial, it does have considerable popular support (Tsuchiya et al., 2003). In this sense, WELLBYs could be considered ageist and certainly are linear in the sense that no distinction is made between a WELLBY early in life than in later in life, that is, they are additive in nature. Layard and colleagues (2022) put forward a Well-being Manifesto, which is based on the ability to measure subjective well-being by asking how satisfied people are in their lives on a scale of 0 to 10 (where 0 means 'not at all satisfied' and 10 means 'very satisfied'). They argue for routine incorporation of such questions and use of such data in the design and evaluation of policy (Layard et al., 2022).

Viewing Public Health Interventions That Can Affect Well-being and Well-becoming as Complex Interventions within Complex Systems

One of the most important developments in health services research and health economics relating to public health and prevention has been the publication of the Medical Research Council (MRC) guide to the evaluation of complex interventions (Craig et al., 2008). Complex interventions include psychological, behavioural, educational, and organizational interventions (Petticrew et al., 2019). Complex interventions are often used within complex systems, such as the health service, public health practice, and areas of social policy such as education, transport, and housing. In 2021, the MRC's guidance for developing and evaluating complex interventions was replaced by a new framework (Skivington et al., 2021). In this new framework, four phases of complex intervention research were identified: development or identification of an intervention; assessment of feasibility of the intervention and evaluation design; evaluation of the intervention; and impactful implementation (see Figure 1.9). These phases are not necessarily sequential and are often associated with multiple interacting components, presenting difficulties to evaluators.

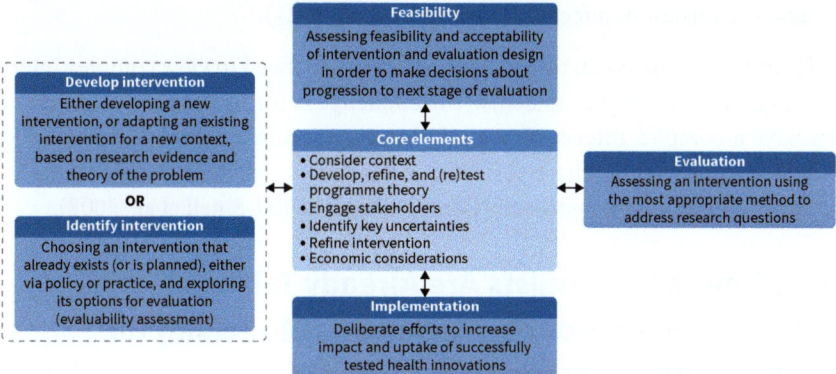

Figure 1.9 Framework for developing and evaluating complex interventions
Reproduced from Skivington, K., Matthews, L., Simpson, S. A., Craig, P., Baird, J., Blazeby, J. M., Boyd, K. A., Craig, N., French, D. P., McIntosh, E., Petticrew, M., Rycroft-Malone, J., White, M., & Moore, L. (2021). A new framework for developing and evaluating complex interventions: Update of Medical Research Council guidance. *BMJ*, *374*(2061), 1–11. http://dx.doi.org/10.1136/bmj.n2061. Licence: Creative Commons BY 3.0 IGO.

The MRC provides the following definitions for terms included in the new framework shown in Figure 1.9:

'context' can be thought of as any feature of the circumstances in which an intervention is conceived, developed, evaluated, and implemented;

'programme theory' describes how an intervention is expected to lead to its effects and under what conditions—the programme theory should be tested and refined at all stages and used to guide the identification of uncertainties and research questions;

'stakeholders' include those who are targeted by the intervention or policy, involved in its development or delivery, or more broadly, those whose personal or professional interests are affected (i.e. who have a stake in the topic)—this includes patients and members of the public as well as those linked in a professional capacity;

'uncertainties' reflects the need to identify the key uncertainties that exist, given what is already known and what the programme theory, research team, and stakeholders identify as being most important to discover—these judgements inform the framing of research questions, which in turn, govern the choice of research perspective;

'refinement' is the process of fine tuning or making changes to the intervention once a preliminary version (prototype) has been developed; and

'economic considerations' can be thought of as determining the comparative resource and outcome consequences of the interventions for those people and organizations affected (Skivington et al., 2021).

Health economists can think about whether they need to view complex interventions within complex systems. The challenge is for us to question whether we have a complex intervention or an intervention in a complex system, and whether the dynamic characteristics of the system matter enough for us to change our evaluation approach (Campbell et al., 2000; Shiell et al., 2008).

How Health Economists Are Already Taking a 'Life-course' Approach in Economic Modelling for Cost-effectiveness Analysis

For those familiar with the principles and methods of economic evaluation, the following sections set out recent developments that are applicable to the evaluation of interventions, programmes, and policies designed to promote well-being and well-becoming. For readers to whom the methods of economic evaluation generally are new, we direct you to Drummond and colleagues

(2015), Morris and colleagues (2007), and specific to the evaluation of public health interventions, Edwards and McIntosh (2019).

The discipline of economics is often subclassified into 'microeconomics' and 'macroeconomics'. Microeconomics tries to understand human choices, decisions, and the allocation of resources. Macroeconomics studies the behaviour of a country and how its policies impact the economy as a whole. Methods of economic evaluation are considered to fall within microeconomic analysis within health economics. Arguably, some econometric analysis relates more to macroeconomic modelling. The following sections cover developments in microeconomic evaluation, macroeconomic evaluation, and developments in CBA and SROI.

Taking a Lifetime or Life-course Time Horizon Perspective in Economic Evaluation

Since 2013, the NICE technical guidance has argued for a 'lifetime' perspective on the measurement of costs and benefits in economic modelling involving the use of life table survival curves and, by definition, taking a long-term perspective:

> The time horizon for estimating clinical effectiveness and value for money should be long enough to reflect all important differences in costs or outcomes between the technologies being compared. Many technologies have effects on costs and outcomes over a patient's lifetime. In these circumstances, a lifetime time horizon is usually appropriate. A lifetime time horizon is needed when alternative technologies lead to differences in survival or benefits that last for the remainder of a person's life. (NICE, 2022, p. 196)

Whilst this has been relatively straightforward for the measurement of benefits, for example, in terms of QALYs, there has been a debate about whether the costs of caring for people who go on to develop other health conditions during their additional years of life they live as a result of a certain treatment, should indeed be factored into the calculations (van Baal et al., 2016). This approach to modelling allows fluctuation of health state of patients through decades, for example, in the treatment of depression, which might be in remission and then return, or declining health states over time as in the case of dementia (Comas-Herrera et al., 2017).

Ultimately, we have to balance time horizon biases with uncertainty of extrapolating into the future. When appraising interventions that impact upon survival, it is important to accurately estimate the survival benefit associated with the new treatment. However, survival data is often censored, meaning that extrapolation techniques are used to obtain estimates of the full survival benefit (Latimer, 2011). Types of extrapolation methods available include exponential,

Weibull, Gompertz, log-logistic, or log normal parametric models, as well as more complex and flexible models. Where such analyses are not completed estimates of the survival, benefit will be restricted to that observed directly in the relevant clinical trial(s) and this is likely to represent an underestimate of the true survival gain. This leads to underestimates of the QALYs gained, and therefore results in inaccurate estimates of cost-effectiveness. Latimer (2011) provided recommendations for how survival analysis can be undertaken more systematically in the form of a Survival Model Selection Process algorithm. This involves fitting and testing a range of survival models and comparing these based upon internal validity and external validity. He argued that this Survival Model Selection Process should improve the likelihood that appropriate survival models are chosen, leading to more robust economic evaluations (Latimer, 2011).

Whether or Not to Include Future Health Care Costs

Back in 1997, David Meltzer from the University of Chicago, argued that if future costs of medical care for all future conditions are not included in an economic evaluation of any specific condition, particularly if it extends life expectancy, then cost-effectiveness estimates will be overstated (Meltzer, 1997). This controversial approach has not been widely adopted: why would we stop anyone smoking using this argument, as they will live longer and cost society more? We can instead think about the extent to which a preventative intervention that can improve well-being across the life-course should really try to take a life-course approach, and take account of a wider range of future benefits across a number of domains relating to well-being that may be positively impacted on by a preventative intervention such as improving resilience, reducing depression or anxiety, and the wider spill-over effects in families and communities.

Advances in the Capability Paradigm that Address Well-being and Well-becoming

At a microeconomic level, there is an interesting programme of work developing in the capability paradigm of outcome in health economics. This centres around a framework based on conceiving capabilities as evolving across the life-course. It seeks to contribute to the modelling of health outcomes across the life-course (Helter et al., 2020; Mitchell et al., 2021). Concerning children and young people, the terms 'well-being' and 'well-becoming' are not used, rather the term 'capability' is used. There is definitely a synergy of ideas evolving and the

Table 1.4 ICEpop CAPability (ICECAP) measures relevant to different life-course stages

Life-course stage	Measure	Link to instruments
Children	ICECAP for Children and Young People (ICECAP-CYP)	https://www.bristol.ac.uk/population-health-sciences/projects/icecap/icecap-cyp/
Adults	ICECAP for Adults (ICECAP-A)	https://www.bristol.ac.uk/population-health-sciences/projects/icecap/icecap-a/
Older adults	ICECAP for Older People (ICECAP-O)	https://www.bristol.ac.uk/population-health-sciences/projects/icecap/icecap-o/
People at the end of life	ICECAP Supportive Care Measure (ICECAP-SCM)	https://www.bristol.ac.uk/population-health-sciences/projects/icecap/icecap-scm/
People close to the person at the end of life	ICECAP Close Person Measure (ICECAP-CPM)	https://www.bristol.ac.uk/population-health-sciences/projects/icecap/icecap-cpm/

need for expanding the evaluative space beyond health functioning towards broader capabilities, and we would argue measurement of well-being and well-becoming. The capability movement in outcome measurement in health economics is addressing the challenge of measuring outcomes within a life-course model. This approach allows for the development of an economic evaluation framework that places different capabilities at the centre of attention depending on where an individual is at in their life-course trajectory (Mitchell et al., 2021). Table 1.4 summarizes how the ICEpop CAPability (ICECAP) measures are being designed to reflect what outcomes are important for people at different life-course stages. This research group has also produced the Carer Experience Scale (Goranitis et al., 2014).

A good example of a public health prevention cost-effectiveness study was undertaken by Deidda and colleagues (2022) which used both QALYs and well-being capabilities in the area of reducing sedentary behaviour across four European countries. Using CUA, from the base-case perspective of the NHS and personal and social services, Deidda and colleagues found that self-management strategies plus exercise referral schemes were highly cost-effective compared to exercise referral schemes alone (ICER €4,270 per QALY), but not compared to usual care. Participants allocated to the self-management strategies plus exercise referral schemes group also showed an improvement in years in full capability compared to exercise referral schemes alone and usual care (Deidda et al., 2022). In the study, years in full capability was calculated from the EQ-5D-5L (EuroQol Research Foundation, 2019) and ICECAP-O measures (Grewal et al., 2006).

Moving Beyond the EQ-5D Towards the EQ Health and Well-being Measure

Again, at a microeconomic level, in health economics the EQ-5D has for decades been the generic preference-based, health-related, quality of life measure supported by NICE (Devlin & Krabbe, 2013; NICE, 2013). Preference-based instruments used in economic evaluation such as the EQ-5D often have a restricted scope to capture wider impacts on informal carers or outcomes in other sectors such as social care (Peasgood et al., 2021). Although sector-specific instruments can be utilized, they can cause issues, such as double-counting, when being used to measure the value and benefits of interventions that overlap across different sectors. In consequence, researchers from the University of Sheffield, in collaboration with the EuroQol Research Foundation and other organizations, have recently developed a new measure called the EQ health and well-being (EQ-HWB) that is sufficiently broad enough to capture benefits of health and social care interventions (Peasgood et al., 2021). This new measure was developed from the Extending the QALY research project. The intention was to incorporate all domains relevant to health and social care interventions within the measure, such as impacts on patients, social care users, and informal carers. The EQ-HWB is a standardized measure that comprises twenty-five items that capture the broader state of well-being that goes beyond conventional measures of health. The purpose of the measure is to capture three distinct concepts: health-related quality of life, social care-related quality of life, and carer-related quality of life. The measure encapsulates all facets that could be impacted by health conditions (physical and mental), treatments, self-management, disability, the use and need of social care, and the experience of being a carer (Peasgood et al., 2021).

The strengths of the Extending the QALY project included best practice with regards to clear theoretical underpinnings and the inclusion of qualitative work as part of the instrument development process (Peasgood et al., 2021). Further strengths included transparency regarding decisions made through the development process and engagement with a wide range of stakeholders. However, Peasgood and colleagues acknowledged that there is a limit to what can be included in a generic measure and that the methods of valuation used means that there is a boundary to the number of domains that can be included. They also advocate for further work to understand whether proxy completion of this measure is feasible and how the EQ-HWB compares with existing measures. In addition, the new measure should be sufficiently generic to be used to evaluate health and social care interventions consistently, while also sensitive enough to measure important changes in quality of life in patients, social care users, and carers (Peasgood et al., 2021). What would also be interesting to ask is how this new measure could be used to capture concepts of well-becoming from one life-course stage to the next, for example, with respect for the need for social care support later in life depending on health and well-being in mid-life.

The 'One Health Economics' Movement

The 'One Health economics' movement acknowledges the interrelated nature of human and animal health (Häsler et al., 2021). In February 2017, experts in economics, environment, data science, policy, and human and veterinary medicine, as well as public health, participated in a workshop on One Health economics (Machalaba et al., 2017). The workshop considered multiple aspects of economic assessment methodologies for One Health approaches, producing recommended guiding principles. The recommendations included: 1) systems thinking to identify risks and mitigation options for decision-making under uncertainty; 2) multisectoral economic impact assessment to identify wider relevance and possible resource-sharing; and 3) consistent integration of environmental considerations. The One Health economics movement is focused on the prevention of disease, but its systems approach and inter-disciplinary, intersectoral nature is of great interest to the ideas of well-being and well-becoming going forward.

Increased Use of Cost-benefit Analysis and Social Return on Investment Analysis in the Evaluation of Interventions to Promote Well-being and Well-becoming

Below are brief descriptions of a number of methods of economic evaluation which are increasingly being advocated in the evaluation of public health interventions. With respect to the evaluation of public health interventions—with potential costs and benefits spanning a range of sectors beyond the health sector, and with multiple policy goals—NICE has over the last decade recommended the use of CBA and disaggregated cost consequence analysis (CCA), developed a range of ROI tools, and explored the use of SROI (NICE, 2011, 2012). Probably the most interesting developments in health and well-being measurements have been put forward by HM Treasury relating to identification, measurement, and valuation of well-being changes across

Table 1.5 The taxonomy of sameness and difference for return on investment, social return on investment, cost-benefit analysis, social cost-benefit analysis, and behavioural cost-benefit analysis

Approach	Origins	Reporting guidance	Publication checklist of quality of reporting/critique	Who is wanting that information	Policy decision rule present
ROI	F. Donaldson Brown developed the expanded ROI measure, or DuPont formula, in 1914	Public Health England (2021)	NICE (2011)	Local authorities and their public health commissioners in England, Public Health Wales, and Public Protection Scotland	Positive ROI or highest ROI
SROI	Developed in 1996 by REDF in the US Developed from traditional CBA and social accounting	Nicholls et al. (2009) NEF Consulting (2023)	Fujiwara (2014, 2015) Hutchinson et al. (2019) Banke-Thomas et al. (2015)	Local authorities and their public health commissioners in England, Public Health Wales, and Public Protection Scotland; the third sector (i.e. voluntary sector)	Positive SROI ratio
CBA	French engineer and economist Jules Dupuit introduced the concept of CBA in 1848; later formalized by Alfred Marshall	McIntosh et al. (2010)	Sanghera et al. (2015)	HM Treasury	Positive net benefit or highest net benefit
Social CBA	Little and Mirrlees (1974) and UNIDO developed social CBA techniques in the late 1960s	HM Treasury (2022) *The Green Book*	HM Treasury (2022) *The Green Book*	HM Treasury	Positive net benefit or highest net benefit
Behavioural CBA	Behavioural economics theory (Edwards, 1954; Simon, 1955)	Hölzinger and Grayson (2019)	Not available	HM Treasury and the Behavioural Insights Team	Positive benefit cost ratio or highest benefit cost ratio

CBA = cost-benefit analysis
HM Treasury = Her Majesty's Treasury
NEF = New Economics Foundation
NICE = National Institute for Health and Care Excellence
REDF = Roberts Enterprise Development Fund
ROI = return on investment
SROI = social return on investment
UNIDO = United Nations Industrial Development Organization
US = United States of America

prospective government policy cross-sectorally (HM Treasury, 2021b). The following sections complement: the taxonomy of the origins; the reporting guidance; the publication checklist of quality reporting; who is wanting that information; the measurement units of inputs and outputs; and the policy decision rule present for CBA and SOI (shown in Table 1.5; Edwards & Lawrence, 2021).

Cost-benefit analysis

CBA was formalized in the US Flood Control Act of 1936, which asserted that the federal government had a responsibility to support flood control activities 'if the benefits to whomsoever they may accrue are in excess of the estimated costs, and if the lives and social security of people are otherwise adversely affected' (Arnold, 1988, p. 71). The Kaldor-Hicks criteria of hypothetical compensation argued that a public policy was justified if it produced social gains in excess of social losses so that it was possible for winners from the policy to compensate losers even if compensation did not actually take place—the foundation of new applied welfare economics from the 1950s onwards. Hicks argued that the business of the economist is 'to estimate as far as he [or she] can the gains and losses that are likely to accrue, to various classes, or sections of the population, from the proposed action' (Hicks, 1983, p. 366) with a view to hypothetical compensation being possible. Adler and Posner (1999) rejected the Kalder-Hicks approach, emphasized the social objective of improving overall well-being with considerable emphasis on distributional issues, for example, by statistical averaging of group gains and losses over time and space. There is growing interest, particularly in environmental economics, in the inclusion of equity weights in CBA and that it may make a considerable difference to policy recommendations, but much mainstream CBA has been reluctant to use such weights because of the uncertainty about their values and the wide range they could take (Atkinson & Mourato, 2008).

Social cost-benefit analysis

Little and Mirrlees (1974) and United Nations Industrial Development Organization (UNIDO) developed social CBA techniques in the late 1960s. Social CBA is a marginal analysis technique that assesses the impact of different options on social welfare (HM Treasury, 2020), taking into account the social, economic, environmental, and financial impacts. This technique can be used to express the social costs and social benefits of government policies to society in monetary terms so that the consequences of a range of policies can be compared using a common metric. Change in welfare is measured as the aggregate willingness-to-pay (WTP) for the effects of a certain policy intervention. Social

CBA has been championed in the Netherlands with respect to the evaluation of transport and road system planning including congestion charges, tobacco policy, and alcohol pricing and availability policy (de Kinderen et al., 2019; de Wit et al., 2019; van Meerkerk et al., 2015). This approach is now advocated by HM Treasury (2022) in *The green book*, which provides guidance on how to appraise policies, programmes, and projects.

Behavioural cost-benefit analysis

CBA is based on the neoclassical welfare economics paradigm which assumes that people maximize their long-term best interest, have stable preferences, and are consistent rational actors. Behavioural CBA involves bringing insights from behavioural economics into CBA to reflect the fact that people actually do not always behave rationally (Weimer, 2017). Behavioural economics can provide an empirically informed perspective on CBA, including the important realization that even subtle features of the environment or the design of public health interventions can have meaningful impacts on behaviour (Matjasko et al., 2016). As such, behavioural economics underpins 'nudge theory' which argues the case for positive reinforcement and indirect suggestions as ways to influence the behaviour and decision-making of groups or individuals (Thaler & Sunstein, 2009).

With respect to the economic evaluation of public health interventions, it has proved challenging sometimes to capture economic benefits, for example, the CBA of the Sure Start Programme in the UK for young families (Martin & Pearson, 2004). Public health interventions can fail to be effective due to assumptions about rationality which may be limited or bounded as a result of limited opportunities to take up the offer, addiction, social norms, and the context in which choices are made (Matjasko et al., 2016). The behavioural economics approach, applied to CBA, draws on related fields of psychology and neuroscience.

Behavioural economics has implications for how we conduct CBA as a result of this, particularly whether we should actually use WTP estimates as a basis for shadow prices where no market values exist, for example in the case of a public good such as prevention. Asking people to state their preference for what they would pay for a hypothetical public health intervention to which they may not respond rationally may lead to misleading non-market values which could influence CBA calculations. This applies equally to the argument that a distinction should be made between decision-utility and experienced-utility, making the normative assumption that the allocation of resources should be based on experienced-utility rather than decision-utility. This approach favours 'prospect theory' as a basis for CBA because decision-making under uncertainty departs from 'expected utility theory' (Kahneman & Tversky, 1979; Tversky & Kahneman, 1986). Prospect theory, developed by Daniel Kahneman and Amos Tversky in 1979, underpins behavioural economics and aims to describe the actual behaviour of people and challenges expected utility theory developed by von Neumann and Morgenstern. Prospect theory involves individuals weighing up their potential losses and gains of an action and does not require the assumptions of expected utility theory, that is, rationality (Kahneman & Tversky, 1979; Tversky & Kahneman, 1986). This has implications for what discount rates are chosen in CBA because of present-bias due to irrational impatience. Overall, behavioural economics cautions health economists to the framing of WTP questions and how these might influence the outcome of applying CBA in the evaluation of public health interventions where health and other benefits are often accrued far into the future. Field experiments are becoming more common beyond laboratory experiments to test out whether irrational behaviour as found in the laboratory would influence the calculation of shadow prices representing people's behaviour in real life. This is an effort to use evidence to improve the conduct of CBA (Weimer, 2017). The UK Government has recognized the importance of behavioural economics in establishing the Behavioural Insights Team (The Behavioural Insights Team, n.d.).

Return on investment

ROI was developed by F. Donaldson Brown, who worked at DuPont Company in 1908 as a sales representative in the Explosive Department, and later in the Treasurer's Office in the US. He developed a formula for monitoring business performance that included earnings, working capital, and investments into a single measure, termed ROI. ROI is a performance measure used to evaluate the efficiency of an investment or compare the efficiency of a number of different investments. It tries to directly measure the amount of financial return on a particular investment relative to the investment's cost. To calculate ROI, the benefit (or return) of an investment is divided by the cost of that investment. The result is expressed as a percentage or ratio. ROI analysis has been advocated and is being used in public health to quantify the impact of relatively recent disinvestment in public health, during a decade of austerity and coinciding with a move out of the NHS and into local authority in England. In a systematic review to examine the ROI of public health interventions in high-income countries with universal health care, Masters and colleagues (2017) included fifty-two studies and found a median ROI of 14.3 to 1, and a median cost-benefit ratio (CBR) of 8.3. The median ROI for all twenty-nine local public health interventions was 4.1 to 1, and the median CBR was 10.3. Even larger benefits were reported in twenty-eight studies analysing nationwide public health interventions: the median ROI was 27.2, and the median CBR was 17.5 (Masters et al., 2017). The authors interpreted these results as demonstrating public health interventions as highly cost saving and that cuts to local spending on public health represented a false economy. There were a handful of studies in the review with a negative median or negative ROI or CBR, for example, those provided by Nichol (2001). To address the limitation of defining what constitutes a 'public health intervention', Masters and colleagues used Acheson's (1988) broad definition of public health when considering their search strategy. By including the various fields of public health, the authors established that these fifty-two included studies were representative of public health interventions in general. ROI, and to a lesser extent SROI analysis, do not explicitly reflect 'opportunity cost'. This concept of opportunity cost is absolutely central to the main methods of economic evaluation in the health economics toolbox.

Public Health England (2021) has published resources to help local commissioners achieve value for money by estimating the ROI and cost-effectiveness (cost per QALY) of public health programmes, including how to:

- assess which interventions provide the best value for money, by calculating their costs, benefits, and ROI;
- make the most of a budget by deciding how to split resources across different public health programmes; and
- compare costs, savings, and clinical outcomes.

Public Health England (2021) has produced interactive tools for the following health conditions and services: contraceptive services; Best Start in Life; oral health in pre-school children; older adults; end of life care; mental health; musculoskeletal conditions; NHS Diabetes Prevention Programme; weight management; cardiovascular disease; colorectal cancer; falls prevention; movement into employment; and air pollution. For example, the development of the older adults' NHS and social care ROI tool presents ROI for four different analytical perspectives: NHS financial ROI (where benefits are measured exclusively as gross NHS savings for every £1 spent by commissioners on the intervention); social care financial ROI (where benefits are measured exclusively as gross social care savings for every £1 spent by commissioners on the intervention); financial ROI (where benefits are measured as gross NHS and social care savings for every £1 spent by commissioners on the intervention), and SROI (where benefits include gross NHS and social care savings in addition to monetized QALYs for every £1 spent by commissioners on the intervention; Public Health England, 2020). We could not find evidence on how well these are working and how they could be used in local natural experiments.

Social return on investment

SROI was developed by the Roberts Enterprise Development Fund (REDF) in 1996 (Krlev et al., 2013). Since then, there has been a gradual revision of the original methodology (Tuan, 2008), which has led to the 'triple bottom line' (Norman & MacDonald, 2004), underpinned by the 'blended value accounting' theory (Emerson, 2003). SROI is an evaluative framework that helps organizations to quantify the social, environmental, and economic value being created by producing a ratio that states how much social value (in monetary terms) is created for every £1 of investment (NEF Consulting, 2023; Nicholls et al., 2009). In the UK, SROI has been championed by NEF. NEF offers consultancy and training on the methodology and practice needed to conduct an SROI analysis to clients such as local authorities, universities, public health services, charities, and community groups. Over the last twenty years, a perceived lack of methodological rigour has led health economists amongst others to question the robustness of SROI methods. There is greater acceptance more recently that value judgements required in SROI about the range of stakeholders, range of outcomes, and best proxy financial measures for outcomes also exist in the conduct of CBA. Interestingly, the place of SROI in some organizational settings has been questioned. In consideration of the use of SROI of methods in non-profit organizations and social enterprises, Nielsen and colleagues (2021) concluded that SROI may not be the most appropriate method where organizations have fuzzy purposes, broad value creation goals, broad target groups, very individual or subjective proxies, strongly lagged outcomes, complex or unobservable causality, and lack of legitimacy among stakeholders.

Econometric approaches

Health economists are undertaking novel life-course dynamic microsimulation modelling. In a paper by Skarda and colleagues (2021), they describe the 'LifeSim' model of developmental, economic, social, and health outcomes from birth to death for each child in the Millennium Cohort Study (MCS) in England. LifeSim is a flexible and policy-relevant model which can be easily implemented to carry out long-term childhood policy analysis. New policy-relevant variables of interest, including childhood variables, can be easily incorporated within LifeSim, and the input datasets can be updated as required. Skarda and colleagues (2021) designed a model that links together a diverse set of individual-level life outcomes of interest to policymakers. They consulted with experts in childhood development and childhood policy, demography, epidemiology, human capital economics, and labour economics. They made use of interdisciplinary theory on human capital formation in childhood and how this influences educational attainment, earnings, physical illness, mental illness, mortality, and other outcomes with important impacts on individual well-being through the life-course and other associated public cost.

The Precautionary Principle in Public Health, the COVID-19 Pandemic, and How We Approach the Economics of Well-being and Well-becoming

The precautionary principle emerged during the 1970s in German environmental law, where it was referred to as 'Vorsorgeprinzip'. The precautionary principle enables decision-makers to adopt precautionary measures when scientific information is uncertain and there is potential for causing harm. While science can improve our knowledge base, it can rarely provide certainty, so decisions must be made based on the best available information while erring on the side of caution. We have seen the use of the precautionary principle in the handling internationally of the COVID-19 pandemic (Greenhalgh et al., 2020; Hanna et al., 2020). As put forward by Fischer and Ghelardi (2016), the precautionary principle in the evaluation of public health interventions reverses the onus of proof of effectiveness and cost-effectiveness in interventions designed to reduce harm and seems particularly relevant at the time of the COVID-19 pandemic. The UK Government acted without full evidence, but was aware that the direct health effects of COVID-19 on society would be amplified by the wider economic impacts on health resulting from economic hardship through: 1) public and private indebtedness; 2) an uneven impact of lockdown across regions and countries; and 3) poverty and subsequent effects on health and access to health and social care (Begg, 2020). Fisher and Ghelardi stated that, 'The expectation in Public Health is that interventions employed to reduce harm will not actually increase harm, where "harm" in this context does not include opportunity cost' (Fisher & Ghelardi, 2016, p. 1). This is contrary to the evidence-based medicine paradigm where the onus is to demonstrate clinical effectiveness and cost-effectiveness with sufficient certainty before introducing a new drug or device. These authors consider the cost of society taking precautions to protect public health or mitigate the effects of poverty, for example, and that these precautions are not costless. Looking more broadly across health and the environment, the Rio Declaration on Environment and Development states that, 'In order to protect the environment, the precautionary approach shall be widely applied by States according to their capabilities. Where there are threats of serious or irreversible damage, lack of full scientific certainty shall not be used as a reason for postponing cost-effective measures to prevent environmental degradation' (UN, 1992, principle 15, p. 3).

The problem is that its wider application across different sectors has no agreement about the definition of the degree of precaution and appropriate costs, who bears those costs and who may reap the subsequent benefits. It can be argued that CBA and SROI are actually more closely aligned to the decision theory Bayesian approach to the evaluation of public health interventions put forward by Fischer and colleagues (2013) than CEA and CUA based on RCT evidence (see Figure 1.10). The use of a posterior combination of existing and new updated evidence from a range of sources as well as, or in the absence of, RCT evidence, and awareness of potential 'bias', along the lines of Kahneman's WYSIATI principle (Kahneman, 2012), describes how analysts might take a viewpoint of society or a local community in the case of CBA and SROI. Analysts could then build up a balance sheet of inputs, outputs, and outcomes, and then attempt in both cases to place a monetary value on them. Kahneman used the term WYSIATI to describe the cognitive bias we use when we try to automatically make sense of partial information in a complex world. Fischer and colleagues argued that decision theory aims to forecast the likely impact of a public health intervention and that then it is up to policymakers to weigh up wider costs and outcomes beyond the direct health impacts desired. The processes of CBA and SROI aim to capture these and place monetary values on them where possible.

In Bayesian decision theory, the best estimate of the health effect of an intervention need not depend exclusively on evidence from RCTs but can also depend on prior beliefs based on theory, observation and experience. The basic idea is that one starts with an initial set of beliefs and then updates those beliefs as new evidence becomes available. The initial beliefs are called the 'prior distribution' and the updated beliefs are called the 'posterior distribution'. In some cases it may be appropriate to use a 'null' or 'uninformative' prior and rely exclusively on RCT evidence. In other cases, however, one can use 'informative prior beliefs'—as illustrated below.

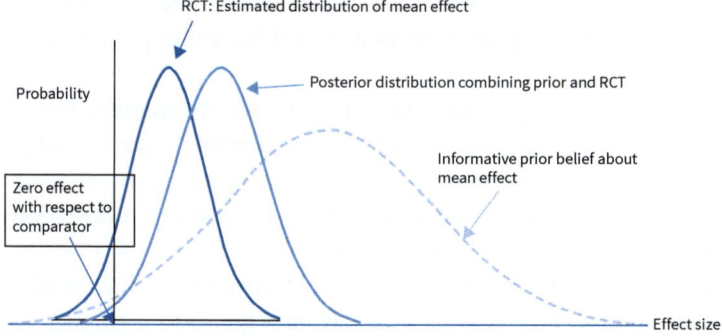

Figure 1.10 Informative prior beliefs

However, we need to be careful. In a US non-profit setting of the evaluation of social enterprises, Cordes alluded to the danger of thinking 'fast' using readily available values in a heuristic sense (Cordes, 2017). He argued that, 'because of difficulties in monetization, attempting to quantify non-profit performance with either SROI analysis or CBA will tend to favour activities with outcomes that are readily translated into dollars, and/or create incentives for non-profits to focus more on those activities that can be monetized' (Cordes, 2017, p. 104). The acknowledgement of the importance of different forms and levels of evidence in science and social science has manifested itself in developments in systematic reviewing, realist reviewing, and the production of rapid reviews for the needs of decision-makers (Khangura et al., 2012). A rapid review study is defined as 'a type of knowledge synthesis in which components of the systematic review process are simplified or omitted to produce information in a short period of time' (Tricco et al., 2015). As this book covers the whole life-course we make use of rapid review methodology.

How We Present Evidence of Value for Money in This Book

In this book, we present and discuss examples at each life-course stage of interventions, policies, or services, some provided by the NHS, social care, employers, schools, and third or charitable sectors, or by communities themselves, that provide 'good value for money' from a payer's perspective. On one side of this equation is what the intervention, policy, or service costs the payer, and this is often in the public sector. On the other side of the equation is how we measure outcome, effectiveness, and, more importantly, how we value these outcomes. It is important to recognize that charities accumulate statistics relevant to a particular issue and are a lobbying body. We draw on evidence they put forward in the absence of other sources.

Some of the evidence we present is in terms of cost-effectiveness. For example, how many people might successfully quit smoking from a given smoking cessation advertising campaign, or how many mothers continue to breastfeed beyond six months as a result of increased midwife support or a more family-friendly public environment per pound spent. Some of the evidence we present is in terms of the additional life years gained from a policy, intervention, or service. For example, reducing salt intake from 8 grams to 6 grams a day is estimated to prevent over 8,000 premature deaths and saves the NHS over £570 million annually (Public Health England, 2016).

One of the most important contributions health economists have made to enable the measurement of value for money of using scarce health care resources through the NHS has been the concept of the QALY (Spencer et al., 2022). For a full in-depth analysis of the historical development and place of QALYs, see the article by MacKillop and Sheard (2018). Based on values from a sample of the UK population, additional years of life at a population level are weighted to reflect the health-related quality of those additional years of life. This is a hypothetical concept along the lines of saving a statistical life on the road from reducing traffic speed. This concept has underpinned the decision-making process of NICE in the UK. This approach taken by NICE has shaped the way most countries internationally (with a public health care system), either tax funded or based on social insurance, have tackled the problem of rising demand for health care and limited resources.

We present evidence of how economists have used the pound (or any relevant currency) as a common denominator for weighing up the costs and outcomes or benefits, or the financial ROI of policies, interventions, or services to promote well-being and well-becoming. CBA has its theoretical roots in welfare economics. It can include only that to which a financial value can be assigned, and at its centre is the principle that something is worth what a person is 'willing to pay' for it, and where no market exists, a shadow price has to be found. CBA has proved useful in enabling the evaluation of public health interventions and policies that can impact the health of the population across sectors. An example of this would be a CBA of introducing cycle paths across cities in Norway, where costs and benefits to health, transport, commerce, and the environment are all weighed up in a single calculation (TemaNord, 2005).

We also present examples of evidence that economists have produced on the SROI or triple bottom line of the financial, economic, and environmental impact of policies, programmes, and services that can improve well-being and well-becoming. This methodology challenges the view that value is the narrow concept of what someone is willing to pay for something through markets; instead, we build on estimates of the 'social value' of, for example, increased community confidence, pride, and shared activities from increased security from crime in a particular neighbourhood. Dolan and colleagues (2007, 2005) provided a methodology for estimating the economic and social costs associated with victimization in relation to violent crime. They conceptualized losses from the fear of crime as all costs in anticipation of possible victimization. Using data from Farrall and Gadd (2004), valuing health loss from episodes of fearfulness gave a mean health annual loss of 0.00065 QALYs. If valued at £30,000 per QALY (as was the case at the time), this would represent an intangible cost of £19.50 per capita per year (Dolan et al., 2007).

We present case studies of published estimates of the costs to society of not addressing health and well-being harming factors across the life-course.

Additionally, we present estimates of the economic benefits to society of policies and programmes that aim to mitigate harming factors or enhance health, well-being, and well-becoming. We include examples of cost-utility, cost-effectiveness, and cost-benefit, or SROI estimates of the relative returns from spending at a microeconomic or programme level on various interventions. This strategy for presenting evidence feels messy and it reflects the state of the application of health economics to the field of public health and prevention.

An elephant in the room is the clear blue water that lies between methods of economic evaluation within the field of health economics and increased interest in adoption of value-based health care methods in the NHS. The concept of cost-effectiveness in health economics is an incremental concept of marginal benefit relative to marginal cost from a payer perspective, often the NHS, but sometimes the public sector or wider society. In value-based health care, often but not always, the concept of value is a calculation based on averages taking a patient-informed perspective. By analysing the concept of value for individuals and society as a whole, we gain insight into how we can enhance the ways in which we can improve value and the tools for accomplishing that (Lewis, 2022). Muir Gray explained the concept of value from a medical perspective: 'Obsessional improvements in quality and safety continue to be important, but even those meritorious activities must add value, not simply improve performance. . . . What is emerging is a new paradigm: better value through population and personalized medicine' (Gray, 2013, p. 201).

This book is an attempt to apply a well-becoming lens on the practice of economic evaluation of public health and preventative interventions through the life-course. Its scope is wide and by default a systematic review approach of evidence would be too great to cover this landscape. What we have tried to do is review the following databases—Web of Science, Medline, CINAHL, PsycInfo, and Cochrane Library—in order to provide up-to-date examples of systematic reviews relevant to each chapter to guide the interested reader.

Structure of the Book

This book follows a life-course model with chapters aligned to pregnancy and early years; adolescence; working age; older age phases of life; and death. The ethos of the book is similar to the book *Extra time* by Camilla Cavendish (2019), which enables people to think about older age in a different way. In this book, we ask the reader to think about the life-course and where we should be investing in cost-effective interventions to support the prevention of chronic disease, disability, and premature death.

The following chapters in this book focus on the evidence of how we can be healthy and happy at each life-course stage, but it is important to acknowledge that we do not, as a society, all have the same opportunities to live healthy and happy lives. This is an argument made by Paul Dolan with respect to social class, an argument that resonates with Michael Marmot's focus on neighbourhoods in terms of where we live, work, and seek our opportunities for recreation. These are fundamental to well-being and well-becoming in the context of this book.

Chapter 2, 'Cross-cutting themes influencing well-being and well-becoming across the life-course', considers the following themes: good work; our surrounding; money and resources; housing; education and skills; the food we eat; transport; and family, friends, and communities. We have chosen to focus on these cross-cutting themes because they have been identified as protective factors and factors that can help individuals and society to maintain good health and well-being (Health Foundation, 2020b; Public Health England, 2019).

Chapter 3, 'Well-being in the early years and childhood', explores the economic case for investing in the critical window of the first few years of life. This chapter focuses on topics such as ACEs; maternal mental health; growing up in poverty; housing; preschool experience; early years vaccinations; dental health; and free school meals.

Chapter 4, 'The well-being and well-becoming of adolescents and young adults', focuses on the challenges for the Millennium generation, and is structured around the following five domains of well-being: good health and optimum nutrition; connectedness, positive values, and contribution to society; safety and a supportive environment; learning, competence, education, skills, and employability; and agency and resilience (Ross et al., 2020). This chapter presents examples of economic evidence of effective and cost-effective interventions to promote resilience and prevent long-term effects of a number of issues such as social media and obesity.

Chapter 5, 'Well-being of the workforce', focuses on the economic arguments relevant to keeping healthy through working age; valuing employees; opportunities for good quality employment; reducing absenteeism and presenteeism due to physical and mental ill-health; and worklessness and returning to work.

Chapter 6, 'Living well for longer', focuses on how to create an environment in which older adults can flourish and is organized around themes identified by the WHO (2007) as important for creating age-friendly environments: transportation; housing; social participation; respect and social inclusion; civic participation and employment; communication and information; community support and health services; and outdoor spaces and buildings.

Chapter 7, 'Dying well', focuses on agency in decision-making relating to how and where people die, and explores dying well across the life-course. This chapter considers the factors that can influence what might be considered a 'good death': place of death; one's company in death; cause of death; and one's manner of facing death (Campbell, 2020).

Chapter 8, 'Diversifying health economics to provide a life-course lens on health, well-being, and well-becoming', revisits concepts of well-being and well-becoming, how they are beginning to be used in health economics, and puts forward a range of ideas for future research and policy support. We also present a new infographic: 'The well-being and well-becoming wheel' (Edwards, 2022). This infographic explains the concept of well-becoming for the purpose of health economics research and policy support within a life-course model. This chapter calls for the need to take a public health and prevention economics lens and a behaviour lens to improve health, well-being, and well-becoming, and explores how we can shift towards a 'well-being economy'.

This book was written during the COVID-19 pandemic, the impact of which has been felt across the life-course. Throughout this book we draw on available evidence documenting the challenges this has brought about, examples of cost-effective interventions, and important questions to consider going forward. We have called these questions 'curiosity questions' because we remain curious and want to see more work done in this area.

Curiosity Questions

- Where does well-being and the concept of well-becoming fit into our traditional collective understanding of what the discipline of health economics is and could be in the future?

- What is the relationship between well-being as part of health economics applied to a wider evaluative space, and well-being in the sense of life satisfaction measurement by economists interested in measuring societal happiness?

- How does taking a 'life-course' perspective change the way we design, undertake, and report economic evaluation studies of individual clinical or public health interventions, or policies and programmes?

- What trade-offs are health economists willing to make between horizon bias and managing uncertainty in modelling future costs and benefits of preventative interventions that could have an impact on health and well-being throughout the life-course?

References

Acheson, D. (1988). *Public health in England: The report of the committee of inquiry into the future development of the public health function.* HM Stationery Office.

Adams-Prassl, A., Boneva, T., Golin, M., & Rauh, C. (2020). *IZA DP No. 13183: Inequality in the impact of the coronavirus shock: Evidence from real time surveys.* IZA Institute of Labor Economics. https://www.iza.org/publications/dp/13183/inequality-in-the-impact-of-the-coronavirus-shock-evidence-from-real-time-surveys

Adler, M. D., Dolan, P., & Kavetsos, G. (2017). Would you choose to be happy? Tradeoffs between happiness and the other dimensions of life in a large population survey. *Journal of Economic Behavior & Organization*, **139**, 60–73. https://doi.org/10.1016/j.jebo.2017.05.006

Adler, M. D., & Posner, E. A. (1999). Rethinking cost-benefit analysis. *The Yale Law Journal*, **109**, 165–247. https://doi.org/10.2307/797489

All Party Parliamentary Group on Social Integration. (2020). *Social connection in the COVID-19 crisis. Initial report from the COVID-19 inquiry by the All Party Parliamentary Group on Social Integration.* British Future. https://www.britishfuture.org/wp-content/uploads/2020/05/Social-Connection-in-the-COVID-19-Crisis.pdf

Arnold, J. L. (1988). *The evolution of the 1936 Flood Control Act.* Office of History, US Army Corps of Engineers.

Ashton, K., Schröder-Bäck, P., Clemens, T., Dyakova, M., Stielke, A., & Bellis, M. A. (2020). The social value of investing in public health across the life course: a systematic scoping review. *BMC Public Health*, **20**(1), 1–18. https://doi.org/10.1186/s12889-020-08685-7

Atkinson, G., & Mourato, S. (2008). Environmental cost-benefit analysis. *Annual Review of Environment and Resources*, **33**, 317–344. https://doi.org/10.1146/annurev.environ.33.020107.112927

Banke-Thomas, A. O., Madaj, B., Charles, A., & van den Broek, N. (2015). Social return on investment (SROI) methodology to account for value for money of public health interventions: A systematic review. *BMC Public Health*, **15**, 582–595. https://doi.org/10.1186/s12889-015-1935-7

Begg, I. (2020, 6 April). *The economic consequences of Covid-19.* The London School of Economics and Political Science. https://blogs.lse.ac.uk/europpblog/2020/04/06/the-economic-consequences-of-covid-19/

Bibby, J., Everest, G., & Abbs, I. (2020, 7 May). *Will COVID-19 be a watershed moment for health inequalities?* The Health Foundation. https://www.health.org.uk/sites/default/files/2020-05/Will%20COVID-19%20be%20a%20watershed%20moment%20for%20health%20inequalities.pdf

Blundell, R., Costa Dias, M., Joyce, R., & Xu, X. (2020). COVID-19 and inequalities. *Fiscal Studies*, **41**(2), 291–319. https://doi.org/10.1111/1475-5890.12232

Brazier, J., Peasgood, T., Mukuria, C., Marten, O., Kreimeier, S., Luo, N., Mulhern, B., Pickard, S., Augustovski, F., Greiner, W., Engel, L., Belizan, M., Yang, Z., Monteiro, A., Kuharic, M., Gibbons, L., Ludwig, K., Carlton, J., Connell, J., . . . & Rejon-Parrilla, J. C. (2022). The EQ-HWB: Overview of the development of a measure of health and wellbeing and key results. *Value in Health*, **25**(4), 482–491. https://doi.org/10.1016/j.jval.2022.01.009

Brien, P., & Keep, M. (2023, 12 September). *Public spending during the Covid-19 pandemic.* House of Commons Library, UK Parliament. https://commonslibrary.parliament.uk/research-briefings/cbp-9309/

Bu, F., Steptoe, A., & Fancourt, D. (2020). Who is lonely in lockdown? Cross-cohort analyses of predictors of loneliness before and during the COVID-19 pandemic. *Public Health, 186,* 31–34. https://doi.org/10.1016/j.puhe.2020.06.036

Buck, D., & Maguire, D. (2015). *Inequalities in life expectancy: Changes over time and implications for policy.* The King's Fund. https://www.kingsfund.org.uk/sites/default/files/field/field_publication_file/inequalities-in-life-expectancy-kings-fund-aug15.pdf

Butland, B., Jebb, S., Kopeman, P., McPherson, K., Thomas, S., Mardell, J., & Parry, V. (2007). *Foresight. Tackling obesities: Future choices—project report* (2nd ed.). Government Office for Science. https://assets.publishing.service.gov.uk/media/5a759da7e5274a4368298a4f/07-1184x-tackling-obesities-future-choices-report.pdf

Campbell, S. M. (2020). Well-being and the good death. *Ethical Theory and Moral Practice, 23*(3), 607–623. https://doi.org/10.1007/s10677-020-10101-3

Campbell, M., Fitzpatrick, R., Haines, A., Kinmonth, A. L., Sandercock, P., Spiegelhalter, D., & Tyrer, P. (2000). Framework for design and evaluation of complex interventions to improve health. *BMJ, 321,* 694–696. https://doi.org/10.1136/bmj.321.7262.694

Cassidy, C. (2017). Wellbeing, being well or well becoming: Who or what is it for and how might we get there? In M. Thorburn (Ed.), *Wellbeing, education and contemporary schooling* (pp. 13–26). Routledge.

Cavendish, C. (2019). *Extra time: 10 lessons for an ageing world.* Harper Collins.

Children's Commissioner. (2020). *We're all in this together? Local area profiles of child vulnerability.* Children's Commissioner for England. https://assets.childrenscommissioner.gov.uk/wpuploads/2020/04/cco-were-all-in-this-together.pdf

Chrysopoulou, A. (2020, 16 December). *The vision of a well-being economy.* Stanford Social Innovation Review. https://ssir.org/articles/entry/the_vision_of_a_well_being_economy

Cicchetti, D., & Toth, S. L. (2005). Child maltreatment. *Annual Review of Clinical Psychology, 1,* 409–438. https://doi.org/10.1146/annurev.clinpsy.1.102803.144029

Coast, J. (2019). Assessing capability in economic evaluation: a life course approach? *The European Journal of Health Economics, 20,* 779–784. https://doi.org/10.1007/s10198-018-1027-6

Coast, J., Kinghorn, P., & Mitchell, P. (2015). The development of capability measures in health economics: opportunities, challenges and progress. *The Patient-Patient-Centered Outcomes Research, 8*(2), 119–126. https://doi.org/10.1007/s40271-014-0080-1

Comas-Herrera, A., Knapp, M., Wittenberg, R., Banerjee, S., Bowling, A., Grundy, E., Jagger, C., Farina, N., Lombard, D., Lorenz, K., & McDaid, D. (2017). MODEM: A comprehensive approach to modelling outcome and costs impacts of interventions for dementia [Protocol paper]. *BMC Health Services Research, 17*(1), 1–8. https://doi.org/10.1186/s12913-016-1945-x

Cookson, R., & Claxton, K. (Eds.). (2012). *The humble economist: Tony Culyer on health, health care and social decision making.* University of York Centre for Health Economics.

Cookson, R., Griffin, S., Norheim, O. F., & Culyer, A. J. (Eds.). (2020). *Distributional cost-effectiveness analysis: Quantifying health equity impacts and trade-offs.* Oxford University Press.

Cordes, J. J. (2017). Using cost-benefit analysis and social return on investment to evaluate the impact of social enterprise: Promises, implementation, and limitations. *Evaluation and Program Planning, 64*, 98–104. https://doi.org/10.1016/j.evalprogplan.2016.11.008

COVID-19 Critical Intelligence Unit. (2020, 23 April). *Evidence check: Domestic and family violence and COVID-19*. NSW Government Health. https://aci.health.nsw.gov.au/__data/assets/pdf_file/0010/579493/Evidence-Check-Domestic-and-family-violence-and-COVID-19.pdf

Craig, P., Dieppe, P., Macintyre, S., Michie, S., Nazareth, I., & Petticrew, M. (2008). Developing and evaluating complex interventions: The new Medical Research Council guidance. *BMJ, 337*, a1655. https://doi.org/10.1136/bmj.a1655

Culyer, A. J. (1989). The normative economics of health care finance and provision. *Oxford Review of Economic Policy, 5*(1), 34–58. https://doi.org/10.1093/oxrep/5.1.34

Dalziel, P., Saunders, C., & Saunders, J. (2018). *Wellbeing economics: The capabilities approach to prosperity*. Springer Nature.

Dawson, S., Campbell, S. M., Giles, S. J., Morris, R. L., & Cheraghi-Sohi, S. (2018). Black and minority ethnic group involvement in health and social care research: A systematic review. *Health Expectations, 21*(1), 3–22. https://doi.org/10.1111/hex.12597

de Kinderen, R. J. A., Wijnen, B. F. M., Evers, S. M. A. A., Hiligsmann, M., Paulus, A. T. G., de Wit, G. A., van Gils, P. F., Over, E. A. B., Suijkerbuijk, A. W. M, & Smit, F. (2019). Social cost-benefit analysis of tobacco control policies in the Netherlands. *European Journal of Public Health, 29*(Suppl. 4). https://doi.org/10.1093/ eurpub/ckz185.793

de Wit, G. A., van Gils, P. F., Over, E. A. B., Suijkerbuijk, A. W. M., Lokkerbol, J., Smit, F., Spit, W. J., Evers, S. M. A. A., & de Kinderen, R. J. A. (2019). Social cost-benefit analysis of regulatory policies to reduce alcohol use in The Netherlands. *European Journal of Public Health, 29*(Suppl. 4). https://doi.org/10.1093/eurpub /ckz185.794

Deidda, M., Geue, C., Kreif, N., Dundas, R., & McIntosh, E. (2019). A framework for conducting economic evaluations alongside natural experiments. *Social Science & Medicine, 220*, 353–361. https://doi.org/10.1016/j.socscimed.2018.11.032

Deidda, M., Coll-Planas, L., Tully, M. A., Giné-Garriga, M., Kee, F., Roqué i Figuls, M., Blackburn, N. E., Guerra-Balic, M., Rothenbacher, D., Dallmeier, D., & Caserotti, P. (2022). Cost-effectiveness of a programme to address sedentary behaviour in older adults: Results from the SITLESS RCT. *European Journal of Public Health, 32*(3), 415–421. https://doi.org/10.1093/eurpub/ckac017

Department of Health. (2012). *Long-term conditions compendium of information* (3rd digital ed.). Long Term Conditions Team. https://assets.publishing.service.gov.uk/government/uploads/system/uploads/attachment_data/file/216528/dh_134486.pdf

Devlin, N. J., & Krabbe, P. F. (2013). The development of new research methods for the valuation of EQ-5D-5L. *The European Journal of Health Economics, 14*(Suppl. 1), 1–3. https://doi.org/10.1007/s10198-013-0502-3

Diabetes UK. (2019, 25 February). *Number of people with diabetes reaches 4.7 million*. https://www.diabetes.org.uk/node/12167

Dodge, R., Daly, A., Huyton, J., & Sanders, L. (2012). The challenge of defining wellbeing. *International Journal of Wellbeing, 2*(3), 222–235. https://doi.org/10.5502/ijw.v2i3.4

Dolan, P. (2014). *Happiness by design: Finding pleasure and purpose in everyday life*. Penguin Books Limited.

Dolan, P. (2019). *Happy ever after: A radical new approach to living well*. Penguin Random House.

Dolan, P., & Kahneman, D. (2008). Interpretations of utility and their implications for the valuation of health. *The Economic Journal*, **118**(525), 215–234. https://doi.org/10.1111/j.1468-0297.2007.02110.x

Dolan, P., Layard, R., O'Donnell, G., Delaney, L., Krekel, C., Sanders, J., Blanco-Jimenez, C., Laffan, K., Kavetsos, G., & Kudrna, L. (2021). *Shaping the post-Covid world: Moving towards wellbeing over the lifetime as the unit of analysis in policy.* London School of Economics and Political Science. https://www.lse.ac.uk/PBS/assets/documents/SPCW-WELLBEING-FINAL.pdf

Dolan, P., Loomes, G., Peasgood, T., & Tsuchiya, A. (2005). Estimating the intangible victim costs of violent crime. *British Journal of Criminology*, **45**(6), 958–976. https://doi.org/10.1093/bjc/azi029

Dolan, P., & Peasgood, T. (2007). Estimating the economic and social costs of the fear of crime. *British Journal of Criminology*, **47**(1), 121–132. https://doi.org/10.1093/bjc/azl015

Drummond, M. F., Sculpher, M. J., Claxton, K., Stoddart, G. L., & Torrance, G. W. (2015). *Methods for the economic evaluation of health care programmes* (4th ed.). Oxford University Press.

Early Intervention Foundation. (2020, 11 June). *The impact of COVID-19 on education and children's services. Written evidence submitted to the Education Committee Inquiry by the Early Intervention Foundation.* https://www.eif.org.uk/files/blog/eif-covid19-children-education-submission.pdf

Eaton, G. (2020, 16 April). Will the UK pay for this pandemic with another decade of austerity? *The New Statesman.* https://www.newstatesman.com/politics/economy/2020/04/coronavirus-uk-economy-cuts-austerity-bank-of-england

Edwards, R. T. (2001). Paradigms and research programmes: Is it time to move from health care economics to health economics? *Health Economics*, **10**(7), 635–649. https://doi.org/10.1002/hec.610

Edwards, R. T. (2022). Well-being and well-becoming through the life-course in public health economics research and policy: A new infographic. *Frontiers in Public Health*, **10**, 1035260. https://doi.org/10.3389/fpubh.2022.1035260

Edwards, R. T., Bryning, L., & Lloyd-Williams, H. (2016). *Transforming young lives across Wales: The economic argument for investing in early years.* Centre for Health Economics and Medicines Evaluation, Bangor University. https://cheme.bangor.ac.uk/documents/transforming-young-lives/CHEME%20transforming%20Young%20Lives%20Full%20Report%20Eng%20WEB%202.pdf

Edwards, R. T., & Lawrence, C. L. (2021). 'What you see is all there is': The importance of heuristics in cost-benefit analysis (CBA) and social return on investment (SROI) in the evaluation of public health interventions. *Applied Health Economics and Health Policy*, **19**(5), 653–664. https://doi.org/10.1007/s40258-021-00653-5

Edwards, R.T., & McIntosh, E. (Eds.). (2019). *Applied health economics for public health practice and research.* Oxford University Press.

Edwards, R. T., Spencer, L. H., Anthony, B. F., & Bryning, L. (2019). *Wellness in work: The economic arguments for investing in the health and wellbeing of the workforce in Wales.* Centre for Health Economics and Medicines Evaluation, Bangor University. https://cheme.bangor.ac.uk/documents/Wellness-in-Work-Report.pdf

Edwards, R. T., Spencer, L. H., Bryning, L., & Anthony, B. F. (2018). *Living well for longer: The economic argument for investing in the health and wellbeing of older people in Wales*. Centre for Economic Health and Medicines Evaluation, Bangor University. https://cheme.bangor.ac.uk/documents/livingwell2018.pdf

Edwards, W. (1954). The theory of decision making. *Psychological Bulletin*, 51, 380–417. https://doi.org/10.1037/h0053870

Elwell-Sutton, T., Finch, D., & Bibby, J. (2019). *The nation's health: Priorities for the next government*. The Health Foundation. https://www.health.org.uk/sites/default/files/2019-11/ge01-_the_nations_health.pdf

Emerson, J. (2003). The blended value proposition: Integrating social and financial returns. *California Management Review*, 45(4), 35–51https://doi.org/10.2307/41166187

Erman, M., & Wingrove, P. (2023, 10 March). *Bayer plans to spend $1 bln on US pharma R&D in 2023-US pharma head*. Reuters. https://www.reuters.com/business/hea lthcare-pharmaceuticals/bayer-plans-spend-1-bln-us-pharma-rd-2023-us-pha rma-head-2023-03-09/

EuroQol Research Foundation. (2018, December). *EQ-5D-3L: User guide. Basic information on how to use the EQ-5D-5L instrument. Version 6.0.* https://euroqol.org/ publications/user-guides/

EuroQol Research Foundation. (2019, September). *EQ-5D-5L User guide. Version 3.0.* https://euroqol.org/publications/user-guides/

Farrall, S., & Gadd, D. (2004). Evaluating crime fears: A research note on a pilot study to improve the measurement of the 'fear of crime' as a performance indicator. *Evaluation*, 10(4), 493–502. https://doi.org/10.1177/1356389004050216

Ferguson, B. (2016, 22 February). *Investing in prevention: The need to make the case now*. UK Health Security Agency. https://publichealthmatters.blog.gov.uk/2016/02/22/investing-in-prevention-the-need-to-make-the-case-now/

Fischer, A. J., & Ghelardi, G. (2016). The precautionary principle, evidence-based medicine, and decision theory in public health evaluation. *Frontiers in Public Health*, 7(4), 107. https://doi.org/10.3389/fpubh.2016.00107

Fischer, A. J., Threlfall, A., Meah, S., Cookson, R., Rutter, H., & Kelly, M. P. (2013). The appraisal of public health interventions: An overview. *Journal of Public Health*, 35(4), 488–494. https://doi.org/10.1093/pubmed/fdt076

Fujiwara, D. (2014). *Measuring the social impact of community investment: The methodology paper*. Housing Associations Charitable Trust (HACT). https://hact.org.uk/publicati ons/measuring-the-social-impact-of-community-investment-methodology-paper/

Fujiwara, D. (2015). *The seven principle problems of SROI*. Simetrica. https://socialvalueuk. org/wp-content/uploads/2023/01/The-Seven-Principle-Problems-with-SROI_Daniel-Fujiwara-4.pdf

Garcia, L., Pearce, M., Abbas, A., Mok, A., Strain, T., Ali, S., Crippa, A., Dempsey, P. C., Golubic, R., Kelly, P., Laird, Y., McNamara, E., Moore, S., de Sa, T. H., Smith, A. D., Wijndaele, K., Woodcock, J., & Brage, S. (2023). Non-occupational physical activity and risk of cardiovascular disease, cancer and mortality outcomes: A dose–response meta-analysis of large prospective studies. *British Journal of Sports Medicine*, 57(15), 979–989. http://dx.doi.org/10.1136/bjsports-2022-105669

Giannetti, B. F., Agostinho, F., Almeida, C. M. V. B., & Huisingh, D. (2015). A review of limitations of GDP and alternative indices to monitor human wellbeing and to manage eco-system functionality. *Journal of Cleaner Production*, 87, 11–25. https://doi.org/ 10.1016/j.jclepro.2014.10.051

Goranitis, I., Coast, J., & Al-Janabi, H. (2014). An investigation into the construct validity of the Carer Experience Scale (CES). *Quality of Life Research*, **23**, 1743–1752. https://doi.org/10.1007/s11136-013-0616-1

Gray, J. M. (2013). The shift to personalised and population medicine. *The Lancet*, **382**(9888), 200–201. https://doi.org/10.1016/S0140-6736(13)61590-1

Greenhalgh, T., Schmid, M. B., Czypionka, T., Bassler, D., & Gruer, L. (2020). Face masks for the public during the Covid-19 crisis. *BMJ*, **369**, m1435. https://doi.org/10.1136/bmj.m1435

Grewal, I., Lewis, J., Flynn, T., Brown, J., Bond, J., & Coast, J. (2006). Developing attributes for a generic quality of life measure for older people: Preferences or capabilities? *Social Science & Medicine*, **62**(8), 1891–1901. https://doi.org/10.1016/j.socscimed.2005.08.023

Hanna, T. P., Evans, G. A., & Booth, C. M. (2020). Cancer, COVID-19 and the precautionary principle: Prioritizing treatment during a global pandemic. *Nature Reviews Clinical Oncology*, **17**(5), 268–270. https://doi.org/10.1038/s41571-020-0362-6

Häsler, B., Cuevas, S., Canali, M., Aragrande, M., Shaw, A., & Zinsstag, J. (2021). One health economics. In J. Zinsstag, E. Schelling, L. Crump, M. Whittaker, M. Tanner, & C. Stephen (Eds.), *One health: The theory and practice of integrated health approaches* (2nd ed., pp. 118–134). CABI.

Hawkes, H. (2021, 6 September). *GDP alternatives: 8 ways of measuring economic health*. In the Black. https://www.intheblack.com/articles/2021/09/06/8-ways-of-measuring-economic-health

Health and Equity in Recovery Plans Working Group. (2020). *Direct and indirect impacts of COVID-19 on health and wellbeing*. https://www.ljmu.ac.uk/~/media/phi-reports/2020-07-direct-and-indirect-impacts-of-covid19-on-health-and-wellbeing.pdf

Heckman, J. J. (2008). The case for investing in disadvantaged young children. *CESifo DICE Report*, **6**(2), 3–8. http://hdl.handle.net/10419/166932

Heckman, J. J. (2012, 7 December). *Invest in early childhood development: Reduce deficits, strengthen the economy*. The Heckman Equation. https://heckmanequation.org/wp-content/uploads/2013/07/F_HeckmanDeficitPieceCUSTOM-Generic_052714-3.pdf

Helliwell, J. F. (2019). Determinants of well-being and their implications for health care. *Annals of Nutrition and Metabolism*, **74**(2), 8–14. https://doi.org/10.1159/000499141

Helliwell, J. F., Layard, R., Sachs, J., & De Neve. J.-E. (Eds.). (2020). *World happiness report 2020*. Sustainable Development Solutions Network. https://happiness-report.s3.amazonaws.com/2020/WHR20.pdf

Helter, T. M., Coast, J., Łaszewska, A., Stamm, T., & Simon, J. (2020). Capability instruments in economic evaluations of health-related interventions: A comparative review of the literature. *Quality of Life Research*, **29**(6), 1433–1464. https://doi.org/10.1007/s11136-019-02393-5

Hicks, J. (1983). *Classics and moderns: Collected essays on economic theory* (Vol. 3). Harvard University Press.

Hill, S. (2019). *An investigation of economic evaluation methods for public health interventions: Meeting the needs of public health decision-makers* [Doctoral thesis, Newcastle University]. Newcastle University Theses Repository. https://theses.ncl.ac.uk/jspui/bitstream/10443/4908/1/Hill%20SR%202019.pdf

HM Treasury. (2020). *Magenta Book: Central government guidance on evaluation*. https://assets.publishing.service.gov.uk/government/uploads/system/uploads/attachment_data/file/879438/HMT_Magenta_Book.pdf

HM Treasury. (2021a). *Build back better: Our plan for growth.* https://assets.publishing.serv ice.gov.uk/government/uploads/system/uploads/attachment_data/file/968403/PfG_F inal_Web_Accessible_Version.pdf

HM Treasury. (2021b). *Wellbeing guidance for appraisal: Supplementary Green Book guidance.* Social Impacts Task Force. https://assets.publishing.service.gov.uk/governm ent/uploads/system/uploads/attachment_data/file/1005388/Wellbeing_guidance_for_ appraisal_-_supplementary_Green_Book_guidance.pdf

HM Treasury. (2022). *The Green Book: Central government guidance on appraisal and evaluation.* https://assets.publishing.service.gov.uk/government/uploads/system/uplo ads/attachment_data/file/1063330/Green_Book_2022.pdf

Hölzinger, O., & Grayson, N. (2019). *Birmingham health economic assessment and natural capital accounts: Revealing the true value of council-managed parks and greenspaces.* Birmingham City Council. Consultancy for Environmental Economics & Policy. https://www.birmingham.gov.uk/download/downloads/id/13452/birmingham_natura l_capital_accounts_-_july_2019.pdf

Home Affairs Select Committee. (2020). *Home Office preparedness for Covid-19 (Coronavirus): Domestic abuse and risks of harm within the home. Second report of session 2019–21.* House of Commons. https://committees.parliament.uk/publications/ 785/documents/5040/default/

Hughes, K., Bellis, M. A., Hardcastle, K. A., Sethi, D., Butchart, A., Mikton, C., Jones, L., & Dunne, M. P. (2017). The effect of multiple adverse childhood experiences on health: A systematic review and meta-analysis. *The Lancet Public Health*, 2(8), e356– e366. https://doi.org/10.1016/S2468-2667(17)30118-4

Hutchinson, C. L., Berndt, A., Forsythe, D., Gilbert-Hunt, S., George, S., & Ratcliffe, J. (2019). Valuing the impact of health and social care programs using social return on investment analysis: How have academics advanced the methodology? A systematic review. *BMJ Open*, 9, e029789. https://doi.org/10.1136/bmjopen-2019-029789

Ipsos MORI and The Fawcett Society. (2020, 20 May). *6 in 10 women finding it harder to stay positive day-to-day due to Coronavirus.* Women more likely to bearing the emotional and impact of the pandemic. https://www.fawcettsociety.org.uk/Handlers/ Download.ashx?IDMF=f173fde3-4edb-4c51-8453-7244e867ed90

Isba, R., Edge, R., Jenner, R., Broughton, E., Francis, N., & Butler, J. (2020). Where have all the children gone? Decreases in paediatric emergency department attendances at the start of the COVID-19 pandemic of 2020. *Archives of Disease in Childhood*, 105(7), 704–704. https://doi.org/10.1136/archdischild-2020-319385

Kahneman, D. (2012). *Thinking, fast and slow.* Macmillan.

Kahneman, D., Diener, E., & Schwarz, N. (Eds.). (1999). *Well-being: The foundations of hedonic psychology.* Russell Sage Foundation.

Kahneman, D., & Tversky, A. (1979). Prospect theory: An analysis of decision under risk. *Econometrica*, 47, 263–291. https://doi.org/10.2307/1914185

Kane, P. (2007, 26 February). Not wellbeing, but wellbecoming. *The Guardian.* https://www. theguardian.com/commentisfree/2007/feb/26/theresbeensomuchthats

Karoly, L. A., & Bigelow, J. H. (2005). *The economics of investing in universal preschool education in California.* Rand Corporation. https://www.rand.org/content/dam/rand/ pubs/monographs/2005/RAND_MG349.pdf

Kessler, R. C., Berglund, P., Demler, O., Jin, R., Merikangas, K. R., & Walters, E. E. (2005). Lifetime prevalence and age-of-onset distributions of DSM-IV disorders in the national comorbidity survey replication. *Archives of General Psychiatry*, **62**(6) 593–602. https://doi.org/10.1001/archpsyc.62.6.593

Khan, L. (2016). *Missed opportunities: A review of recent evidence into children and young people's mental health*. Centre for Mental Health. https://www.consaludmental.org/publicaciones/Missed-Opportunities.pdf

Khangura, S., Konnyu, K., Cushman, R., Grimshaw, J., & Moher, D. (2012). Evidence summaries: The evolution of a rapid review approach. *Systematic Reviews*, **1**(1), 1–9. https://doi.org/10.1186/2046-4053-1-10

Khunti, K., & Farooqi, A. (2020, 1 July). *Ensuring ethnic diversity in COVID-19 research*. National Institute for Health and Care Research. https://www.nihr.ac.uk/blog/ensuring-ethnic-diversity-in-covid-19-research/25160

Krlev, G., Münscher, R., & Mülbert, K. (2013). *Social return on investment (SROI): State-of-the-art and perspectives. A meta-analysis of practice in Social Return on Investment (SROI) studies published 2002–2012*. Centre for Social Investment, University of Heidelberg. https://d-nb.info/1195630204/34

Kubiszewski, I., Costanza, R., Franco, C., Lawn, P., Talberth, J., Jackson, T., & Aylmer, C. (2013). Beyond GDP: Measuring and achieving global genuine progress. *Ecological Economics*, **93**, 57–68. https://doi.org/10.1016/j.ecolecon.2013.04.019

Kuruvilla, S., Sadana, R., Montesinos, E. V., Beard, J., Vasdeki, J. F., de Carvalho, I. A., Thomas, R. B., Drisse, M.-N. B., Daelmans, B., Goodman, T., Koller, T., Officer, A., Vogel, J., Valentine, N., Wootton, E., Banerjee, A., Magar, V., Neira, M., Bele., J. M. O., . . . Bustreo, F. (2018). A life-course approach to health: Synergy with sustainable development goals. *Bulletin of the World Health Organization*, **96**(1), 42–50. https://doi.org/10.2471/BLT.17.198358

Latimer, N. (2011). *NICE DSU technical support document 14: Undertaking survival analysis for economic evaluations alongside clinical trials—extrapolation with patient-level data*. Decision Support Unit, ScHARR, University of Sheffield. https://www.ncbi.nlm.nih.gov/books/NBK395885/pdf/Bookshelf_NBK395885.pdf

Layard, R., Graham, C., De Neve, J.-E., & O'Donnell, G. (2022, 8 July). *A wellbeing manifesto*. https://cep.lse.ac.uk/textonly/people/layard/papers/0598_WellbeingManifesto.pdf

Layard, R., & Ward, G. (2020). *Can we be happier?: Evidence and ethics*. Penguin Books Limited.

Le, L. K. D., Esturas, A. C., Mihalopoulos, C., Chiotelis, O., Bucholc, J., Chatterton, M. L., & Engel, L. (2021). Cost-effectiveness evidence of mental health prevention and promotion interventions: A systematic review of economic evaluations. *PLoS Medicine*, **18**(5), e1003606. https://doi.org/10.1371/journal.pmed.1003606

Levell, P., Sampson, T., Crowley, M. A., & Winters, L. A. (2020). *What is the likely impact of Brexit on inequality in household earnings?* Economics Observatory. https://www.economicsobservatory.com/what-likely-impact-brexit-inequality-household-earnings

Lewis, S. (2022). Value-based healthcare: Is it the way forward? *Future Healthcare Journal*, **9**(3), 211–215. https://www.ncbi.nlm.nih.gov/pmc/articles/PMC9761467/

Lindsay, W. A., Murphy, M. M., Almghairbi, D. S., & Moppett, I. K. (2020). Age, sex, race and ethnicity representativeness of randomised controlled trials in peri-operative medicine. *Anaesthesia*, **75**(6), 809–815. https://doi.org/10.1111/anae.14967

Little, I., & Mirrlees, J. (1974). *Project appraisal and planning for developing countries.* Heinemann Educational.

Local Government Association. (2020). *Coronavirus: LGA responds to Children's Commissioner report on vulnerable children.* https://www.local.gov.uk/about/news/coro navirus-lga-responds-childrens-commissioner-report-vulnerable-children

Local Government Association. (2023). *Public mental health and wellbeing and COVID-19.* https://www.local.gov.uk/public-mental-health-and-wellbeing-and-covid-19

Machalaba, C., Smith, K. M., Awada, L., Berry, K., Berthe, F., Bouley, T. A., Bruce, M., Cortiñas Abrahantes, J., El Turabi, A., Feferholtz, Y., Flynn, L., Fournié, G., Andre, A., Grace, D., Jonas, O., Kimani, T., Le Gall, F., Jose Miranda, J., Peyre, M., . . . Karesh, W. B. (2017). One Health Economics to confront disease threats. *Transactions of The Royal Society of Tropical Medicine and Hygiene,* 111(6), 235–237. https://doi.org/10.1093/trs tmh/trx039

MacKillop, E., & Sheard, S. (2018). Quantifying life: Understanding the history of quality-adjusted life-years (QALYs). *Social Science & Medicine,* 211, 359–366. https://doi.org/10.1016/j.socscimed.2018.07.004

Marmot, M., Allen, J., Boyce, T., Goldblatt, P., & Morrison, J. (2020a). *Health equity in England: The Marmot review 10 years on.* Institute of Health Equity. https://www.health.org.uk/publications/reports/the-marmot-review-10-years-on

Marmot, M., Allen, J., Goldblatt, P., Boyce, T., McNeish, D., Grady, M., & Geddes, I. (2010). *Fair society, healthy lives: The Marmot review. Strategic review of health inequalities in England post-2010.* https://www.instituteofhealthequity.org/resources-reports/fair-society-healthy-lives-the-marmot-review

Marmot, M., Allen, J., Goldblatt, P., Herd, E., & Morrison, J. (2020b). *Build back fairer: The COVID-19 Marmot review.* Institute of Health Equity. https://www.health.org.uk/publi cations/build-back-fairer-the-covid-19-marmot-review

Marmot, M., & Wilkinson, R. (Eds.). (2005). *Social determinants of health* (2nd ed.). Oxford University Press.

Martela, F., & Sheldon, K. M. (2019). Clarifying the concept of well-being: Psychological need satisfaction as the common core connecting eudaimonic and subjective well-being. *Review of General Psychology,* 23(4), 458–474. https://doi.org/10.1177/10892 68019880886

Martin, S., Lomas, J., & Claxton, K. (2019). *Is an ounce of prevention worth a pound of cure? Estimates of the impact of English public health grant on mortality and morbidity.* Centre for Health Economics Discussion Papers, University of York. https://www.york.ac.uk/media/che/documents/papers/researchpapers/CHERP166_Impact_Public_Hea lth_Mortality_Morbidity.pdf

Martin, A., & Pearson, M. (2004). *Kirklees district Sure Start Thornhill evaluation report.* University of Huddersfield. http://www.ness.bbk.ac.uk/support/AnnualReports/documents/906.pdf

Mason, A., & Towse, A. (Eds.). (2008). *The ideas and influence of Alan Williams: Be reasonable, do it my way!* Radcliffe Publishing.

Masten, A. S. (2018). Resilience theory and research on children and families: Past, present, and promise. *Journal of Family Theory & Review,* 10(1), 12–31. https://doi.org/10.1111/jftr.12255

Masters, R., Anwar, E., Collins, B., Cookson, R., & Capewell, S. (2017). Return on investment of public health interventions: A systematic review. *Journal of Epidemiology and Community Health*, 71, 827–834. https://doi.org/10.1136/jech-2016-208141

Matjasko, J. L., Cawley, J. H., Baker-Goering, M. M., & Yokum, D. V. (2016). Applying behavioral economics to public health policy: Illustrative examples and promising directions. *American Journal of Preventive Medicine*, 50(5), S13–S19. https://doi.org/10.1016/j.amepre.2016.02.007

McDaid, D., Sassi, F., & Merkur, S. (Eds.). (2015). *Promoting health, preventing disease: The economic case*. Open University Press & McGraw-Hill.

McIntosh, E., Clarke, P., Frew, E., & Louviere, J. J. (2010). *Applied methods of cost-benefit analysis in health care* (Vol. 4). Oxford University Press.

Meltzer, D. (1997). Accounting for future costs in medical cost-effectiveness analysis. *Journal of Health Economics*, 16(1), 33–64. https://doi.org/10.1016/S0167-6296(96)00507-3

Ministry of Housing and Urban Affairs. (2019). *Ease of Living Index 2019: Assessment framework*. Government of India. http://amplifi.mohua.gov.in/assets/html-landing/pdf/eol.pdf

Mishra, G., Hardy, R., & Kuh, D. (Eds.). (2023). *A life course approach to women's health* (2nd ed.). Oxford University Press.

Mitchell, P. M., Husbands, S., Byford, S., Kinghorn, P., Bailey, C., Peters, T. J., & Coast, J. (2021). Challenges in developing capability measures for children and young people for use in the economic evaluation of health and care interventions. *Health Economics*, 30(9), 1990–2003. https://doi.org/10.1002/hec.4363

Morgan, D., & James, C. (2022). *Investing in health systems to protect society and boost the economy: Priority investments and order-of-magnitude cost estimates* (OECD Health Working Papers No. 144). https://dx.doi.org/10.1787/d0aa9188-en

Morgan, A., & Ziglio, E. (2007). Revitalising the evidence base for public health: An assets model. *Promotion & Education*, 14(Suppl. 2), 17–22. https://doi.org./10.1177/10253823070140020701x

Morris, S., Devlin, N., & Parkin, D. (2007). *Economic analysis in health care*. John Wiley & Sons.

National Health Service England. (2014). *Five year forward view*. https://www.england.nhs.uk/wp-content/uploads/2014/10/5yfv-web.pdf

National Health Service England. (2022, 28 March). *NHS Prevention Programme cuts chances of Type 2 diabetes for thousands*. https://www.england.nhs.uk/2022/03/nhs-prevention-programme-cuts-chances-of-type-2-diabetes-for-thousands/

National Health Service Business Services Authority. (2021, 26 August). *Prescribing for diabetes—England 2015/16 to 2020/21*. https://www.nhsbsa.nhs.uk/statistical-collections/prescribing-diabetes-england/prescribing-diabetes-england-201516-202021

National Institute for Health and Care Excellence. (2011). *Supporting investment in public health: Review of methods for assessing cost effectiveness, cost impact and return on investment* (Proof of concept report). https://www.nice.org.uk/media/default/About/what-we-do/NICE-guidance/NICE-guidelines/Public-health-guidelines/Additional-publications/Cost-impact-proof-of-concept.pdf

National Institute for Health and Care Excellence. (2012). *Methods for the development of NICE public health guidance* (PMG4). https://www.nice.org.uk/process/pmg4

National Institute for Health and Clinical Excellence. (2013). *Guide to the methods of technology appraisal 2013* (PMG9). https://www.nice.org.uk/process/pmg9/

National Institute for Health and Clinical Excellence. (2022). *NICE health technology evaluations: The manual* (PMG36). www.nice.org.uk/process/pmg36

New Economics Foundation Consulting. (2023). *Social return on investment (SROI)*. https://www.nefconsulting.com/what-we-do/evaluation-impact-assessment/sroi/

Nichol, K. L. (2001). Cost-benefit analysis of a strategy to vaccinate healthy working adults against influenza. *Archives of Internal Medicine, 161*, 749–795. https://doi.org/10.1001/archinte.161.5.749

Nicholls, J., Lawlor, E., Neitzert, E., & Goodspeed, T. (2009). *A guide to social return on investment*. Office of the Third Sector, Cabinet Office. https://neweconomics.org/uplo ads/files/aff3779953c5b88d53_cpm6v3v71.pdf

Nielsen, J. G., Lueg, R., & Van Liempd, D. (2021). Challenges and boundaries in implementing social return on investment: An inquiry into its situational appropriateness. *Nonprofit Management and Leadership, 31*(3), 413–435. https://doi.org/10.1002/nml.21439

Norman, W., & MacDonald, C. (2004). Getting to the bottom of 'triple bottom line'. *Business Ethics Quarterly, 14*, 243–262. https://doi.org/10.5840/beq200414211

Nsamenang, A. B. (2010). Fathers, families, and children's well-becoming in Africa. In M. E. Lamb (Ed.), *The role of the father in child development* (5th ed., pp. 388–412). John Wiley & Sons Inc.

Office for Budget Responsibility. (2022). *Fiscal risks and sustainability*. HM Government. https://obr.uk/docs/dlm_uploads/Fiscal_risks_and_sustainability_2022-1.pdf

Office for Budget Responsibility. (2023, 17 April). *Brexit analysis*. https://obr.uk/forecasts-in-depth/the-economy-forecast/brexit-analysis/#assumptions

Office for National Statistics. (2018a, 26 September). *Surveys using our four personal well-being questions*. https://www.ons.gov.uk/peoplepopulationandcommunity/wellbeing/methodologies/surveysusingthe4officefornationalstatisticspersonalwellbeingquestions

Office for National Statistics. (2018b, 13 August). *Living longer: How our population is changing and why it matters*. https://www.ons.gov.uk/peoplepopulationandcommunity/birthsdeathsandmarriages/ageing/articles/livinglongerhowourpopulationischanging andwhyitmatters/2018-08-13

Office for National Statistics. (2019, 15 March). *Living longer: Caring in later working life*. https://www.ons.gov.uk/peoplepopulationandcommunity/birthsdeathsandmarriages/ageing/articles/livinglongerhowourpopulationischangingandwhyitmatters/2019-03-15

Office for National Statistics. (2020a, 9 April). *Coronavirus and the social impacts on Great Britain: 9 April 2020*. https://www.ons.gov.uk/peoplepopulationandcommunity/heal thandsocialcare/healthandwellbeing/bulletins/coronavirusandthesocialimpactsongreat britain/9april2020

Office for National Statistics. (2020b, 8 June). *Coronavirus and loneliness, Great Britain: 3 April to 3 May 2020*. https://www.ons.gov.uk/releases/coronavirusandlonelinessgreat britain3april2020to3may2020

Office for National Statistics. (2020c, 11 June). *Coronavirus and the social impacts on disabled people in Great Britain (14 May to 24 May 2020)*. https://www.gov.uk/governm ent/statistics/coronavirus-and-the-social-impacts-on-disabled-people-in-great-brit ain-14-may-2020-to-24-may-2020

Office for National Statistics. (2020d, 24 April). *Coronavirus and the social impacts on disabled people in Great Britain (27 March to 13 April 2020)*. https://www.ons.gov.uk/peoplepopulationandcommunity/healthandsocialcare/disability/articles/coronavirusanddthesocialimpactsondisabledpeopleingreatbritain/2020-04-24

Office for National Statistics. (2020e, 28 April). *Healthcare expenditure, UK health accounts: 2018*. https://www.ons.gov.uk/peoplepopulationandcommunity/healthandsocialcare/healthcaresystem/bulletin s/ukhealthaccounts/2018

Office for National Statistics. (2021, 1 February). *International comparisons of GDP during the coronavirus (COVID-19) pandemic*. https://www.ons.gov.uk/economy/grossdomesticproductgdp/articles/internationalcomparisonsofgdpduringthecoronaviruscovid19pandemic/2021-02-01

Office for National Statistics. (2022, 12 January). *Past and projected period and cohort life tables: 2020-based, UK, 1981 to 2070*. https://www.ons.gov.uk/peoplepopulationandcommunity/birthsdeathsandmarriages/lifeexpectancies/bulletins/pastandprojecteddatafromtheperiodandcohortlifetables/2020baseduk1981to2070

Office for National Statistics. (2023, 31 July). *UK Government debt and deficit: December 2022*. https://www.ons.gov.uk/economy/governmentpublicsectorandtaxes/publicspending/bulletins/ukgovernmentdebtanddeficitforeurostatmaast/december2022

Osberg, L. (1985). The measurement of economic welfare. In D. Laidler (Ed.), *Approaches to economic well-being* (Vol. 26, pp. 49–89). Royal Commission of the Economic Union and Development Prospects for Canada (MacDonald Commission). University of Toronto Press. http://hdl.handle.net/10222/72989

Osberg, L., & Sharpe, A. (2001). Comparisons of trends in GDP and economic well-being – The impact of social capital. In J. F. Helliwell (Ed.), *The contribution of human and social capital to sustained economic growth and well-being: International Symposium Report* (pp. 310–351). Human Resources Development Canada and OECD.

Osuafor, C. N., Golubic, R., & Ray, S. (2021). Ethnic inclusivity and preventative health research in addressing health inequalities and developing evidence base. *EClinicalMedicine*, *31*, 1–3. https://doi.org/10.1016/j.eclinm.2020.100672

Owen, L. & Fischer, A. (2019). The cost-effectiveness of public health interventions examined by the National Institute for Health and Care Excellence from 2005 to 2018. *Public Health*, *169*, 151–162. https://doi.org/10.1016/j.puhe.2019.02.011

Peasgood, T., Mukuria, C., Carlton, J., Connell, J., Devlin, N., Jones, K., Lovett, R., Naidoo, B., Rand, S., Rejon-Parrilla, J. C., Rowen, D., Tsuchiya, A., & Brazier, J. (2021). What is the best approach to adopt for identifying the domains for a new measure of health, social care and carer-related quality of life to measure quality-adjusted life years? Application to the development of the EQ-HWB? *The European Journal of Health Economics*, *22*(7), 1067–1081. https://doi.org/10.1007/s10198-021-01306-z

Perez, C. C. (2019). *Invisible women: Exposing data bias in a world designed for men*. Chatto & Windus.

Peterman, A., Potts, A., O'Donnell, M., Thompson, K., Shah, N., Oertelt-Prigione, S., & van Gelder. N. (2020). *Pandemics and violence against women and children*. Center for Global Development. https://www.cgdev.org/sites/default/files/pandemics-and-vawg-april2.pdf

Petticrew, M., Knai, C., Thomas, J., Rehfuess, E. A., Noyes, J., Gerhardus, A., Grimshaw, J. M., Rutter, H., & McGill, E. (2019). Implications of a complexity perspective for systematic reviews and guideline development in health decision making. *BMJ Global Health*, 4(Suppl. 1), e000899. https://doi.org/10.1136/bmjgh-2018-000899

Pitchforth, J., Fahy, K., Ford, T., Wolpert, M., Viner, R. M., & Hargreaves, D. S. (2018). Mental health and well-being trends among children and young people in the UK,1995–2014: Analysis of repeated cross-sectional national health surveys. *Psychological Medicine*, 48, 1275–1285. https://doi.org/10.1017/S0033291718001757

Portas, M. (2020, January). *Welcome to the kindness economy* [Video]. TED Conferences. https://www.ted.com/talks/mary_portas_welcome_to_the_kindness_economy

Public Health England. (2016, 22 March). *New PHE data on salt consumption levels*. https://www.gov.uk/government/news/new-phe-data-on-salt-consumption-levels

Public Health England. (2019, 23 May). *Health matters: Prevention—a life course approach*. https://www.gov.uk/government/publications/health-matters-life-course-approach-to-prevention/health-matters-prevention-a-life-course-approach

Public Health England. (2020). *The older adults' NHS and social care return on investment tool: Final report*. https://assets.publishing.service.gov.uk/government/uploads/sys tem/uploads/attachment_data/file/860613/Older_adults_NHS_and_social_care_ret urn_on_investment_tool_-_Final_report.pdf

Public Health England. (2021, 14 August). *Health economics: A guide for public health teams*. https://www.gov.uk/guidance/health-economics-a-guide-for-public-health-teams#the-cost-effectiveness-of-specific-topic-areas

Rajan, A. (Host). (2021, 7 January). Rethink fairness: Health (Episode 4) [Audio podcast]. In *BBC Rethink*. https://www.bbc.co.uk/programmes/m000qxzl

Rea, D., & Burton, T. (2020). New evidence on the Heckman curve. *Journal of Economic Surveys*, 34(2), 241–262. https://doi.org/10.1111/joes.12353

Rethink Mental Illness. (2020). *Mental Health Policy Group: 2020 Comprehensive spending review*. https://www.rethink.org/campaigns-and-policy/campaign-with-us/resources-and-reports/mental-health-policy-group-2020-comprehensive-spending-review/

Richards, D., Enrique, A., Eilert, N., Franklin, M., Palacios, J., Duffy, D., Earley, C., Chapman, J., Jell, G., Sollesse, S., & Timulak, L. (2020). A pragmatic randomized waitlist-controlled effectiveness and cost-effectiveness trial of digital interventions for depression and anxiety. *Nature Partner Journals Digital Medicine*, 3(1), 1–10. https://doi.org/10.1038/s41746-020-0293-8

Ross, D. A., Hinton, R., Melles-Brewer, M., Engel, D., Zeck, W., Fagan, L., Herat, J., Phaladi, G., Imbago-Jácome, D., Anyona, P., Sanchez, A., Damji, N., Terki, F., Baltag, V., Patton, G., Silverman, A., Fogstad, H., Banerjee, A., & Mohan, A. (2020). Adolescent well-being: A definition and conceptual framework. *Journal of Adolescent Health*, 67(4), 472–476. https://doi.org/10.1016/j.jadohealth.2020.06.042

Roubinov, D., Bush, N. R., & Boyce, W. T. (2020). How a pandemic could advance the science of early adversity. *JAMA Pediatrics*, 174(12), 1131–1132. https://doi.org/10.1001/jamapediatrics.2020.2354

Roy, E. (2019, 11 November). *How cuts are affecting social care performance: What the data says*. Community Care. https://www.communitycare.co.uk/2019/11/11/making-social-care-priority/

Rutter, H. (2018). The complex systems challenge of obesity. *Clinical Chemistry*, **64**(1), 44–46. https://doi.org/10.1373/clinchem.2017.272831

Rutter, H., Savona, N., Glonti, K., Bibby, J., Cummins, S., Finegood, D. T., Greaves, F., Harper, L., Hawe, P., Moore, L., Petticrew, M., Rehfuess, E., Shiell, A., Thomas, J., & White, M. (2017). The need for a complex systems model of evidence for public health. *The Lancet*, **390**(10112), 2602–2604. https://doi.org/10.1016/S0140-6736(17)31267-9

Ryan, R. M., & Deci, E. L. (2001). On happiness and human potentials: A review of research on hedonic and eudaimonic well-being. *Annual Review of Psychology*, **52**(1), 141–166. https://doi.org/10.1146/annurev.psych.52.1.141

Ryff, C. D., & Singer, B. (1998). The contours of positive human health. *Psychological Inquiry*, **9**(1), 1–28. https://doi.org/10.1207/s15327965pli0901_1

Sanghera, S., Frew, E., & Roberts, T. (2015). Adapting the CHEERS statement for reporting cost-benefit analysis. *Pharmacoeconomics*, **33**, 533–534. https://doi.org/10.1007/s40273-015-0265-z

Sen, A .K. (1999). *Development as freedom*. Random House.

Seymour, R. (2020, 23 January). *Can we be happier? by Richard Layard review—a breathless tribute to the 'science of happiness'*. The Guardian. https://www.theguardian.com/books/2020/jan/23/can-we-be-happier-richard-layard-review

Shiell, A., Hawe, P., & Gold, L. (2008). Complex interventions or complex systems? Implications for health economic evaluation. *BMJ*, **336**(7656), 1281–1283. https://doi.org/10.1136/bmj.39569.510521.AD

Shuttleworth, K., & Nicholson, E. (2020, 18 August). *Devolution and the NHS*. Institute for Government. https://www.instituteforgovernment.org.uk/explainers/devolution-nhs

Simon, H. A. (1955). A behavioral model of rational choice. *The Quarterly Journal of Economics*, **69**(1), 99–118. https://doi.org/10.2307/1884852

Skarda, I., Asaria, M., & Cookson, R. (2021). LifeSim: A lifecourse dynamic microsimulation model of the Millennium Birth Cohort in England. *medRxiv*, 1–37. https://doi.org/10.1101/2021.02.12.21251642

Skivington, K., Matthews, L., Simpson, S. A., Craig, P., Baird, J., Blazeby, J. M., Boyd, K. A., Craig, N., French, D. P., McIntosh, E., Petticrew, M., Rycroft-Malone, J., White, M., & Moore, L. (2021). A new framework for developing and evaluating complex interventions: Update of Medical Research Council guidance. *BMJ*, **374**(2061), 1–11. http://dx.doi.org/10.1136/bmj.n2061

Spencer, A., Rivero-Arias, O., Wong, R., Tsuchiya, A., Bleichrodt, H., Edwards, R. T., Norman, R., Lloyd, A., & Clarke, P. (2022). The QALY at 50: One story many voices. *Social Science & Medicine*, **296**, 114653. https://doi.org/10.1016/j.socscimed.2021.114653

Stansfield, J., Mapplethorpe, T., & South, J. (2020, 1 June). *The community response to coronavirus (COVID-19)*. UK Health Security Agency. https://ukhsa.blog.gov.uk/2020/06/01/the-community-response-to-coronavirus-covid-19/

Sugden, R., & Williams, A. (1978). *The principles of practical cost-benefit analysis*. Oxford University Press.

Swann, S., & Shaw, D. (2020, 12 May). *Coronavirus: Lockdown could bring hope for drugs gang teens*. BBC News. https://www.bbc.co.uk/news/uk-52535549

Taylor-Gooby, P., Petricek, T., & Cunliffe, J. (2021). Covid19, charitable giving and collectivism: A data-harvesting approach. *Journal of Social Policy*, 1–22. https://doi.org/10.1017/S0047279421000714

TemaNord. (2005). *CBA of cycling*. Nordic Council of Ministers.

Thaler, R. H., & Sunstein, C. R. (2009). *Nudge: Improving decisions about health, wealth and happiness*. Penguin Books Limited.

Thapar, A., Collishaw, S., Pine, D. S., & Thapar, A. K. (2012). Depression in adolescence. *The Lancet*, **379**(9820), 1056–1067. https://doi.org/10.1016/S0140-6736(11)60871-4

The Behavioural Insights Team. (n.d.). *The Behavioural Insights Team*. https://www.bi.team

The Health Foundation. (2020a, 15 December). *Government must put health at heart of nation's pandemic recovery* [Press release]. https://www.health.org.uk/news-and-comment/news/government-must-put-health-at-heart-of-nations-pandemic-recovery

The Health Foundation. (2020b). *What makes us healthy?* https://www.health.org.uk/what-we-do/a-healthier-uk-population/what-makes-us-healthy

The Health Foundation. (2023, 17 March). *Public health grant: What it is and why greater investment is needed*. https://www.health.org.uk/news-and-comment/charts-and-infographics/public-health-grant-what-it-is-and-why-greater-investment-is-needed

Treanor, M. (2019). *ACEs—repackaging old problems in shiny new (Emperor's) clothes*. The University of Edinburgh. https://blogs.ed.ac.uk/CRFRresilience/2019/08/01/repackaging-old-problems/

Tricco, A. C., Antony, J., Zarin, W., Strifler, L., Ghassemi, M., Ivory, J., Perrier, L., Hutton, B., Moher, D., & Straus, S. E. (2015). A scoping review of rapid review methods. *BMC Medicine*, **13**(1), 1–15. https://doi.org/10.1186/s12916-015-0465-6

Tsuchiya, A., Dolan, P., & Shaw, R. (2003). Measuring people's preferences regarding ageism in health: Some methodological issues and some fresh evidence. *Social Science & Medicine*, **57**(4), 687–696. https://doi.org/10.1016/S0277-9536(02)00418-5

Tuan, M. T. (2008). *Measuring and/or estimating social value creation: Insights into eight integrated cost approaches*. Bill & Melinda Gates Foundation. https://docs.gatesfoundation.org/documents/wwl-report-measuring-estimating-social-value-creation.pdf

Tversky, A., & Kahneman, D. (1986). Rational choice and the framing of decisions. *The Journal of Business*, **59**(4), pt. 2, S251–S278. https://www.jstor.org/stable/2352759

United Kingdom Government. (2023, 20 April). *Deaths in United Kingdom*. https://coronavirus.data.gov.uk/details/deaths

United Nations. (1992). *Report of the United Nations conference on environment and development. Annex I: Rio declaration on environment and development*. https://www.un.org/en/development/desa/population/migration/generalassembly/docs/globalcompact/A_CONF.151_26_Vol.I_Declaration.pdf

United Nations Development Programme. (2020). *Human Development Index (HDI)*. Human Development Reports. http://hdr.undp.org/en/content/human-development-index-hdi

van Baal, P., Meltzer, D., & Brouwer, W. (2016). Future costs, fixed healthcare budgets, and the decision rules of cost-effectiveness analysis. *Health Economics*, **25**(2), 237–248. https://doi.org/10.1002/hec.3138

van Meerkerk, J., Verrips, A., & Hilbers, H. (2015). *A social cost benefit analysis of road pricing in the Netherlands*. CPB Netherlands Bureau for Economic Policy Analysis.

https://www.cpb.nl/sites/default/files/publicaties/download/cpb-background-docum ent-social-cost-benefit-analysis-road-pricing-netherlands.pdf

Vardakoulias, O. (2013, April). *Economics in policy making. Social CBA and SROI*. The New Economics Foundation. https://www.nefconsulting.com/wp-content/uploads/2014/10/ Briefing-on-SROI-and-CBA.pdf

Vemuri, A. W., & Costanza, R. (2006). The role of human, social, built, and natural capital in explaining life satisfaction at the country level: Toward a National Well-Being Index (NWI). *Ecological Economics*, 58(1), 119–133. https://doi.org/10.1016/j.ecole con.2005.02.008

von Hippel, C. (2018). A next generation assets-based public health intervention development model: The public as innovators. *Frontiers in Public Health*, 6, 248. https:// doi.org/10.3389/fpubh.2018.00248

Weatherly, H., Drummond, M., Claxton, K., Cookson, R., Ferguson, B., Godfrey, C., Rice, N., Sculpher, M., & Sowden, A. (2009). Methods for assessing the cost-effectiveness of public health interventions: Key challenges and recommendations. *Health Policy*, 93(2-3), 85–92. https://doi.org/10.1016/j.healthpol.2009.07.012

Weimer, D. (2017). *Behavioural economics for cost benefit analysis*. Cambridge University Press.

Welsh Government. (2015). *Well-being of Future Generations (Wales) Act 2015*. https://gov. wales/sites/default/files/publications/2021-10/well-being-future-generations-wales-act-2015-the-essentials-2021.pdf

Welsh Government. (2023). *Welsh Government's Well-being of Future Generations continuous learning and improvement plan for 2023 to 2025*. https://www.gov.wales/ sites/default/files/pdf-versions/2023/3/2/1680013197/continuous-learning-and-impr ovement-plan-for-2023-to-2025.pdf

Wiking, M. (2019). *The key to happiness: How to find purpose by unlocking the secrets of the world's happiest people*. Penguin Life.

Williams, A. (1987). Health economics: The cheerful face of the dismal science? In A. Williams (Ed.), *Health and economics. Proceedings of section F (economics) of the British Association for the Advancement of Science, Bristol, 1986* (pp. 1–11). Palgrave Macmillan.

Wilson, H., & Waddell, S. (2020). *Covid-19 and early intervention: Understanding the impact, preparing for recovery*. Early Intervention Foundation. https://www.eif.org.uk/ files/pdf/covid-19-services-impact-recovery.pdf

World Health Organization. (1995). *Constitution of the World Health Organization*. https:// apps.who.int/iris/bitstream/handle/10665/121457/em_rc42_cwho_en.pdf

World Health Organization. (2005). *Preventing chronic diseases: A vital investment*. WHO global report. https://iris.who.int/bitstream/handle/10665/43314/9241563001_eng.pdf

World Health Organization. (2007). *Global age-friendly cities: A guide*. Community Health. https://apps.who.int/iris/handle/10665/43755

Xu, K., Soucat, A., Kutzin, J., Brindley, C., Maele, N. v., Touré, H., Garcia, M. A., Li, D., Barroy, H., Flores, G., Roubal, T., Indikadahena, C., Cherilova, V., & Siroka, A. (2018). *Public spending on health: A closer look at global trends*. World Health Organization. https://apps.who.int/iris/rest/bitstreams/1165184/retrieve

Chapter 2

Cross-cutting Themes Influencing Well-being and Well-becoming across the Life-course

Llinos H. Spencer, Ned Hartfiel, Mary Lynch,
Nathan Bray, Bethany F. Anthony,
Catherine L. Lawrence, and
Rhiannon T. Edwards

Introduction: Why Health Economists Need to Understand the Mechanisms of Health and Well-being

For years it has felt like, as health economists, we have been parachuted in to join multidisciplinary clinical trial groups, or use existing data or estimates from the literature to identify, measure, and value costs and outcomes relevant to a medicine, diagnostic test, or health care intervention. As some health economists have turned to evaluating the cost-effectiveness or return on investment (ROI) of public health interventions, it has become more necessary to understand mechanisms of how interventions end up being effective and potentially cost-effective or not, particularly where these require co-production or behaviour change by patients, or in the case of preventative interventions, by all of us. There are parallels in pharmacoeconomics in considerations of compliance with the taking or not of medications where behaviour change is of interest (De Geest et al., 2019; Gwadry-Sridhar et al., 2009). In public health economics we have seen the characterization of public health interventions as 'complex interventions' (Skivington et al., 2021), the increased use of logic models to illustrate context (Public Health England, 2018a; Rehfuess et al., 2018), and the increased use of realist synthesis methods to document what works, how, and in what context (Emmel et al., 2018; HM Treasury, 2020; Public Health England, 2018). To this end, it is perhaps helpful to explore in this chapter various models that underpin our understanding of well-being and well-becoming that are integral to the following chapters of this book.

Llinos H. Spencer, Ned Hartfiel, Mary Lynch, Nathan Bray, Bethany F. Anthony, Catherine L. Lawrence, and Rhiannon T. Edwards, *Cross-cutting Themes Influencing Well-being and Well-becoming across the Life-course* In: *Health Economics of Well-being and Well-becoming across the Life-course*. Edited by: Rhiannon T. Edwards and Catherine L. Lawrence, Oxford University Press. © Oxford University Press 2024. DOI: 10.1093/9780191919336.003.0002

How We Think about Well-being Today

In the United Kingdom (UK), the Office for National Statistics (ONS) defines well-being as, 'how we are doing as individuals, as communities and as a nation, and how sustainable this is for the future' (ONS, 2021a, p. 2). The ONS has created the Measures of National Well-being Dashboard which monitors and reports how the UK is doing by producing accepted and trusted measures for different areas of life that matter most to the UK population. These areas include personal well-being, our relationships, health, what we do, where we live, personal finance, economy, education and skills, governance, and environment (ONS, 2021a).

This chapter highlights a number of historical models of the basic needs we all share across the life-course and how they reflect the wider determinants of our health, well-being and well-becoming. These models are by Maslow (1943, 2017), Dahlgren and Whitehead (2006), and more recently, The Health Foundation (Bibby & Lovell, 2018). As outlined in Chapter 1, well-being, happiness, and health are distinct concepts, but they overlap. You can be unhappy in good health, and happy in poor health. Several studies have documented links between happiness and health that are maintained even after negative emotions are taken into account, implying that associations between happiness and health may be distinctive (Steptoe, 2019). Based on these models, the aim of this chapter is to consider aspects that are associated with good positive well-being and well-becoming through the life-course and set out some of the economic costs to society of not investing in those key areas, amplified by the coronavirus disease 2019 (COVID-19) pandemic and its outcomes. Barriers and enablers of well-being and well-becoming for economic benefit in the future are also discussed.

Maslow's Hierarchy of Needs Model

Maslow's (1943, 2017) hierarchy of needs model is still useful today as it introduces the concept that basic needs have to be fulfilled first before psychological needs or self-fulfilment. Although Maslow's hierarchy of needs is believed by many to be static, he asserted that the order of needs is not rigid and that there is some fluidity between the levels. This model can be divided into deficiency needs and growth needs (see Figure 2.1). The first four levels are often referred to as 'deficiency needs' (D-needs), and the top level is known as 'growth or being needs' (B-needs) (Noltemeyer et al., 2012). Deficiency needs have to be satisfied before growth needs. Growth needs relate to the concepts of reaching full potential and well-becoming. The next section develops the theme of human

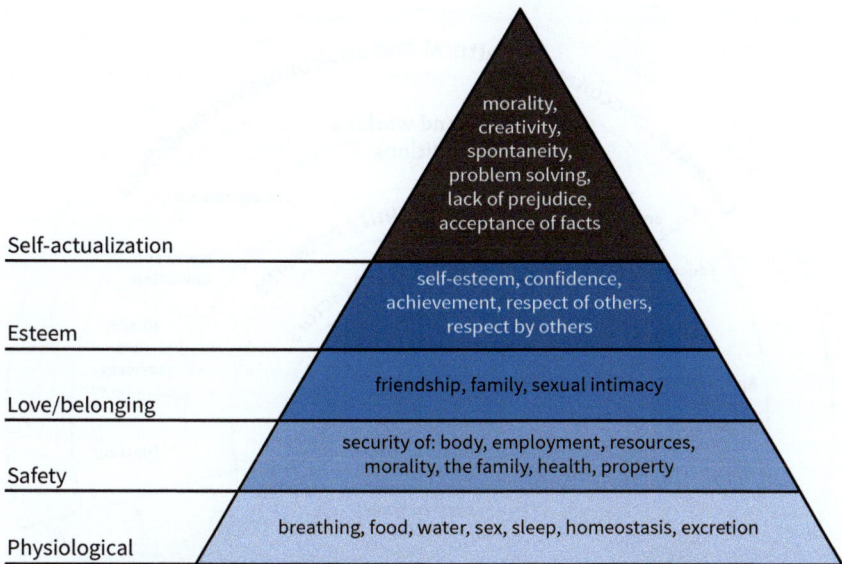

Figure 2.1 Maslow's (2017) hierarchy of needs model
Reproduced with permission from Maslow, A. H. (2017). *A theory of human motivation*. BN
Publishing. © Maslow 2017. All rights reserved.

needs and relates these to the person within society and the economy through
the Dahlgren and Whitehead (2006) rainbow model of determinants of health.

The Dahlgren and Whitehead Rainbow Model of Determinants of Health

The Dahlgren and Whitehead (2006) rainbow model of determinants of health
was originally developed in 1991 to show how environmental, social, and economic factors can shape health and inequalities in health (see Figure 2.2).
Economic, environmental, and social inequalities can determine people's risk
of becoming ill, their ability to prevent sickness, or their access to effective treatments. The Dahlgren and Whitehead model maps the relationship between the
individual, their environment, and health. Individuals are placed in the centre
and surrounding them are the various layers of influences on health, such as individual lifestyle factors, community influences, living and working conditions,
and more general social conditions. This model has helped researchers and
policymakers construct a host of hypotheses about the determinants of health
and explore the relative influence of these determinants on different health outcomes and the interactions between the various determinants.

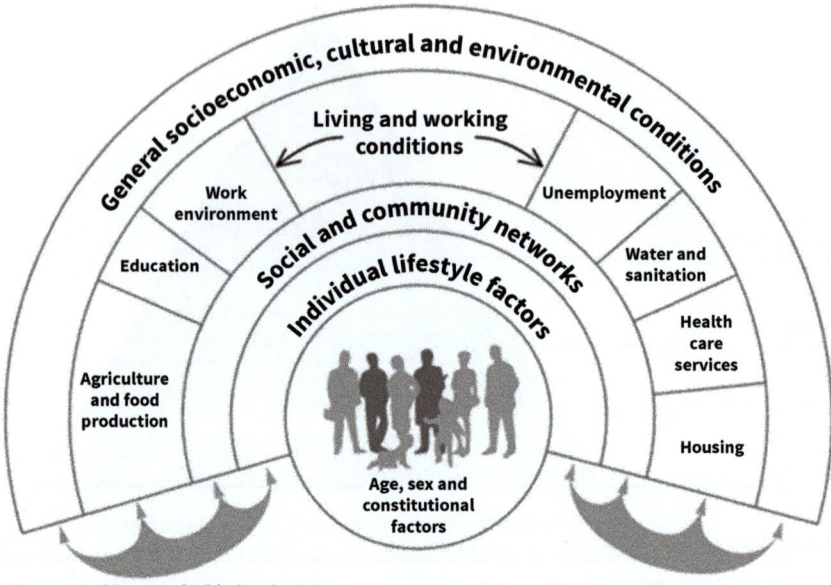

Source: Dahlgren and Whitehead, 1993

Figure 2.2 Dahlgren and Whitehead's (2006) rainbow model of determinants of health
Reproduced from Dahlgren, G., & Whitehead, M. (2006). *European strategies for tackling social inequities in health: Levelling up Part 2.* World Health Organization. Copyright © 2006. https://iris.who.int/bitstream/handle/10665/107791/E89384.pdf

The Dahlgren and Whitehead (2006) rainbow model remains one of the most well-known and effective illustrations of health determinants and has had a widespread impact in research on health inequality. Psychosocial explanations are considered at the individual (micro) and social (macro) levels. At the micro-level it is argued that 'cognitive processes of comparison', in particular perceived relative deprivation, contribute to heightened levels of stress and subsequent ill-health. At the macro-level, psychosocial explanations focus on impairment of social bonds and limited civic participation, so-called social capital, that flows from income inequalities. The Dahlgren and Whitehead model provides an insight into the fact that social and economic factors are part of health disparities (see Figure 2.2).

The Health Foundation Model of What Makes Us Healthy

The Health Foundation (2017) developed the 'What makes us healthy?' model shown in Figure 2.3. This is arguably a roadmap of health and well-being, which includes the following themes: good work; our surroundings; money

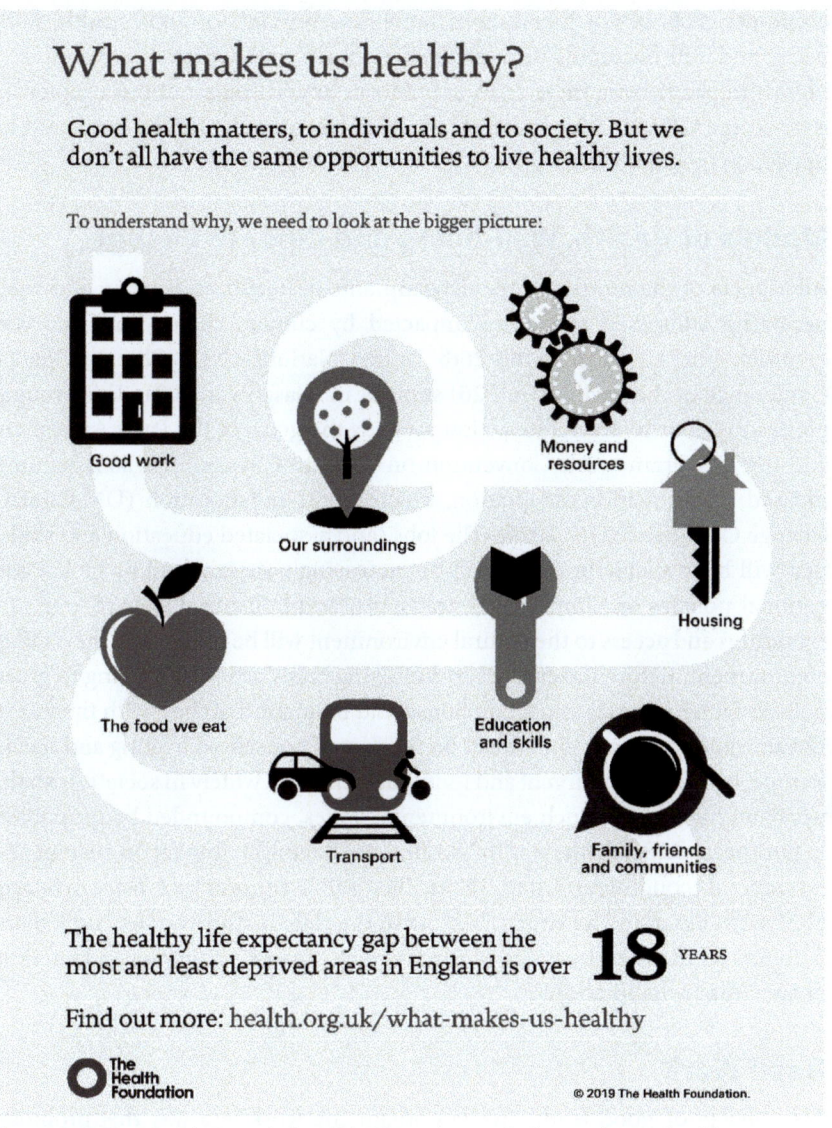

Figure 2.3 The Health Foundation (2017) roadmap of what makes us healthy
Reproduced with permission from The Health Foundation. (2017, 29 June). *Infographic: What makes us healthy?*. https://www.health.org.uk/infographic-what-makes-us-healthy. Copyright © The Health Foundation 2019. All rights reserved.

and resources; housing; education and skills; the food we eat; transport; and family, friends, and communities. We use this model to provide a framework for Chapter 2 and discuss cross-cutting themes that may influence our life-time health and well-being opportunity architecture. We give a case study of economic costs of not investing in these determinants of good health, well-being, and well-becoming through the life-course, and potential economic savings from prioritizing these areas in public policy. Throughout this chapter we refer to the COVID-19 pandemic, where it has amplified these costs and its impact on inequalities.

Models of Health, Well-being and Climate Change

All aspects of the models of the determinants of health, well-being and well-becoming addressed above are impacted by climate change in some way or other. The UK hosted the 26th United Nations (UN) Climate Change Conference of the Parties (COP26) summit in Glasgow in 2021. This brought parties together to accelerate action towards the goals of the Paris Agreement and the UN Framework Convention on Climate Change. The 2021 summit focused on mitigation, adaptation, finance, and collaboration (UN Climate Change Conference UK, 2021). The jobs (and associated education and skills) that will be available in future will be increasingly determined by global and national policies on climate, fuel, transport, and housing. Likewise, our surroundings and access to the natural environment will be affected by the COP26 commitment. Before the current cost of living crisis, we were looking to green policies which have an impact on household finances. This has, with the war in Ukraine and the knock-on impact on the cost of household heating and fuel in Europe, become more urgent and its impact felt more widely in society, with the worst-off hardest hit. Such environmental issues, compounded by geopolitics in Europe, specifically the war in Ukraine, are having an impact on current and future food economies (Orhan, 2022). The COP27 summit took place in Sharm El-Sheikh, Egypt in November 2022, with the slogan 'Together for implementation' as its focus and continued the four key themes: mitigation, adaptation, finance, and collaboration.

Good Work

The concept of 'good work' involves organizing work in a way that promotes good physical and mental health. The UK Government's Industrial Strategy set out five functional principles of good quality work: satisfaction; fair pay; participation and progression; well-being, safety and security; and voice and autonomy (HM Government, 2017b; UK Government, 2018). Good employment, especially paid employment, is important for quality of life (Edwards et al., 2019; Welsh et al., 2016). Good quality work contributes to the well-being of workers by meeting the basic psychological needs of respect, self-efficacy, self-esteem, sense of belonging, and meaningfulness (Hunter, 2010).

The relationship between work and health was the subject of seminal work by Marmot and colleagues (Marmot et al., 1991). The Whitehall studies investigated social determinants of health, particularly cardiovascular disease prevalence and mortality rates among British civil servants. The first prospective cohort study began in 1967 and examined over 17,500 male civil servants aged between twenty and sixty-four years over a ten-year period. Findings showed a steep inverse association between social class, as assessed by grade of employment, and mortality from a wide range of diseases. The second cohort study, conducted from 1985 to 1988, investigated the degree and causes of social gradient in morbidity in a new cohort of 10,300 civil servants, aged between thirty-five and fifty-five years (two-thirds male and one-third female). Self-perceived health status and symptoms were worse in participants in lower status jobs (Marmot et al., 1991).

Since the Whitehall studies, higher paid work has remained associated with better health outcomes (Marmot et al., 2010). The nature of work can adversely affect health through poor physical conditions such as exposure to chemicals or other hazards, long hours, and shift work. Adverse psychosocial conditions may include conflict, lack of autonomy or control, and poor pay or insufficient hours (e.g. zero-hours contracts) (Goods et al., 2019). Temporary work and the risk of redundancy can affect stress levels, job satisfaction, and the well-being of employees (Durcan, 2015). Public Health England have promoted good quality jobs for good health, with some of the key characteristics of good work being autonomy, fair pay, a good work-life balance, and the absence of bullying or harassment (Durcan, 2015; Farmer & Stevenson, 2017).

Before the COVID-19 pandemic, it was estimated that one million people were on zero-hours contracts out of a workforce of thirty-two million people in the UK (Datta et al., 2019). Although zero-hours contracts may suit some employers and employees, this type of employment is not seen as sustainable over time. Many of these zero-hours contracts are in industries that are generally low-paid sectors, such as retail, health and social care, and hospitality (Datta et al., 2019). Zero-hours contracts (also known as 'no guaranteed hours contracts') can lead to 'in-work' poverty. In-work poverty occurs when a working person's income, after housing costs, is less than 60 per cent of the national average, and the person does not earn enough to meet the cost of living (Chartered Institute of Personnel and Development (CIPD), 2023). In 2022 there were 14.5 million people (more than one in five) who were living in poverty in the UK. This figure is made up of 8.1 million working-age adults, 4.3 million children, and 2.1 million pensioners (Joseph Rowntree Foundation, 2022).

In the UK, a person no longer has to retire from work at a certain age and can carry on working for as long as they want to (UK Government, 2021a). The percentage of those aged over fifty in employment has increased over time as more older people are encouraged to work into later life (Sewdas et al., 2017). The employment rate of people aged fifty to sixty-four increased from 56 per cent in 1984 to 72 per cent in 2020. For those aged sixty-five and over, the employment rate increased from 5 per cent in 1984 to 10 per cent in 2020 (Department for Work & Pensions, 2020). Although there are benefits to working longer, such as passing on experience to future generations of workers, older employees have higher rates of chronic disease than younger employees. Older employees may also be more vulnerable to work-related health risks such as injuries and fatigue (Jones et al., 2013). A systematic review of studies on the health effects of employment in those aged over sixty-four years identified seventeen relevant studies (sixteen studies had a cohort or cross-sectional design and one study evaluated an intervention; Baxter et al., 2021). The findings suggested that working into later life has beneficial or neutral effects on overall health status and physical health, and mixed effects on mental health. Male workers, those working part-time or reducing to part-time hours, and people working in jobs which are not low quality or low reward reported greater benefits to extending their working life. Adverse effects were found for those working in high demand or low reward jobs. Baxter and colleagues (2021) discussed the potential for widening health inequalities between those older adults who are in a position to reduce their working hours and those who need to continue working into later life full-time for financial reasons.

Our Surroundings

The environment in which we live and work is an important determinant of our quality of life and life expectancy. The importance of neighbourhoods has been emphasized in Chapter 1 where we presented the Marmot curve of life expectancy and quality-adjusted life expectancy by level of neighbourhood income deprivation (see Figure 1.2). We can operationalize nature in terms of 'green space' (e.g. parks, woodlands, street trees, and vegetation cover) and 'blue space' (e.g. rivers, lakes, beaches, canals, and promenades; White et al., 2021). Interventions that encourage engaging with green and blue spaces can positively promote health and well-being (Calogiuri & Chroni, 2014). Access to green and blue space has been shown to reduce the risk of chronic diseases such as cardiovascular diseases (Pereira et al., 2012), obesity (Swinburn & Egger, 2002), cancer (Li, 2010), and type 2 diabetes (Maas et al., 2009). See Box 2.1 for a case study on parkrun, an organized free, community event where people can walk, jog or run a timed 5 kilometre route that takes place in various counties across the UK and globally.

Box 2.1 Case study: parkrun

parkrun is an organized free, weekly timed 5 kilometre run/walk that takes place in various counties across the UK and globally (www.parkrun. com; see Figure 2.4). The majority of parkrun events are intended to be inclusive of all abilities (Wiltshire & Stevinson, 2018). parkrun welcomes walkers, joggers, runners, and volunteers (Reece et al., 2019). Uptake of the parkrun offer appears to have largely been organic across countries supported by the parkrun administration. The global parkrun philosophy is to enable everyone to be active and foster a community spirit to achieve a healthier, happier population (Reece et al., 2019). parkrun was halted as part of the social distancing restrictions in the UK in March 2020 and re-started in August 2021.

Over four million people have participated in parkrun events across five continents to date (www.parkrun.com/countries). A scoping review of the evidence of the reach and impact of parkrun identified fifteen eligible studies: twelve from the UK and three from Australia (Grunseit et al., 2020). According to the studies reviewed, mechanisms to improve health and well-being included: the timed component of parkrun (Wiltshire & Stevinson, 2018); undertaking exercise in green space (Rogerson et al., 2016); the physical activity itself (Stevinson & Hickson, 2014); developing fitness (Stevinson et al., 2015); and making social connections (Sharman et al., 2019). Feeling valued and disrupting accepted dialogues about

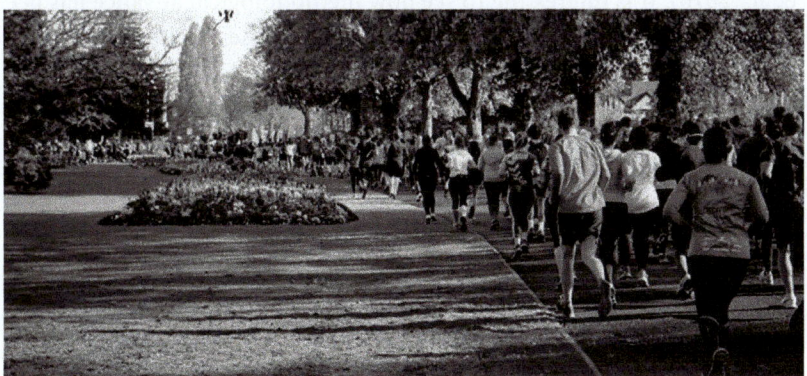

Figure 2.4 Runners taking part in a parkrun event
Reproduced with permission from parkrun Group. (2021, 13 August). *UK update—13 August.* https://blog.parkrun.com/uk/2021/08/13/uk-update-13-august/ Copyright © parkrun Group. All rights reserved.

gender and physical competence were also relevant when considering the volunteering aspect of the parkrun administration (Sharman et al., 2019; Stride et al., 2020).

Despite numerous studies looking at the health effects of parkrun, there has been little economic evaluation of parkrun in terms of its costs relative to health benefits measured by preference-based quality of life measures. This is a good example of the need to understand the mechanism of how a public health intervention such as parkrun may be effective and potentially cost-effective. Grunseit and colleagues recognized the potential for economic evaluation of the parkrun movement, saying that, 'as a multi-component intervention with a range of interacting parts and with multiple local adaptations, future research could examine the emergent properties of parkrun' (Grunseit et al., 2020, p. 8). For the health economist interested in the evaluation of parkrun, the intervention is often adapted locally to suit local communities so may not constitute a generic intervention (Skivington et al., 2021; Craig et al., 2008). Health economists have the opportunity to learn from environmental and natural resource accounting economists about estimation of value in use of the natural environment. These economists have for some time quantified the non-market value of, for example, marine or parkland space, particularly in its use for promoting physical activity and well-being. They have developed standardized methods for capturing and valuing the health benefits of, for example, aquatic physical activities, and the potential savings by the NHS from individuals, such as using the blue gym (Papathanasopoulou et al., 2016). It is interesting to see how methodological advance has been two-way and how environmental economists use quality-adjusted life years (QALYs) to estimate health gains within a wide cost-benefit analysis (CBA), for example, use of marine environments where a spectrum of outcomes are of interest, such as the provision of food, regulation of climate, and the provision of settings for cultural gains, along with health benefits (Papathanasopoulou et al., 2016).

Researchers have noted that economic evaluation, which is a key component of health investment decision-making, would quantify the cost-benefit of parkrun (Ding et al., 2020; Grunseit et al., 2020). A social return on investment (SROI) methodology could also be used to quantify the wider benefits of parkrun in the manner used by other sport studies (Davies et al., 2019). An SROI analysis would allow potential funders, local authorities, and those wishing to set up similar interventions to understand the true health and social impact of parkrun (Quirk et al., 2021).

Due to increased physical activity in green space, it is estimated that £2.1 billion per year could be saved in health care costs if everyone in England had good access to green space (Public Health England, 2020). Physical activity is viewed as an essential health-improving input in the health production process. Moderate/intense exercise and/or exercise training in healthy children and adolescents are associated with a reduction in the incidence of infection and a faster recovery of the immune system (Simpson et al., 2020). Physical activity in green and blue spaces are beneficial for physical and mental health outcomes (Dadvand et al., 2016). For example, green and blue spaces are resources that can be used to promote health and well-being by reducing stress and risk of poor mental health (Bowler et al., 2010; Buhnik, 2010; Mitchell, 2013; Thompson Coon et al., 2011). The positive benefits of green and blue spaces are now advocated in land-use planning (Barton et al., 2009; Grinde & Patil, 2009). Investing in new urban and rural environmental infrastructures could help improve health and well-being and result in social and economic gains while saving on health care resource use (Lynch et al., 2020). Parks and green spaces are estimated to save the UK National Health Service (NHS) around £111 million per year (£3.16 per person), based only on a reduction in the number of visits to the general practitioner (GP) and excluding other costs such as prescriptions and referrals (Watt et al., 2018).

A systematic review found that the public is willing to pay between £5.72 and £15.64 for not postponing or losing an outdoor experience and for walking in local environments under current and improved environmental conditions, respectively (Lynch et al., 2020). Spencer and colleagues (2020) reviewed the literature on how household income affects access to green space and showed that access and availability of green space in local residential environments can promote and encourage participation in physical activity and support active living (e.g. Bedimo-Rung et al., 2005; Gladwell et al., 2013). Spending time in green space can enhance social interaction and cognitive development (Kabisch et al., 2017), and reduce aggressive behaviours in both adults and children (e.g. Amoly et al., 2015; Gascon et al., 2015; Younan et al., 2016). During 2020 and 2021, the UK Government imposed restrictions during a number of national lockdowns in an attempt to control the spread of the COVID-19 virus, for example, by closing gyms and restricting travel (Freeman & Eykelbosh, 2020; Institute for Government, 2022). This disrupted many people's daily routines and limited their access to physical exercise. The government emphasized the importance of daily exercise on health and well-being.

In 2008, the Centre for Well-being at the New Economics Foundation developed the Five Ways to Wellbeing programme, which is a public health message promoting evidence-based practices for improving personal well-being

(Aked & Thompson, 2011; Bragg et al., 2015; Mackay et al., 2019; Pretty et al., 2007). Contact with nature and involvement in nature-based interventions have been shown to facilitate each of the five ways to well-being: connecting with others; being active; taking notice; keep learning; and giving. The delivery of health-related therapeutic interventions in natural environments such as wilderness therapy is becoming an increasingly accepted approach in treating mental health conditions (Bowen et al., 2016). Exercise outdoors in natural environments is associated with higher levels of well-being and lower levels of stress and anxiety (Thompson Coon et al., 2011). A meta-narrative evidence synthesis of environmental, health, well-being, social, and equity effects of urban green space interventions found that green spaces do have a role to play in creating a culture of health and well-being in urban settings (Hunter et al., 2019). These researchers highlighted that the true potential of urban green settings has not yet been realized as studies often do not take account of the multifunctional nature of these spaces (Hunter et al., 2019). For example, the provision of urban street trees may have a positive impact on mental well-being and biodiversity in the area, but also increase air pollution levels due to reduced air circulation from canopy density (Jin et al., 2014). Hunter and colleagues also called for policymakers to ensure that any provision or improvement of urban green spaces is done through an 'equity lens' to minimize negative consequences of gentrification and unequal access to urban green space.

Money and Resources

Higher income is associated with better health (see Figure 2.5). For example, people in the bottom 40 per cent of the income distribution are almost twice as likely to report poor health as those in the top 20 per cent (Tinson, 2020). Lower income is associated with more life stresses, which can harm health and allow fewer opportunities for good health. Poor health, in turn, can limit the opportunity to obtain stable employment and a higher income (Tinson, 2020).

In 2019/2020, there were 11.7 million people (18 per cent) in the UK in relative low income before housing costs and 14.5 million people (22 per cent) in poverty after accounting for housing costs. This includes 3.2 million children (23 per cent) in relative low income before housing costs and 4.3 million children (31 per cent) in poverty after accounting for housing costs (Department for Work and Pensions, 2021). During 2020/2021, inflation was at or below 1 per cent. Since then, inflation has increased more than earnings growth and so the cost of living has risen, squeezing household budgets (Joseph Rowntree Foundation, 2022). With respect to households that are working but poor, 56

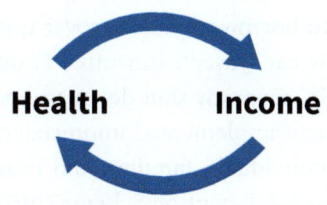

Better health

- allows people to gain and sustain employment
- can reduce the costs people face from ill-health
- allows people to have more options, such as a more active life.

Health **Income**

Higher income

- means people face fewer stresses
- allows people to meet more of their needs
- can be spent on health-promoting assets, such as better-quality housing or food.

○ The Health Foundation © 2020

Figure 2.5 The relationship between health and income
Reproduced with permission from Tinson, A. (2020, 25 July). *Living in poverty was bad for your health long before COVID-19*. The Health Foundation. https://www.health.org.uk/publications/long-reads/living-in-poverty-was-bad-for-your-health-long-before-COVID-19

per cent of people were in a working family in 2019/2020, compared with 39 per cent in 2000. Seven in ten children in poverty were part of a family where at least one parent works in 2019/2020. Such poverty is explained in part by rising housing, food, and energy costs and falling benefit incomes (Goulden, 2020).

The risk of poverty is higher for workers with disabilities, people from ethnic minority backgrounds, part-time workers, those in families with children, and those in single-adult families, especially lone parents working in the hospitality and food services (Joseph Rowntree Foundation, 2021). These groups already struggling to stay afloat have borne the brunt of the economic and health impacts of the COVID-19 pandemic. Working single parents have seen the fastest rise in poverty, from two in ten in 2010 to three in ten in 2020, prior to the COVID-19 pandemic (Goulden, 2020). The cost of living in the UK increased significantly during 2021 and 2022. In October 2022, the annual rate of inflation reached 11.1 per cent, a forty-one-year high, before gradually subsiding in the following months, for example, to 8.7 per cent in May 2023. High inflation has an impact on the affordability of goods and services for households. Energy prices are a major contributor to high inflation, with both household energy tariffs and road fuel costs increasing. As a result of Russia's invasion of Ukraine, gas prices increased to record levels during 2022 due to Russian supply cuts. Between May 2022 and May 2023, domestic gas prices increased by 36 per cent, while domestic electricity prices rose by 17 per cent (Harari et al., 2023). The cost of food and non-alcoholic beverages rose by 18.4 per cent in the year to May 2023 (ONS, 2023).

People receiving income-related benefits tend to have higher debts and lower savings than those who are not receiving income-related benefits, and are more likely to have to borrow money to cover unexpected expenses, such as a new boiler or a new car (Joseph Rowntree Foundation, 2021). In 2020, with large parts of the UK economy shut down and people required to stay at home, the UK Government implemented unprecedented economic measures to provide support for individuals, families, and businesses. These measures included the Coronavirus Job Retention Scheme (furlough) and increased existing financial support such as the £20 weekly Universal Credit uplift (Joseph Rowntree Foundation, 2021). Despite the scale of action, 28 per cent of adults saw their family finances deteriorate by September 2020. Many families had to rely on savings or debt to get by, with more than half (54 per cent) of those in the poorest fifth seeing their debts rise compared with 31 per cent of the wealthiest fifth (Suleman et al., 2021). High-income families were more likely to have seen a strengthening of the household's financial position (e.g. by working from home and not spending money on commuting and eating out). The implications of the COVID-19 pandemic were more serious for the living standards of lower-income (working-age) families than higher-income families (Brewer & Gardiner, 2020). Further to this, the cost of living crisis, including the rise in fuel bills, has had serious consequences for families with unpredictable income from work and benefits (Hill & Webber, 2022). The Joseph Rowntree Foundation has recommended policies to address rising living costs for low-income families (Hill & Webber, 2022). These include:

- Increase the adequacy of social security benefits in line with inflation to reduce child poverty.
- Improve the system of local welfare support—making broad support automatic was beneficial (e.g. the Universal Credit uplift, free COVID-19 testing, free school meal vouchers in school holidays to those eligible), but there has been relatively low awareness of local support such as the Household Support Fund.
- Giving immediate access to Statutory Sick Pay from the first day of sickness (which was introduced during the pandemic) has since been revised back to payment from day four.
- Easier channels of communication about health and financial support as some families do not have access to technology or are not confident using technology.
- Improving mental health support for both adults and children.

(Hill & Webber, 2022)

Housing

Housing conditions have a major impact on health and well-being. 'Poor housing' is defined as a dwelling that fails to meet the statutory minimum standard of housing in England (i.e. contains one or more Category 1 Hazards under the Housing Health and Safety Rating System), which poses a serious and immediate risk to the health and safety of occupants. Excess cold resulting from poor building construction, lack of insulation, and inadequate heating is one of the most prevalent hazards in the home and can contribute to death and ill-health (Chartered Institute of Environmental Health, 2011). Just before the COVID-19 pandemic reached the UK, there were 28,300 excess winter deaths in England and Wales (December 2019 to March 2020). This was 19.6 per cent higher than in winter 2018/2019. Respiratory diseases continued to be the leading cause of excess winter deaths that occurred from 2019 to 2020 (ONS, 2020a).

In England, 1.6 million (10 per cent) owner-occupied homes had a Category 1 hazard in 2019, which, if not addressed, would result in an annual cost to the NHS of £783 million (Garrett et al., 2023). With a mean cost of £3,434 to make an individual home safer, it would take seven years for the investment to pay back if the investment to mitigate all the hazards occurred at once, based on the saving to the NHS for first year treatment costs (Garrett et al., 2023). Around 619,000 (13 per cent) private rented homes had a Category 1 hazard in 2019, which, if not addressed, would result in an annual cost to the NHS of £290 million, while 217,000 (5 per cent) of social rented homes had a Category 1 hazard in 2019, which, if not addressed, would result in an annual cost to the NHS of £65 million (Garrett et al., 2023). The most prevalent Category 1 hazards in England are excessive cold and falls associated with stairs.

In Wales, a report by Public Health Wales, Community Housing Cymru, and the Building Research Establishment found that poor housing costs the NHS £95 million per year (Watson et al., 2019). Addressing causes of ill-health associated with poor housing, such as cold, damp, and fall hazards, could lead to 39 per cent fewer hospital admissions for circulatory and respiratory illness, and every £1 spent improving warmth for vulnerable households could result in a £4 ROI. The report also highlighted the importance of adapting homes and providing services that reduce falls for older people and people with disabilities, and that such services provide value for money and could generate £7.50 savings for health and social care for every £1 spent (Watson et al., 2019).

The term 'fuel poverty' refers to the inability to keep a home adequately warm due to the cost of energy bills (Hills, 2012). Government schemes such as the

Affordable Warmth grants (replacing the Warm Front scheme) have been implemented to help low-income households increase indoor warmth and energy efficiency. In 2021, 25 per cent of households in Scotland were in fuel poverty, 24 per cent in Northern Ireland, 14 per cent in Wales, and 13 per cent in England (Hinson et al., 2023). Over 530,000 pensioners over sixty-five years are living in poor housing, which costs the NHS £624 million per year (Connolly, 2018). A Joseph Rowntree Foundation report found that since the start of 2022, seven million low-income households (households that have an income in the bottom 40 per cent of all household incomes, adjusted for household size and composition) have either gone without enough food in the previous thirty days or gone without at least one essential, such as a warm enough home or basic toiletries, because they were unable to afford it (Schmuecker & Earwaker, 2022). The report also found that 5.2 million low-income households have either cut down on or skipped meals, or gone hungry, due to lack of money or food in the previous thirty days. Up from a fifth since October 2021, 4.6 million low-income households are in arrears on at least housing-related bill, such as rent, council tax or utilities, or they are behind on borrowing repayments (Schmuecker & Earwaker, 2022). Housing improvements related to increasing warmth and reducing fuel poverty can be a cost-effective way of improving the health of social housing tenants (e.g. Bray et al., 2017). See Box 2.2 for a case study on a historical cohort study seeking to determine the impact of warmth-related housing improvements on the health, well-being, and quality of life of families living in social housing.

Maintenance of the property of older people is another housing initiative that has potential savings to the taxpayer through reducing accidents within the home, potentially leading to the postponement of residential care fees. Postponing entry into residential care by just one year through adapting homes saves £39,480 per person (Berg, 2023). Home modifications can include adapted toilets, showers, lifting equipment, and new heating systems. Several research studies have evaluated the impact of housing improvements, such as energy-efficiency improvements, high-quality heating, and the fitting of handrails on stairs (Buck et al., 2016). For example, Nottingham City Homes, in partnership with Nottingham Trent University, conducted a two-year impact study on the wider social benefits of the Secure, Warm, Modern programme (Jones et al., 2016). The aim of the programme was to bring Nottingham's 28,500 council homes up to and above the national Decent Homes standard. Between 2009 and 2011, single-glazed windows were replaced with 'A-rated' double-glazed windows in 13,700 properties and upgraded heating to full central heating systems in 7,380 homes, as well as topping up loft insulation up to 200mm. Following these upgrades, on average, the energy efficiency of the properties increased

Box 2.2 Case study: A historical cohort study to improve population health through better social housing

Gentoo, a social housing contractor in North East England, recruited households for participation in this historical cohort study (Bray et al., 2017). Participants were asked to complete a questionnaire about their well-being, quality of life, and health service use before and twelve months after receiving housing improvements (a new energy-efficient boiler and double-glazing). Two hundred and twenty-eight households took part in the study. The mean cost of the intervention per household was £3,725 (standard deviation = £1,041). At twelve-months post-intervention there was a 16 per cent reduction (–£94.79) in household six-month health service use. Although this was a relatively small change in health service use, there was probably a higher return on investment for society. For example, grandparents being able to look after their grandchildren in their own warm homes, enabling their children to engage in paid employment. Cold homes, particularly those below 16° Celsius, cause a substantially increased risk of cardiovascular and respiratory conditions (Mason & Roys, 2011). Bray and colleagues (2017) found that participants in the over sixty-five year age group experienced significant improvements in health status, while those under sixty-five years did not. Therefore, there is some economic evidence that warm homes may also be a cost-effective way of reducing health service expenditure, particularly in older populations who are more susceptible to respiratory infections and diseases, such as pneumonia and influenza.

from 60 (out of 100) to 68, equating to an average reduction in carbon dioxide emissions of nearly one tonne per year per property. Each tenant could save between £95 and £223 each year on their fuel bill due to fitting double-glazed windows, and £225 a year from upgrading from a 'G-rated' boiler to an 'A-rated' boiler (Jones et al., 2016).

Poor housing can cause problems with childhood development (Lee et al., 2022). The health of a child's lungs has a crucial role in shaping their overall health and life expectancy. During childhood there is a window of opportunity for optimal respiratory maturation. This developmental process can be impaired by inadequate housing conditions, such as exposure to viruses, dust, mould, and pollution, particularly in cold or overcrowded environments.

A longitudinal study in England found that children who lived in cold, damp homes in the previous three years had rates of respiratory illness over twice as high compared with those who had not (Barnes et al., 2008). A systematic review by the World Health Organization (WHO, 2018) found that lung function deteriorated with every 1° Celsius decrease below 9° Celsius of indoor temperature for children with asthma. In regions with temperate or colder climates, WHO (2018) recommends an indoor temperature of 18° Celsius to protect the health of the general population during cold seasons.

The impact of the COVID-19 pandemic was felt unevenly across societies worldwide. A month before the first UK national lockdown during the COVID-19 pandemic in 2020, the report 'Health equity in England: The Marmot review 10 years on' showed that life expectancy had gone into reverse for the most socioeconomically deprived communities, revealing a growing gap in health between wealthy and deprived areas (Marmot et al., 2020). People living in economically deprived areas in the United States (US) were at increased risk of transmission of the COVID-19 virus (Finch & Hernández Finch, 2020). In Spain, districts with the lowest mean income had the highest incidence of COVID-19 per 10,000 inhabitants; in contrast, those with the highest income had the lowest incidence (Baena-Diéz et al., 2020).

The COVID-19 pandemic prompted an unprecedented public health response from the UK Government, local authorities, and the voluntary sector to protect rough sleepers. The Everyone In initiative supported 37,000 vulnerable people into longer-term accommodation during the pandemic. This included people who would not usually be entitled to assistance under homelessness legislation. Funding was increased by 85 per cent compared to 2019, and the number of rough sleepers decreased by over a third (Department for Levelling Up, Housing and Communities et al., 2021). A systematic review of accommodation-based interventions included a network meta-analysis and showed that all types of accommodation which provided support were more effective than no intervention or Basic/Unconditional accommodation in terms of housing stability and health (Keenan et al., 2021). Sourcing accommodation was challenging across all studies. Collaboration between stakeholders and practitioners was shown to be fruitful but difficult to coordinate across different agencies and organizations. Few studies focused on cost or cost-effectiveness (Keenan et al., 2021). In September 2022, the UK Government published the Ending Rough Sleeping for Good strategy, focusing on a four-pronged approach of prevention, intervention, and recovery, and ensuring a joined-up transparent approach supported by £2 billion funding up to 2025 (Department for Levelling Up, Housing and Communities, 2022).

Education and Skills

Good educational attainment is an important protective factor for good health across the life-course (see Figure 2.6). Early years education positively impacts the life chances of disadvantaged children, especially when they can attend pre-school and learn alongside children from different social backgrounds (House of Commons Education Committee, 2019). Good educational attainment starts from birth. Investment in the early years (especially from birth to seven years) has been shown to benefit a child's development and socialization, thus helping to prevent costly social problems later in life (Edwards et al., 2016). Therefore, investment in the early years is not a luxury, but an economic necessity with outcomes realised over time. When considered the same way as national invest-ment in economic development, early years investment contributes to building social capital and promoting economic growth (Edwards et al., 2016).

One of the main goals of primary and secondary education is to equip young people with the skills they need to enter the labour market and build a suc-cessful career. However, many young people, particularly those from disadvan-taged backgrounds, can find it difficult to enter employment due to a lack of basic skills (Newton et al., 2020; Sharp et al., 2015). Fifty-six per cent of UK

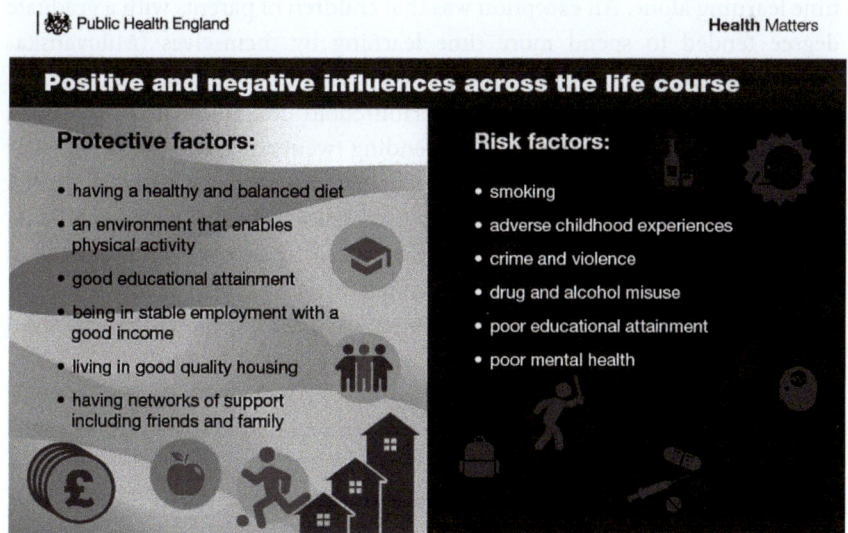

Figure 2.6 Positive and negative influences across the life-course
Reproduced from Public Health England. (2019a, 23 May). *Health matters: Prevention—a life course approach*. https://www.gov.uk/government/publications/health-matters-life-course-approach-to-prevention/health-matters-prevention-a-life-course-approach. Licence: Creative Commons BY 3.0 IGO.

organizations experience skills shortages and 55 per cent struggle to find new employees with the right level of experience (The Open University, 2020). Organizations spent £6.6 billion to address these short-term gaps in 2020, an increase from £4.4 billion in 2019 (The Open University, 2020). There is no doubt that this skills shortage has been exacerbated by Brexit.

The loss of education by children experienced during the COVID-19 pandemic risks widening the gap in future health outcomes. The cohort of children and young people who have missed periods of education could lag behind pre-pandemic cohorts. The loss of education has also been experienced unequally, with children from more disadvantaged backgrounds having experienced a greater deterioration in their educational outcomes (Suleman et al., 2021). Using data from the Household Pulse Survey, collected by the US Census Bureau in collaboration with several federal agencies, Milovanska-Farrington (2021) found that educated parents were more likely to spend time educating their children. The data also showed that Asian and Black parents were more likely to spend time with their children than White parents. Higher income and employment were negatively associated with parental time investment in the child. During the COVID-19 pandemic, fathers were more likely than mothers to educate their children. Parental education, race, and ethnic background were not statistically significant determinants of the likelihood that children spent time learning alone. An exception was that children of parents with a graduate degree tended to spend more time learning by themselves (Milovanska-Farrington, 2021).

In the UK, using data from the UK Household Longitudinal Study, Cheng and colleagues (2021) reported that spending twenty or more hours per week on childcare or home-schooling was associated with poor parental mental health. During the COVID-19 pandemic and school closures, home-schooling had a negative impact on the work-life balance of many working parents. In particular, working parents experienced higher levels of financial distress compared to workers without children. Women experienced more financial insecurity compared to men (Cheng et al., 2021; Etheridge & Spantig, 2020).

At the onset of the COVID-19 pandemic in March 2020, people living in the UK were experiencing stagnant income growth and low levels of financial resilience. At this time, 65 per cent of families in the bottom 20 per cent of the income distribution had either no savings or savings below £1,500 (Tinson, 2020). During the pandemic, the pattern of employment loss and furloughing by income indicated that the long-term economic and health consequences of the pandemic would be felt more acutely by those with lower incomes. Government support to bolster incomes and provide retraining support for those who lost their jobs could help the health and well-being of workers as good jobs are associated with better health outcomes and more health-promoting behaviours, such as increased physical activity (Henseke, 2018).

Funded by the charity Business in the Community, the Ready for Work programme is an example of a successful intervention providing skills training to employees, especially for people from disadvantaged groups, including those who have experienced homelessness. The purpose of the programme was to equip individuals with the skills they need to enter and sustain employment (Inge et al., 2012). A one-year investment in the Ready for Work programme generated £3.2 million of social benefit, and for every £1 invested in the programme, £3.12 of social value was generated (Inge et al., 2012).

Conceptualizing the Commercial Determinants of Health

Commercial entities can have a positive impact on health and society, for example, through producing products and services that are beneficial to health. However, there is growing evidence that the products and practices of some commercial entities, particularly multinational and transnational corporations, are responsible for increasing rates of preventable ill-health, planetary damage, and social and health inequity (Gilmore et al., 2023). These complex (and often negative) links between the commercial sector and health are referred as the 'commercial determinants of health' (Kickbusch et al., 2016). They refer to the conditions, actions, and omissions by commercial entities that affect health. For example, companies make choices in the production, price-setting, and targeted marketing of products, such as ultra-processed foods, tobacco, sugar-sweetened beverages, and alcohol, which can lead to health conditions such as cardiovascular disease, type 2 diabetes, and certain cancers, as well as hypertension and obesity.

In the first paper in a series on the commercial determinants of health in *The Lancet*, Gilmore and colleagues (2023) discuss how the severity of the problem is illustrated by the climate emergency and the non-communicable disease epidemic, and that just four industry sectors (tobacco, ultra-processed food, fossil fuel, and alcohol) are already responsible for a third of global deaths. These authors argue how the transition towards market fundamentalism and the growing influence of transnational corporations have fostered a pathological system where commercial entities are increasingly enabled to cause harm (e.g. to humans and the planet) and externalize the costs of doing so (Gilmore et al., 2023). While commercial sector and commercial power increase, so do harms to humans and the planet. Meanwhile, health care systems struggle to meet the demand on their resources, and individuals, governments, and civil society organizations struggle to cover the costs associated with these human and planetary harms. In their paper, Gilmore and colleagues (2023) present a conceptual model of the commercial determinants of health to help with the understanding of this complex issue. The model identifies key commercial practices that, when inadequately regulated, harm health in often hidden and indirect ways. The model also shows the pathways through which these practices negatively impact on health from upstream (e.g. influencing political and economic systems) to downstream (e.g. directly driving consumption of products damaging to health, limiting access to health-related services and products for those unable to pay). Gilmore and colleagues (2023) call for governments to act to improve the well-being of future generations, development, and economic growth. This can be done by using the model to guide solutions from targeted interventions addressing commercial practices to system changes, and by governments to hold commercial entities to account to meet the true costs of the harm they generate.

The Food We Eat and the Food Industry

Sixty per cent of the calories consumed by people living in the UK comes from ultra-processed food products, which are industrially processed and designed and marketed to be addictive (van Tulleken, 2023). The food system necessary for the production of ultra-processed food is the leading cause of declining biodiversity and the second-largest contributor to global emissions. This is contributing to climate change, malnutrition, and obesity (van Tulleken, 2023). The prevalence of obesity has accelerated in the UK, with 55 per cent of adults now classed as obese (NHS Digital, 2020). Data from the National Child Measurement Programme reported that 14.4 per cent of children in Reception (aged four to five years) are obese and 13.3 per cent are overweight, and 25.5 per cent of year six children (aged ten to eleven years) are obese and 15.4 per cent are overweight (NHS Digital, 2022). The social annual cost of obesity in the UK is £58 billion (Palmer, 2022). This includes the cost of obesity-related diseases to the NHS (including COVID-19 and mental health issues), the loss of QALYs for individuals, and the wider costs to society, such as loss of productivity and cost of social care. The NHS spends £6.5 billion on obesity-related diseases annually (Palmer, 2022). Failing to address the challenges posed by the obesity epidemic places probably the largest impact on NHS resources in future. The cost to the NHS for treating obesity related ill-health is set to rise to £9.7 billion per year by 2050 (NHS Digital, 2021; Public Health England, 2017a).

Diets in the UK tend to predominantly consist of carbohydrates, which contributes to obesity as a leading cause of ill-health and premature mortality. Dieticians encourage people with type 2 diabetes to reduce their carbohydrate intake to reverse type 2 diabetes symptoms and obesity (Kelly et al., 2020). Low-carbohydrate diets are still controversial, but with the absence of large randomized controlled trials (RCTs) with cardiovascular measures and other relevant outcomes, adopting a low-carbohydrate diet is seen by service providers and researchers as a legitimate and potentially effective treatment option for patients with diabetes or obesity (Kelly et al., 2020).

There have been arguments against focusing on individual behaviour as a means of reducing population obesity, placing the focus instead on structural drivers in society that determine and influence the whole food environment. The following are examples of structural drivers: drivers wearing seatbelts; banning smoking in public spaces; reducing salt in bread; minimal alcohol pricing; and the emergency public health measures of the pandemic (Edwards & McIntosh, 2019; Swinburn et al., 2011, 2015). Structural factors such as the built environment, transport systems, active recreation opportunities, cuisines and food culture, and culture around body size can moderate or modulate the impact of the global obesity drivers on population body mass index (BMI) and success or otherwise of interventions to address obesity (Swinburn et al., 2011). Figure 2.7 shows places where it is possible to input structural drivers to shape the food environment in which people live.

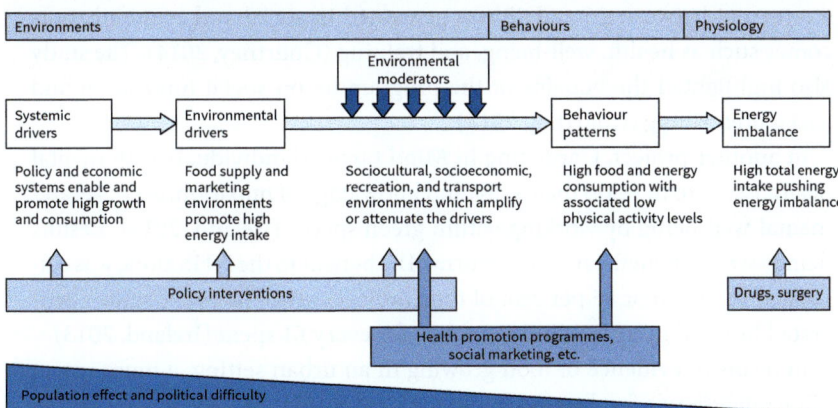

Figure 2.7 A framework to categorize obesity determinants and solutions
Reprinted from Swinburn, B. A., Sacks, G., Hall, K. D., McPherson, K., Finegood, D. T., Moodie, M. L., & Gortmaker, S. L. (2011). The global obesity pandemic: shaped by global drivers and local environments. *The Lancet, 378*(9793), 804–814. Copyright © 2011, with permission from Elsevier.

'Urban farming and gardening' can be defined as the production of fresh local produce grown in busy, populated areas such as inner cities, making use of neighbourhood rooftops, schools, and abandoned areas. Urban farming has grown considerably in recent years and can generate several benefits through the production and access of healthy produce to local communities, and its environmental and social value potential (Aubry & Manouchehri, 2019). The value of horticultural interventions on health and well-being is widely acknowledged (Soga et al., 2017). Previous research has also demonstrated the economic benefits of gardening to support individuals experiencing mental health issues (e.g. Sempik, 2010; Vardakoulias, 2013). Urban gardening contributes to overall community health as social engagement is positively associated with personal attention to health and well-being (Bellows et al., 2004). See Box 2.3 for a case study on the social value of urban food growing.

Box 2.3 Case study: The social value of urban food growing

A number of social return on investment (SROI) studies have demonstrated the social value of community food growing interventions. For example, an SROI analysis of the Local Food programme conducted across three areas in England (Kendal, Cumbria; Borough of Greenwich, London; and Stroud Valleys, Gloucestershire) found that for every £1 invested in the programme, a return of between £6 and £8 was generated in social and economic outcomes such as health, well-being, and training (Courtney, 2014). The study also highlighted the benefits of the programme on social innovation and social prescribing (Courtney, 2014).

In another project, Gardening in Mind targeted individuals with mental health issues to develop their skills and knowledge of nutrition, exercise, and mental well-being by working within green spaces (Ireland, 2013). Results demonstrated beneficial social returns. The benefit to the NHS alone was calculated at £49.26 or 85 per cent of total project costs. The social return generated by Gardening in Mind was £2.04 for every £1 spent (Ireland, 2013).

In terms of evidence of food growing in an urban setting, a more recent SROI analysis of a food growing initiative in a community garden in London yielded an ROI of £3 for every £1 invested (Schoen et al., 2020). This study highlighted the important contribution that community gardens can make to social well-being within cities. Schoen and colleagues (2020) advocated for further acknowledgement of green spaces in urban planning policy.

Addiction and Harmful Consumption Behaviours

'Addiction' is defined as lacking control over doing, taking, or using something to the point where it could be harmful to the individual (NHS, 2021). In this section we consider addictive behaviour in relation to alcohol, drugs, smoking, and gambling—these principles also apply to food.

Alcohol

The effects of harmful alcohol use in the UK costs society £11 billion per annum through alcohol-related crime, £7 billion in lost productivity through un-employment and sickness, and £3.5 billion to the NHS (Public Health England, 2016). Alcohol misuse costs the employee, employer, and workforce in terms of increased accidents in the workplace, greater absenteeism and presenteeism, and premature death (Institute of Alcohol Studies, 2017, 2020). In the UK, more than one in four employees (28 per cent) admit to going to work hungover due to excess alcohol consumption. Most believe this negatively impacts their per-formance at work (Institute of Alcohol Studies, 2017). Specific cognitive func-tions may still be impaired the morning following binge drinking, even when little or no alcohol content is present in the bloodstream (Gunn et al., 2018). Despite many workplaces having clear policies regarding alcohol intoxication at work, few policies consider the effects of alcohol consumption on the fol-lowing day (Health and Safety Executive, 2021).

Drugs

In 2019/2020, one in eleven adults aged sixteen to fifty-nine years in the UK had taken an illicit drug, while one in five adults aged sixteen to twenty-four years reported having taken an illicit drug (ONS, 2020b). Drug misuse can be harmful to the individual, friends and family members, and wider society (Barber et al., 2017). Drug misuse can have a detrimental effect on physical and mental health and lead to unemployment, homelessness, and criminal activity (Barber et al., 2017). In the UK, the societal costs of drug misuse are £20 bil-lion each year. In 2020 to 2021 only £650 million was spent on drug treatment. Every £1 currently spent on harm reduction and treatment gives a combined health and justice ROI of £4 (Department of Health and Social Care, 2021). This figure includes drug-related crime, enforcement, health service use, and deaths linked to eight illicit substances: amphetamines, cannabis, crack cocaine, ec-stasy, heroin, lysergic acid diethylamide (LSD), magic mushrooms, and powder cocaine (Public Health England, 2017b).

Although a working individual may not smoke cannabis or take other toxic substances during working hours, the drug can still have an impact in the workplace. For example, the drug could still be active in their bloodstream from the night before making driving to work dangerous and illegal under the UK's Road Traffic Act 1988. Other adverse effects of illicit drug use include: reduced cognitive abilities, poor timekeeping, poor decision-making, and impaired reaction times, leading to lost productivity, inferior goods/services, errors, and accidents (Nicholson et al., 2016). Illicit drug use may also lead to other health issues, which could, in turn, lead to inappropriate behaviour and absenteeism (Public Health Wales, 2018). Mephedrone, gamma-hydroxybutyrate (GHB), gamma-butyrolactone (GBL), and crystallized methamphetamine are illicit drugs than can increase heart rate and blood pressure, trigger euphoria and sexual arousal, and lead to disinhibition. The prevalence of taking these drugs during sexual intercourse, known as 'chemsex', has been increasing in the UK (McCall et al., 2015; Stuart, 2016). As one of the main effects of GHB is to reduce inhibition, employees going to work with this drug in their bloodstream may speak or behave inappropriately towards their colleagues.

There have been attempts to value the social benefit of drug treatment services. For example, the UK Drug Interventions Programme directs adult drug-misusing offenders out of crime and into treatment programmes. As part of the UK Drug Treatment Outcomes Research Study, a cost-utility analysis (CUA) produced evidence that the Drug Interventions Programme is both effective and cost-effective with an average net cost saving of £668 (average net cost saving including one case of homicide is £6,207) (Collins et al., 2017). The Drug Interventions Programme reduced crime rates, improved quality of life, and reduced subsequent drug use. Langham and colleagues (2018) examined the cost-effectiveness of take-home naloxone for the prevention of overdose fatalities among heroin users in the UK. Naloxone is an opioid antagonist which binds to opioid receptors and can reverse and block the effects of other opioids, such as heroin. A Markov model estimated that the distribution of take-home naloxone would decrease overdose deaths by 6.6 per cent and at an incremental cost per QALY gained of £899 (Langham et al., 2018). This is below the maximum threshold of £20,000 to £30,000 per QALY recommended by the National Institute for Health and Care Excellence (NICE) (Claxton et al., 2015)

Smoking

Smoking cigarettes costs the UK economy in excess of £19 billion a year (International Longevity Centre UK (ILC), 2021). The proportion of adults aged sixteen years and above who reported smoking cigarettes in Great Britain decreased significantly from 14.5 per cent in 2020 to 12.7 per cent in 2021. This downward trend has been observed since 1974 (ONS, 2022). Tobacco smoking is the leading cause of many types of cancer (including cancer of the mouth and throat, cervical cancer, cancer of the colon, liver cancer, lung cancer, stomach cancer, myeloid leukaemia, and pancreatic cancer). Many former smokers live with the long-term effects of smoking, such as cardiovascular conditions and cancer. In the UK, 76,000 people die from smoking every year (NHS, 2022a).

NICE (2021) has published guidance on preventing the uptake of tobacco, promoting quitting, and treating dependence. The guidance refers to priority groups at high risk of tobacco-related harm, such as: people with mental health conditions; people who misuse substances; people with health conditions caused or made worse by smoking; people with a smoking-related illness; communities or groups with high smoking prevalence (e.g. manual workers, travellers, and lesbian, gay, bisexual, transgender and transsexual plus (LGBT+) people); people with a low socioeconomic status; and pregnant women who smoke. The UK Government is also working to minimize the misuse of substances (alcohol, illegal drugs, prescription medication, and new psychoactive substances) at a population level (HM Government, 2017a). In December 2021, the UK Government (2021b) set out its ten-year plan to combat illegal drugs and criminal gangs, and support people with a drug addiction. They have promised to invest £3 billion over the next three years to reduce drug-related crime, death, harm, and overall drug use.

E-cigarettes, also known as vapes, produce an aerosol by heating a liquid that usually contains nicotine, flavourings, and other chemicals (e.g. propylene glycol and vegetable glycerin) (NHS, 2022b). Since e-cigarettes do not burn tobacco or produce tar or carbon monoxide, they are generally regarded as safer alternatives to smoking cigarettes, although the long-term risks of vaping remain unclear (NHS, 2022b). Varenicline (Champix), bupropion (Zyban), and nicotine replacement therapy are licensed aids for quitting smoking in the UK. Smoking cessation services may allow service users to bring their own e-cigarettes, although these are not licensed. In a systematic review, network meta-analysis and cost-effectiveness analysis of smoking cessation medicines and e-cigarettes, Thomas and colleagues (2021) found that combined therapies of medicines were among the most clinically effective, safe, and cost-effective treatment options for smokers. Nicotine replacement therapy standard was most cost-effective, followed by varenicline standard. If the funder is not willing to pay £56 per QALY, then nicotine replacement therapy low dose is estimated to be most cost-effective. If the funder is willing to pay more than £56 per QALY, then e-cigarette low dose is estimated to be most cost-effective (Thomas et al., 2021). As there is currently limited evidence about the safety profile of e-cigarettes, further work is needed to ascertain the long-term effectiveness and safety outcomes of e-cigarettes, particularly in studies with active interventions as comparators.

Gambling

With all potential health-harming activities and products there is a need to consider the contribution that these industries make to jobs in the economy. The Social Market Foundation estimated that largely due to the shift to online gambling in recent years, there are lower economic multiplier effects compared with most parts of the economy and other health-harming activities and products (Corfe et al., 2021).

The annual economic burden of harmful gambling is estimated to be £1.27 billion (Public Health England, 2021). This includes £647 million of direct costs to the UK Government and £619 million of wider societal costs associated with suicide resulting from gambling. Gambling activity is associated with financial distress, lower financial inclusion (e.g. having a credit card, loan, or mortgage), and poor or lack of financial planning (e.g. having insurance, saving money; Muggleton et al., 2021). Spending more money on gambling is associated with smaller amounts spent on insurance and mortgage repayments, total savings, and pension contributions. There is also an association between gambling activity, social isolation, and night-time wakefulness. There is a negative association between gambling and self-care, fitness activities (e.g. gym membership), social activities, and spending on education and hobbies (Muggleton et al., 2021). A systematic review of economic evaluations of public health interventions targeting alcohol, tobacco, illicit drug use, and problematic gambling found fifty-four relevant studies, however, none for problematic gambling (Nystrand et al., 2021). Public Health England (2021) highlighted the need for further research on the effectiveness and cost-effectiveness of interventions to prevent gambling-related harms to help people with gambling problems and people supporting them.

Air Quality and Transport

Transportation plays a key role in economic and social development by facilitating access to resources and markets improving quality of life, connecting individuals with employment, health, education, recreation opportunities, and services (Rassafi & Vaziri, 2005). The movement of individuals and resources has seen a greater shift in dependency on all modes of motorized transportation. In 2019, 99 per cent of the world's population was living in places where WHO air quality guidelines were not being met. The effect of air pollution is associated with 6.7 million premature deaths annually (WHO, 2020). There is a strong relationship between air pollution and coronary heart disease, stroke, lung cancer, and childhood asthma (Public Health England, 2019b). There is an economic implication of air pollution on health, leading to rises in health care expenditures such as increases in the use of prescription medication, accessing and using health care services along with the loss of productivity (Deschênes et al., 2017). In 2017, the cost of air pollution was £42.88 million to the UK society, including the cost of road traffic accidents and road traffic injuries, as well as other illnesses and workdays lost due to injury and ill-health (Public Health England, 2018b).

Accessibility and safety are issues that affect the mode of transport individuals are willing to use (van Soest et al., 2020). A switch from private motor transport to a more active mode of transport can lead to health improvements. Active living and engaging in active transport facilitate individuals to integrate physical activity into daily life. Walking for transport—also known as 'active travel'—along with travel initiatives, are becoming more popular, with some walking groups being part of social prescribing initiatives (Assemi et al., 2020; Patterson et al., 2018) and other well-being initiatives to improve mental health and well-being (Gladwell et al., 2016). Physical activity promotes better sleep (Gladwell et al., 2016), reduced incidence of many non-communicable diseases (Celis-Morales et al., 2017), and a reduction in all-cause mortality (Leitzmann et al., 2007). Although researchers acknowledge other increased risks such as air pollution and road trauma when walking, physical activity benefits outweigh these other health harms (Zapata-Diomedi et al., 2018).

Physical activity plays a vital role in preventing diseases and diminishing the adverse impacts of long-term medical conditions (Hoevenaar-Blom et al., 2011). A Norwegian study explored whether expanding cycling networks in Oslo could impact on overall health and well-being due to increased physical activity, and whether the cycling network was cost-effective (Lamu et al., 2020). The results showed that the new 100 kilometre cycling network produced an additional cost of US$416 per person and yielded 0.019 QALYs per person over the life horizon of the intervention, compared with pre-expansion of the cycling network, and the incremental cost per QALY gained was US$22,350. This suggests that the cycling network was highly cost-effective at a threshold of US$72,550 per QALY. In the UK, NICE (2017) guidance on improving air quality resulting from road traffic-related air pollution and links to ill-health suggested that off-road cycle routes are cost-effective. The cost per QALY was estimated at £5,080, with a benefit-cost ratio of £14 for every £1 invested. This analysis included additional benefits of £64,000 resulting from increased uptake of cycling (NICE, 2017).

Health promotion is a growing responsibility for companies, with more employers now taking part in schemes, such as Cycle to Work (Sustrans, 2021). More bicycle paths are being created either alongside new road developments or alongside existing road infrastructure (Sustrans, 2021). The main disadvantage of active transport (specifically walking) for most people compared to private motor transport is the limited services, especially in rural areas (van Soest et al., 2020). The emphasis on greener transport and sustainability has been a consideration over the past thirty years due to the environmental damage from emissions at both global and local levels (Department for Transport, 2009; Smith, 2020). For the UK to meet its national target of reaching net-zero greenhouse gas emissions as part of the central Paris Agreement, further emphasis needs to be placed on decarbonizing public transport and moving away from personal transport (Conventionally Fuelled Vehicles (CFVs) and Electric Vehicles (EVs); Logan et al., 2020). However, despite the rise in ownership of electric cars in the UK, the main method of transportation still includes personal petrol or diesel driven vehicles, which has a detrimental effect on the cleanliness of the air. Policymakers globally are encouraged to improve air quality to prevent premature deaths for the benefit of society and the economy. Improving air quality in England to be in line with WHO guidelines could save £1.6 billion and 17,000 deaths (Confederation of British Industry (CBI) Economics, 2020; WHO, 2006). During the COVID-19 pandemic lockdowns air quality temporarily improved because of reduced air polluting emissions (specifically nitrogen dioxide and particulate matter; Jephcote et al., 2021).

Getting to Net Zero: Incorporating Health Economics into Carbon Emissions Evaluation and Policy

The UK Government has announced a target of reaching net-zero greenhouse gas emissions by 2050 (ONS, 2019). Air pollution can have damaging impacts on human health, productivity, amenity, and the health of the environment. The policies to reduce carbon emissions in the interest of slowing down adverse climate change are closely linked with the need for policies to reduce air pollution or improve air quality. An example of how health economists have explored interventions to reduce the effects of air quality is provided by Cooper and colleagues (2020). There have been attempts to calculate the QALY gains, for example, of using air purifiers in the homes of children living in London. Home air purifiers aim to reduce indoor air pollution by filtering particulate matter (i.e. dust, dirt, soot, smoke) in the air. Cooper and colleagues (2020) measured particulate matter concentrations over a six-month period in eighteen flats in London where children with asthma lived. They found a 45 per cent reduction of particulate matter when using the home air purifiers over a ninety-minute period. The number of QALYs saved by using home air purifiers in the bedrooms of children during sleep was estimated to be 1,361 additional QALYs per 10,000 children. This research suggests that home air purifiers can reduce the health burdens associated with childhood asthma (Cooper et al., 2020).

In an abridged Cochrane systematic review, Burns and colleagues (2020) reported thirty-eight individual interventions to reduce air pollution and their effects on health from forty-two studies. They identified interventions aiming to address industrial sources (n = 5, e.g. the closure of a factory), residential sources (n = 7, e.g. coal ban), vehicular sources (n = 22, e.g. low emission zones), and multiple sources (n = 4, e.g. tailored measures that target traffic and industrial polluters). Burns and colleagues found that evidence for effectiveness was mixed due to the heterogeneity across interventions, outcomes, and methods employed. There was some evidence to suggest that interventions were associated with improved air quality and human health (Burns et al., 2020).

The detrimental impacts of air pollution have associated economic and/or social costs. We found relatively little published evidence on the cost-effectiveness of air pollution reduction. The UK Department of Environment, Food and Rural Affairs (Defra) has produced guidance for assessing the air quality impact of a policy or project (Defra, 2023).

Family, Friends, and Communities

People who are more socially connected to family, friends, or their community are happier, have better mental and physical health, and live longer, than people who have a smaller social circle with fewer quality relationships (Mental Health Foundation, 2023). Community services such as community transport, public toilets, libraries, leisure facilities, and day centres for older people are known to be beneficial for creating safe communities (Age UK, 2019). Looking after older people in our communities makes it easier for the older generation to look after young grandchildren so that their own children can go to work and contribute to the economy (Edwards et al., 2018). Recognition of the contribution that older people make to the economy, particularly through working and volunteering into older age, fits with the ethos of the 'circular economy'. A circular economy is an alternative to a traditional linear economy (make, use, dispose) in which we keep resources in use for as long as possible (Waste and Resources Action Plan (WRAP) UK, 2019). In the UK, the value of childcare support given by those aged over sixty-five years for their grandchildren was estimated to be worth around £7.7 billion per year (Iparraguirre, 2017).

Social isolation and loneliness are associated with increased anxiety, depression, and cardiovascular disease (Leigh-Hunt et al., 2017). Social isolation and loneliness in older people have a considerable cost impact on public sector resources, and are associated with higher rates of GP visits, hospital admissions, and accident and emergency (A&E) visits compared to older people who self-describe as never feeling lonely (Fulton & Jupp, 2015; Landeiro et al., 2016). In March 2020, in response to the COVID-19 pandemic, the UK Government informed 1.5 million vulnerable people (who were at risk of severe illness and hospital admission) to self-isolate or 'shield' themselves for at least twelve weeks to limit the spread of the virus (Kmietowicz, 2020). A rapid review of interventions to reduce social isolation and loneliness during the COVID-19 pandemic identified the following effective interventions for loneliness: psychological therapies such as mindfulness, Tai Chi Qigong meditation; laughter therapy; lessons on friendships; robotic pets; and social facilitation software (Williams et al., 2021). However, few interventions were found to improve social isolation. For example, a twice weekly activity session decreased social isolation, while telephone befriending, computer training, and exercise programmes had no significant effect on measures of social isolation (Williams et al., 2021).

The impact of loneliness has been compared to other well-known risk factors to health, such as obesity, and has a similar negative influence to that of smoking fifteen cigarettes a day (Holt-Lunstad et al., 2010, 2015). People who experience social isolation and loneliness have a 30 per cent increased risk of heart disease and stroke (Valtorta et al., 2016). There is also strong evidence that older people who experience loneliness are at greater risk of cognitive decline and are 64 per cent more likely to develop dementia (Holwerda et al., 2014). Engagement in social activities and having meaningful social roles has been shown to lead to successful ageing, reduced loneliness, and improved confidence, independence, and quality of life (Adams et al., 2011). In order to mitigate loneliness, social prescribing programmes, such as Together for Health, and the arts and craft-based programme Craft Café, have been estimated to generate high rates of social value of between £4.84 and £8.27 returned for every £1 invested (Social Value Lab, 2011). A cross-sectional study looking at the well-being of older people in six European countries found common and country-specific factors important for life satisfaction (Fagerström et al., 2007). Factors universal across all six countries included the importance of satisfactory social contacts, financial resources, and self-esteem, and feeling hindered by health problems. Targeting these areas in preventative interventions could support older people to live a good life. In 2018, the UK Government's strategy to tackle loneliness supported the implementation of social prescribing initiatives (HM Government, 2018).

Communication technologies (e.g. email, WhatsApp, Messenger, Skype, Zoom, and Teams) can make it easier for older people to maintain friendships and family connections, subject to broadband availability (Women's Royal Voluntary Service (WRVS), 2012). Evidence of the potential value of new technologies on loneliness prevention is mixed. However, internet training may be a cost-effective way to support older people and enable them to maintain good social links, particularly for older people living in very rural communities or all older people abiding by social distancing guidance during a global pandemic (Kinsella, 2014; UK Government, 2020). Internet use can decrease loneliness and help older people retain social ties, particularly among adults in assisted and independent living communities (Cotten et al., 2013). For example, group-based internet and computer training interventions may be cost-effective with an estimated cost per QALY of £15,962 (Owen et al., 2015). Research has shown that older people value help using the internet more than many other forms of practical support such as cleaning or enjoying meals out (Jones et al., 2015).

Having a strong or intimate relationship with a significant other is a growth need as it gives a sense of belonging to the individual, which is apart from other relationships with family members or friends (Maslow, 2017). Living with an abusive partner where intimacy, safety, and respect are missing has individual, social, and economic costs. The social and economic cost for victims of domestic abuse in the year ending March 2017 in England and Wales was £66 billion (Oliver et al., 2019). The cost of physical and emotional harm suffered by the victims themselves was £47 billion. The cost of lost output relating to time taken off work and reduced productivity afterwards was £14 billion. Some of the costs relate to the NHS, some are related to policing, and others include temporary housing or repairs and maintenance to houses damaged by violent behaviour (Oliver et al., 2019).

During the COVID-19 pandemic lockdowns and social restrictions, there was a rise in every kind of domestic abuse (Gibson, 2020). More violent acts were committed within the home. With children out of school, child safeguarding referrals were reduced. One study using data from Birmingham found a 37 per cent decrease in referrals for child protection medical examinations between February and June 2020 than in the same period in 2019, suggesting some children were left exposed to harm (Garstang et al., 2020). The COVID-19 pandemic has magnified domestic violence: the incidence of domestic violence has increased globally; the presence of domestic violence internationally has been revealed more clearly (alongside other adversities and inequalities); and people have had less access to statutory services (Feder, 2021).

Social Prescribing

'Social prescribing', also known as community referral, is a means of enabling health professionals to refer people to a range of local, non-clinical services.

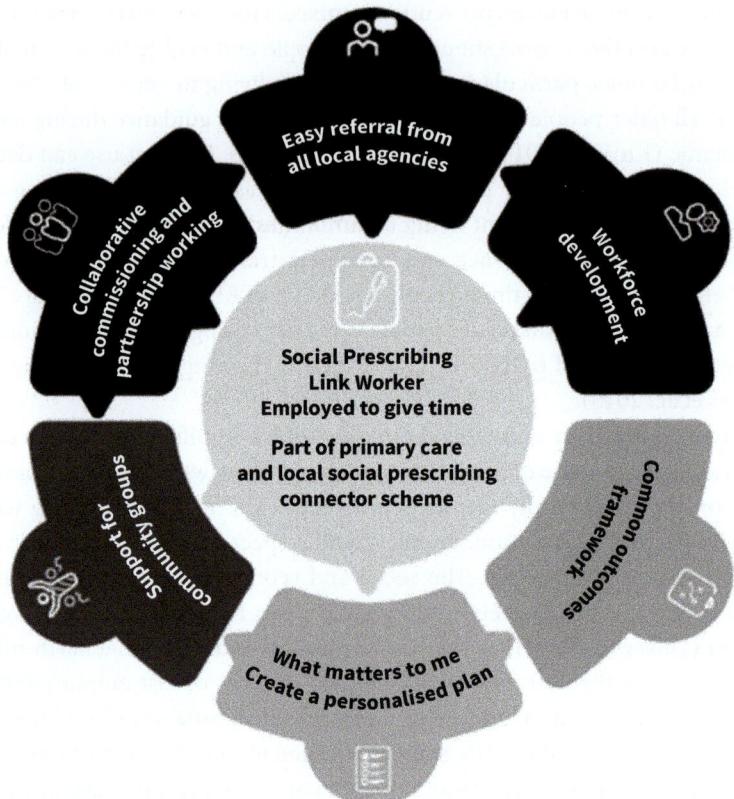

Figure 2.8 Model for social prescribing
Reproduced with permission from NHS England. (2020). *Social prescribing and community-based support: Summary guide*. NHS Improvement. https://www.england.nhs.uk/wp-content/uploads/2020/06/social-prescribing-summary-guide-updated-june-20.pdf. Copyright © 2020 NHS England.

As an alternative to traditional medical intervention (through pharmaceutical prescribing or referring to the secondary hospital sector), social prescribing empowers people to take control of their health and well-being through referral to non-medical 'link workers' who take a holistic approach on what matters to the individual person, connecting people to community groups and statutory services for practical and emotional support (see Figure 2.8; NHS England, 2020).

Social prescribing is designed to support people with social, emotional, or practical needs and aims to improve mental and physical health. For example, people who experience mild or long-term mental health problems, people with complex social needs, people who are lonely or socially isolated, and those with multiple long-term conditions who frequently visit primary or secondary care

are thought to benefit from social prescribing programmes (Buck & Ewbank, 2020). People can be referred to link workers from a wide range of local agencies, including general practice, pharmacies, multidisciplinary teams, hospital discharge teams, allied health professionals, fire services, the police, job centres, social care services, housing associations, and voluntary, community, and social enterprise (VCSE) organizations. Self-referral is also encouraged. Social prescribing fits with the personalized care model developed by NHS England (2020; see Figure 2.9).

A realist review of approaches to social prescribing found that patients are more likely to engage in social prescribing activities if the activity is both accessible and transport to the first session supported (Husk et al., 2019). Adherence to activity programmes can be impacted through having an activity leader who is skilled and knowledgeable or through changes in the patient's conditions or symptoms over time. There is currently a sparse but growing evidence base of the effectiveness and cost-effectiveness of social prescribing programmes (Husk et al., 2019). A report on social prescribing acknowledged the challenge of assessing the cost-effectiveness of social prescribing programmes and the need for the adoption of a broad perspective to capture wider social value (Buck & Ewbank, 2020). A study found that more than half of the outcomes social prescribing can deliver are not being routinely measured in evaluation frameworks (Polley et al., 2019).

In terms of the application of conventional CUA to the evaluation of social prescribing, an example is provided by the evaluation of Doncaster Social Prescribing Service (Dayson & Bennett, 2016). This service was delivered through a partnership between South Yorkshire Housing Association and Doncaster County for Voluntary Services. GPs, community nurses, and pharmacists can refer clients to advisers at the service, who can then provide them with support to access a range of voluntary, community, and statutory services that meet their needs. This generated a cost per QALY of £1,963, much lower than the threshold of £20,000 to £30,000 per QALY recommended by NICE (Claxton et al., 2015). In North Wales, a social return on investment (SROI) approach was undertaken to evaluate the Health Precinct, a community hub that people with chronic conditions were referred to through social prescribing (Jones et al., 2020). The Health Precinct is a partnership between Conwy County Borough Council, Betsi Cadwaladr University Health Board (BCUHB), and Public Health Wales. A treatment plan was developed after a multidisciplinary assessment of the participant's health and well-being needs was undertaken. The treatment plan was typically sixteen weeks long and included achievable exercise goals along with physiotherapy, occupational therapy, or nursing advice. The intervention yielded an SROI ratio of £5.07 of social value generated

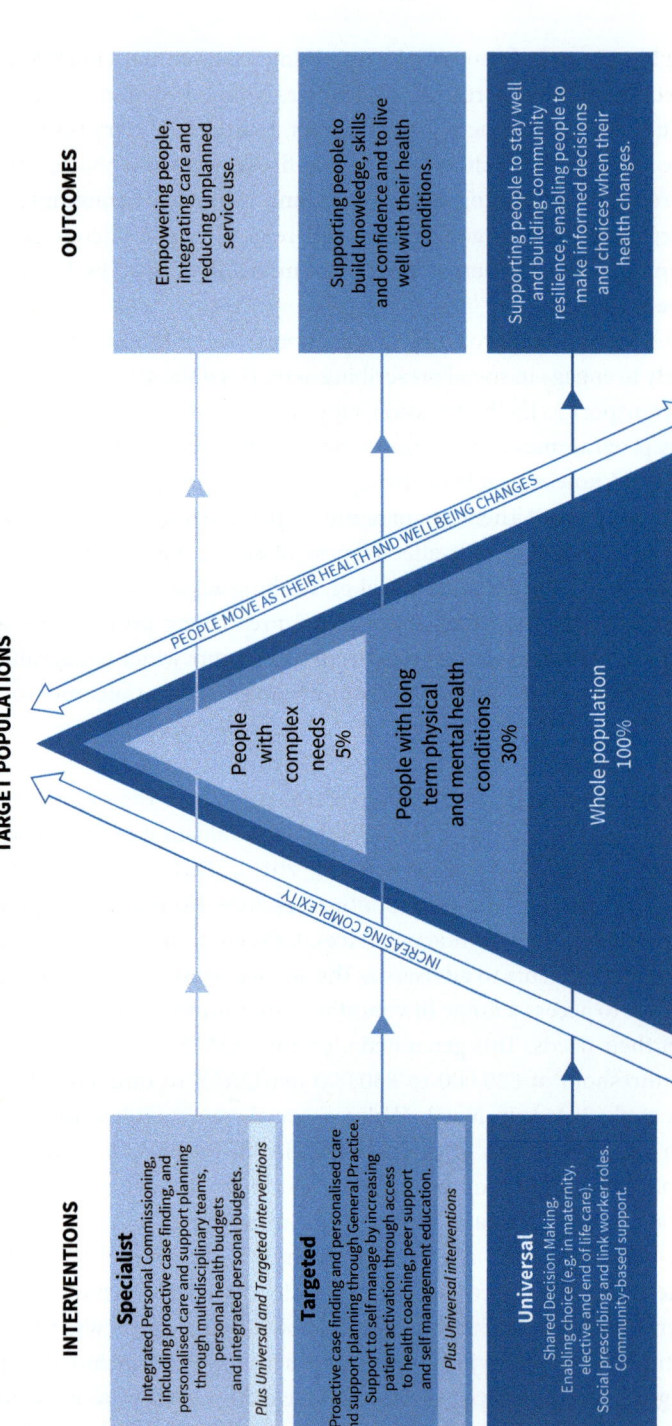

Figure 2.9 Comprehensive model for personalized care

Reproduced with permission from NHS England. (2020). *Social prescribing and community-based support: Summary guide.* NHS Improvement. https://www.engl and.nhs.uk/wp-content/uploads/2020/06/social-prescribing-summary-guide-updated-june-20.pdf. Copyright © NHS England 2020.

for every £1 invested. Sensitivity analysis yielded estimates of between 2.60:1 and 5.16:1 (Jones et al., 2020).

Coed Lleol—Small Woods Wales, a part of the UK-wide charity Small Woods Association, provides nature-based interventions for adults and families. These interventions are particularly aimed at people actively using mental health services, older people in sheltered housing, people with a disability or long-term illness, and people recovering from domestic violence or addictions. Coed Lleol—Small Woods Wales programmes include a diverse range of outdoor activities such as bushcraft, campfire cooking, woodland walks, conservation, foraging, woodland gym, and mindfulness. These programmes are frequently offered in partnership with health or social care organizations, which refer participants as part of social prescribing initiatives. Hartfiel and colleagues (2023) investigated whether nature-based interventions (multi-activity or mindfulness-in-the-woods) for people with mild mental health difficulties could generate a positive SROI. Between May 2017 and January 2019, 120 participants at six outdoor sites participated in a six to twelve-week nature-based intervention, which consisted of weekly two to four-hour sessions. The findings indicated that by the end of the programme, many participants improved in mental well-being, physical activity, self-efficacy, and social trust, and that for every £1 invested in the programme, £2.57 to £4.67 of social value was generated (Hartfiel et al., 2023).

Social Prescribing: An Inadequate Response to the Degradation of Social Care in Mental Health

Psychiatrist Rob Poole and social care researcher Peter Huxley have been amongst few voices to openly criticize the concept of social prescribing (Poole & Huxley, 2023). They argue that social prescribing does not address the social determinants of mental health and it is unlikely to produce lasting change for individuals who experience severe physical and mental health difficulties, who are amongst the most deprived and marginalized members of the population. Poole and Huxley (2023) argue that this situation has coincided with the neglect of social care and the social dimensions of mental health intervention. They state that social prescribing creates a false impression of addressing social factors, and as such is counterproductive. These authors recognize Marmot's (2015) distinction of the social origins of mental ill-health into immediate causes and upstream 'causes of the causes'. However, they emphasize the idea that it is more useful to think in terms of constellations of disadvantage, where structural, environmental, and experiential adversity interact in ways that have a detrimental effect on mental health. In accordance with Tudor Hart's (1971) inverse care law, the people who most benefit from social prescribing are likely to be those with the least severe and complex health needs. Poole and Huxley argue for assertive outreach of public services to support people with more serious mental health challenges, largely a result of their life circumstances.

A Growing Interest in Social Care Economics

In the UK, a decade of austerity prior to the COVID-19 pandemic meant that local authorities had already started looking to shift costs from their services to clients receiving adult social care. The financial and other difficulties of this were compounded by social distancing requirements of lockdowns which meant many people received little or no care over many months. Evaluation of social care policy change or specific social care services and their impact on well-being are challenging for the health economist, mainly because the social care market is split between public statutory provision and private purchasing of services, or a shared contribution model. For the health economist, the perspective of analysis is key. Any one social care service or model may be cost-effective taking a single agency perspective. However, taking a wider social perspective may illuminate great hardship and reduction in well-being as a result of having to make a greater financial contribution in order to receive that social care package of support. With respect to the economic evaluation of social care interventions, Weatherly and colleagues (2017) have undertaken a scoping review highlighting that investment in applied economic evaluations of social care interventions will support more informed recommendations by bodies such as NICE and also develop research capacity in social care economics.

The demand for adult social care increased substantially during the COVID-19 pandemic through an increased number of working-age people with learning difficulties, an ageing population, and increased poverty. Councils in England received 120,000 more requests for support in 2019/2020 than 2015/2016, but provided short or longer-term support to 14,000 fewer people (Bottery & Ward, 2021). The UK Government has allocated £4.6 billion to councils in England following the COVID-19 pandemic, with a large proportion spent on adult social care. An additional £1.9 billion has been allocated for hospital discharge and £1.4 billion in specific grants for adult care. However, it is anticipated that this additional expenditure will not keep pace with costs. Bottery and Ward (2021) from The King's Fund identified six priorities for providing a long-term, wide-ranging reform programme for adult social care:

1. Increase funding: an extra £1.9 billion is needed to meet the demand for adult social care by 2023/2024, along with further funding to meet existing

unmet needs, improve the quality of services, cover the additional costs of the COVID-19 pandemic, support the provider market, fill vacancies, and pay staff a fairer wage.

2. Improve eligibility: initially by easing the financial pressure on local authorities and allowing them to apply existing rules more fairly; in the longer term by changing those rules to make more people entitled to support.

3. Workforce reform: better pay, training, and development to compete with other sectors and deliver the care needed.

4. Re-invigorate personalization: to increase the number and quality of direct payments, to align with the principle of self-directed support outlined in the 2014 Care Act.

5. Prevention is key: local authorities and national government should prioritize reablement services.

6. Carer support needs: a new settlement for carers should be prioritized.

People with disabilities were differentially affected by the COVID-19 pandemic because of three main factors: the increased risk of poor outcomes from the virus itself; reduced access to routine health care and rehabilitation; and the adverse social impacts of efforts to mitigate the pandemic (Shakespeare et al., 2021). People with a learning disability were at an even greater risk of dying from COVID-19 than people with a physical disability. Six out of ten people who died from the virus between January and November 2020 had a disability (Suleman et al., 2021). The place of residence, socioeconomic and geographical circumstances, and pre-existing health conditions all played a part in the raised risk of dying from COVID-19 (ONS, 2021b). People with disabilities are disproportionately exposed to a range of generally disadvantageous circumstances (ONS, 2021b).

Tackling Health Inequalities across the Life-course

Public Health England (2019a) has identified five actions for tackling health inequalities across the life-course: 1) building healthy and resilient communities; 2) adopting a place-based approach to health; 3) tackling housing and fuel poverty; 4) taking action on poverty and health; and 5) taking action on health and justice (see Figure 2.10). The circumstances in which people are born, develop, live, work, and age are the social determinants of health. These fall outside of the health and social care system and can be thought of as the 'causes of the causes' of ill-health (Granger et al., 2022; NHS England, 2019).

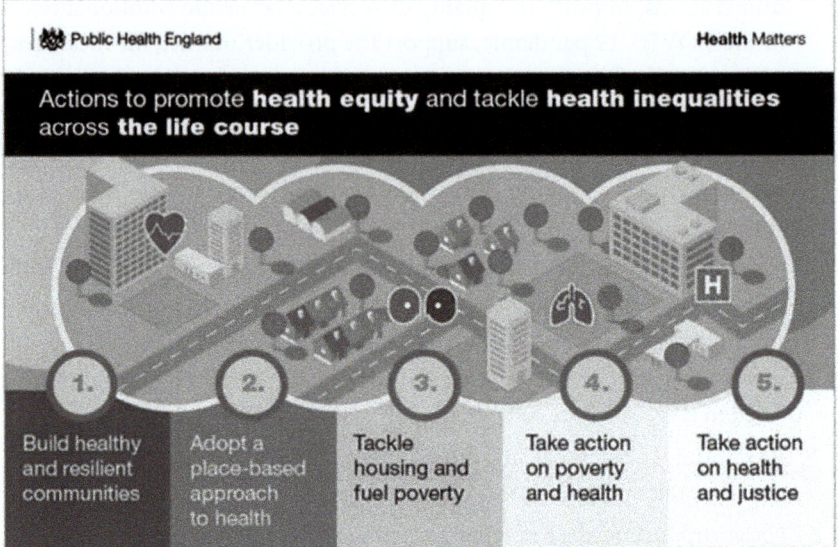

Figure 2.10 Actions to promote health equity and tackle health inequalities across the life-course

Reproduced from Public Health England. (2019a, 23 May). *Health matters: Prevention—a life course approach*. https://www.gov.uk/government/publications/health-matters-life-course-approach-to-prevention/health-matters-prevention-a-life-course-approach. Licence: Creative Commons BY 3.0 IGO.

Summary

In this chapter, we have examined some of the key cross-cutting themes influencing well-being and well-becoming across the life-course, some of the costs to society of health-harming and often addictive behaviours, and given some examples of how economic evaluation has approached these areas to provide evidence of relative cost-effectiveness of interventions within and outside of the health sector to prevent ill-health and premature mortality. The rest of this book is structured around broad life-course stages. The aim is to offer health economists working on economic evaluation and policy research in these life-course stages a context within which to approach their analysis and encourage adoption of a life-course and well-becoming lens. In the following chapter (Chapter 3), we begin our life-course approach by focusing on the economic benefits and returns from investing in early childhood and evidence of the cost-effectiveness of evidence-based programmes in early life.

Curiosity Questions

- Why is it that local government welcomes ROI and SROI methods rather than cost per QALY evidence with respect to public health, prevention, and the promotion of well-being and well-becoming?
- Along the lines of One Health economics (discussed in Chapter 1, The 'One Health Economics' Movement), how can health economics play a greater role in the really big climate change research agenda so that health benefits, including well-being and well-becoming, and potentially avoidable health care and social care costs are factored into government policy considerations?

References

Adams, K. B., Leibbrandt, S., & Moon, H. (2011). A critical review of the literature on social and leisure activity and wellbeing in later life. *Ageing & Society*, **31**, 683–712. https://doi.org/10.1017/S0144686X10001091

Age UK. (2019, July). *Age-friendly communities (England)* [Policy position paper]. https://www.ageuk.org.uk/globalassets/age-uk/documents/policy-positions/housing-and-homes/ppp_age_friendly_neighbourhood_england.pdf

Aked, J., & Thompson, S. (2011). *Five ways to wellbeing. New applications, new ways of thinking*. New Economics Foundation. https://neweconomics.org/uploads/files/d80eba95560c09605d_uzm6b1n6a.pdf

Amoly, E., Dadvand, P., Forns, J., López-Vicente, M., Basagaña, X., Julvez, J., Alvarez-Pedrerol, M., Nieuwenhuijsen, M. J., & Sunyer, J. (2015). Green and blue spaces and behavioral development in Barcelona schoolchildren: The BREATHE project. *Environmental Health Perspectives*, **122**(12), 1351–1358. https://doi.org/10.1289/ehp.1408215

Assemi, B., Zahnow, R., Zapata-Diomedi, B., Hickman, M., & Corcoran, J. (2020). Transport-related walking among young adults: When and why? *BMC Public Health*, **20**(1), 1–13. https://doi.org/10.1186/s12889-020-8338-0

Aubry, C., & Manouchehri, N. (2019). Urban agriculture and health: Assessing risks and overseeing practices. *The Journal of Field Actions*, (S 20), 108–111. https://journals.openedition.org/factsreports/5854

Baena-Diéz, J. M., Barroso, M., Cordeiro-Coelho, S. I., Diáz, J. L., & Grau, M. (2020). Impact of COVID-19 outbreak by income: Hitting hardest the most deprived. *Journal of Public Health (United Kingdom)*, **42**(4), 698–703. https://doi.org/10.1093/pubmed/fdaa136

Barber, S., Harker, R., & Pratt, A. (2017, 21 November). *Human and financial costs of drug addiction*. House of Commons Library. https://researchbriefings.files.parliament.uk/documents/CDP-2017-0230/CDP-2017-0230.pdf

Barnes, M., Butt, S., & Tomaszewski, W. (2008). *The dynamics of bad housing: The impact of bad housing on the living standards of children*. National Centre for Social Research.

Barton, J., Hine, R., & Pretty, J. (2009). The health benefits of walking in greenspaces of high natural and heritage value. *Journal of Integrative Environmental Sciences, 6*(4), 261–278. https://doi.org/10.1080/19438150903378425

Baxter, S., Blank, L., Cantrell, A., & Goyder, E. (2021). Is working in later life good for your health? A systematic review of health outcomes resulting from extended working lives. *BMC Public Health, 21*, 1–11. https://doi.org/10.1186/s12889-021-11423-2

Bedimo-Rung, A. L., Mowen, A. J., & Cohen, D. A. (2005). The significance of parks to physical activity and public health: A conceptual model. *American Journal of Preventive Medicine, 28*(2), 159–168. https://doi.org/10.1016/j.amepre.2004.10.024

Bellows, A., Brown, K., & Smit, J. (2004). *Health benefits of urban agriculture*. Community Food Security Coalition. https://www.csu.edu/cerc/researchreports/documents/HealthBenefitsOfUrbanAgriculture2003.pdf

Berg, V. (2023, 10 August). *Care home fees and costs: How much do you pay?* Care Home. https://www.carehome.co.uk/advice/care-home-fees-and-costs-how-much-do-you-pay

Bibby, J., & Lovell, N. (2018, March). *What makes us healthy? An introduction to the social determinants of health*. The Health Foundation. https://www.health.org.uk/publications/what-makes-us-healthy

Bottery, S., & Ward, D. (2021). *Social care 360*. The King's Fund. https://www.kingsfund.org.uk/sites/default/files/2021-05/social-care-360-2021_0.pdf

Bowen, D. J., Neill, J. T., & Crisp, S. J. (2016). Wilderness adventure therapy effects on the mental health of youth participants. *Evaluation and Program Planning, 58*, 49–59. https://doi.org/10.1016/j.evalprogplan.2016.05.005

Bowler, D. E., Buyung-Ali, L. M., Knight, T. M., & Pullin, A. S. (2010). A systematic review of evidence for the added benefits to health of exposure to natural environments. *BMC Public Health, 10*(1), 456. https://doi.org/10.1186/1471-2458-10-456

Bragg, R., Wood, C., Barton, J., & Pretty, J. (2015). *Wellbeing benefits from natural environments rich in wildlife*. A literature review for the Wildlife Trusts. University of Essex. https://www.wildlifetrusts.org/sites/default/files/2018-05/r1_literature_review_wellbeing_benefits_of_wild_places_lres.pdf

Bray, N., Burns, P., Jones, A., Winrow, E., & Edwards, R. T. (2017). Costs and outcomes of improving population health through better social housing: A cohort study and economic analysis. *International Journal of Public Health, 6*, 1039–1050. https://doi.org/10.1007/s00038-017-0989-y

Brewer, M., & Gardiner, L. (2020). The initial impact of COVID-19 and policy responses on household incomes. *Oxford Review of Economic Policy, 36*, S187–S199. https://doi.org/10.1093/oxrep/graa024

Buck, D., & Ewbank, L. (2020, 4 November). *What is social prescribing?* The King's Fund. https://www.kingsfund.org.uk/publications/social-prescribing

Buck, D., Simpson, M., & Ross, S. (2016). *The economics of housing and health: The role of housing associations*. The King's Fund and the NHS Alliance. https://www.kingsfund.org.uk/sites/default/files/field/field_publication_file/Economics_housing_and_health_Kings_Fund_Sep_2016.pdf

Buhnik, S. (2010). From shrinking cities to Toshi no Shukushō: Identifying patterns of urban shrinkage in the Osaka metropolitan area. *Berkeley Planning Journal*, 23(1), 132–155. https://doi.org/10.5070/BP323111434

Burns, J., Boogaard, H., Polus, S., Pfadenhauer, L. M., Rohwer, A. C., van Erp, A. M., Turley, R., & Rehfuess, E. A. (2020). Interventions to reduce ambient air pollution and their effects on health: An abridged Cochrane systematic review. *Environment International*, 135, 105400. https://doi.org/10.1016/j.envint.2019.105400

Calogiuri, G., & Chroni, S. (2014). The impact of the natural environment on the promotion of active living: An integrative systematic review. *BMC Public Health*, 14(1), 873. https://doi.org/10.1186/1471-2458-14-873

Celis-Morales, C. A., Lyall, D. M., Welsh, P., Anderson, J., Steell, L., Guo, Y., Maldonado, R., Mackay, D. F., Pell, J. P., Sattar, N., & Gill, J. M. R. (2017). Association between active commuting and incident cardiovascular disease, cancer, and mortality: Prospective cohort study. *BMJ*, 357, j1456. https://doi.org/10.1136/bmj.j1456

Chartered Institute of Environmental Health. (2011, July). *CIEH guidance on enforcement of excess cold hazards in England*. https://www.cieh.org/media/1243/cieh-guidance-on-enforcement-of-excess-cold-hazards-in-england.pdf

Chartered Institute of Personnel and Development. (2023, 21 February). *Tackling in-work poverty: Guidance for employers*. https://www.cipd.org/uk/knowledge/guides/in-work-poverty/

Cheng, Z., Mendolia, S., Paloyo, A. R., Savage, D. A., & Tani, M. (2021). Working parents, financial insecurity, and childcare: Mental health in the time of COVID-19 in the UK. *Review of Economics of the Household*, 19(1), 123–144. https://doi.org/10.1007/s11150-020-09538-3

Claxton, K., Martin, S., Soares, M., Rice, N., Spackman, E., Hinde, S., Devlin, N., Smith, P. C., & Sculpher, M. (2015). Methods for the estimation of the National Institute for Health and Care Excellence cost-effectiveness threshold. *Health Technology Assessment*, 19(14), 1. https://doi.org/10.3310/hta19140

Collins, B. J., Cuddy, K., & Martin, A. P. (2017). Assessing the effectiveness and cost-effectiveness of drug intervention programs: UK case study. *Journal of Addictive Diseases*, 36(1), 5–13. https://doi.org/10.1080/10550887.2016.1182299

Confederation of British Industry (CBI) Economics. (2020, 9 September). *Breathing life into the UK economy: Quantifying the economic benefits of cleaner air*. Clean Air Fund. https://www.cleanairfund.org/resource/breathing-life-into-the-uk-economy-cbi-economics-2020/

Connolly, A. M. (2018, 20 March). *Improving health and care through the home*. UK Health Security Agency. https://publichealthmatters.blog.gov.uk/2018/03/20/improving-health-and-care-through-the-home/

Cooper, E., Wang, Y., Stamp, S., & Mumovic, D. (2020). *Health benefits of the use of portable air purifiers that reduce exposure to PM2.5 in residences: The case of childhood asthma in London*. RoomVent 2020. https://discovery.ucl.ac.uk/id/eprint/10129219/1/Cooper_RoomVent_2020_final.pdf

Corfe, S., Bhattacharya, A., & Shepherd, J. (2021). *Double or nothing? Assessing the economic impact of gambling*. Social Market Foundation. https://www.smf.co.uk/wp-content/uploads/2021/03/Double-or-nothing-March-2021.pdf

Cotten, S. R., Anderson, W. A., & McCullough, B. M. (2013). Impact of internet use on loneliness and contact with others among older adults: Cross-sectional analysis. *Journal of Medical Internet Research*, 15(2), e39. https://doi.org/10.2196/jmir.2306

Courtney, P. (2014). *The Local Food programme: A social return on investment approach. Final report.* University of Gloucestershire's Countryside and Community Research Institute. https://eprints.glos.ac.uk/2637/1/The%20Local%20Food%20programme%20-%20A%20Social%20Return%20on%20Investment%20Approach.pdf

Craig, P., Dieppe, P., Macintyre, S., Michie, S., Nazareth, I., & Petticrew, M. (2008). Developing and evaluating complex interventions: The new Medical Research Council guidance. *BMJ*, 337, a1655. https://doi.org/10.1136/bmj.a1655

Dadvand, P., Bartoll, X., Basagaña, X., Dalmau-Bueno, A., Martinez, D., Ambros, A., Cirach, M., Triguero-Mas, M., Gascon, M., Borrell, C., & Nieuwenhuijsen, M. J. (2016). Green spaces and general health: Roles of mental health status, social support, and physical activity. *Environment International*, 91, 161–167. https://doi.org/10.1016/j.envint.2016.02.029

Dahlgren, G., & Whitehead, M. (2006). *European strategies for tackling social inequities in health: Levelling up Part 2.* World Health Organization. https://apps.who.int/iris/bitstream/handle/10665/107791/E89384.pdf

Datta, N., Giupponi, G., & Machin, S. (2019). Zero-hours contracts. *Economic Policy*, 34(99), 369–427. https://doi.org/10.1093/epolic/eiz008

Davies, L. E., Taylor, P., Ramchandani, G., & Christy, E. (2019). Social return on investment (SROI) in sport: A model for measuring the value of participation in England. *International Journal of Sport Policy and Politics*, 11(4), 585–605. https://doi.org/10.1080/19406940.2019.1596967

Dayson, C., & Bennett, E. (2016). *Evaluation of Doncaster social prescribing service: Understanding outcomes and impact.* Sheffield Hallam University. Centre for Regional Economic and Social Research. http://shura.shu.ac.uk/17298/1/eval-doncaster-social-prescribing-service.pdf

De Geest, S., Zullig, L. L., Dunbar-Jacob, J., Hughes, D., Wilson, I. B., & Vrijens, B. (2019). Improving medication adherence research reporting: European Society for Patient Adherence, Compliance and Persistence Medication Adherence Reporting Guideline. *Journal of Cardiovascular Nursing*, 34(3), 199–200. https://doi.org/10.1097/JCN.0000000000000572

Department for Levelling Up, Housing and Communities. (2022). *Ending rough sleeping for good.* https://assets.publishing.service.gov.uk/government/uploads/system/uploads/attachment_data/file/1102408/20220903_Ending_rough_sleeping_for_good.pdf

Department for Levelling Up, Housing and Communities, Department of Health and Social Care, Hughes, E., & Keegan, G. (2021, 29 October). *Government announces support for rough sleepers over winter* [Press release]. https://www.gov.uk/government/news/government-announces-support-for-rough-sleepers-over-winter

Department for Transport. (2009). *Low carbon transport: A greener future.* https://assets.publishing.service.gov.uk/government/uploads/system/uploads/attachment_data/file/228897/7682.pdf

Department for Work and Pensions. (2020, 19 November). *Economic labour market status of individuals aged 50 and over, trends over time: September 2020.* https://www.gov.uk/

government/statistics/economic-labour-market-status-of-individuals-aged-50-and-over-trends-over-time-september-2020/economic-labour-market-status-of-individuals-aged-50-and-over-trends-over-time-september-2020

Department for Work and Pensions. (2021, 25 March). *Households below average income: For financial years ending 1995 to 2020.* National Statistics. https://www.gov.uk/government/statistics/households-below-average-income-for-financial-years-ending-1995-to-2020

Department of Environment, Food and Rural Affairs. (2023, 2 March). *Air quality appraisal: Damage cost guidance.* https://www.gov.uk/government/publications/assess-the-impact-of-air-quality/air-quality-appraisal-damage-cost-guidance

Department of Health and Social Care. (2021, 2 August). *Review of drugs part two: Prevention, treatment, and recovery.* https://www.gov.uk/government/publications/review-of-drugs-phase-two-report/review-of-drugs-part-two-prevention-treatment-and-recovery

Deschênes, O., Greenstone, M., & Shapiro, J. S. (2017). Defensive investments and the demand for air quality: Evidence from the NOx budget program. *American Economic Review, 107*(10), 2958–2989. https://doi.org/10.1257/aer.20131002

Ding, D., Ramirez Varela, A., Bauman, A. E., Ekelund, U., Lee, I. M., Heath, G., Katzmarzyk, P. T., Reis, R., & Pratt, M. (2020). Towards better evidence-informed global action: Lessons learnt from the Lancet series and recent developments in physical activity and public health. *British Journal of Sports Medicine, 54*(8), 462–468. http://dx.doi.org/10.1136/bjsports-2019-101001

Durcan, D. (2015). *Local action on health inequalities: Promoting good quality jobs to reduce health inequalities.* Public Health England. https://fingertips.phe.org.uk/documents/Promoting-good-quality-jobs-to-reduce-health-inequalities-briefing.pdf

Edwards, R. T., Bryning, L., & Lloyd-Williams, H. (2016). *Transforming young lives across Wales: The economic argument for investing in early years.* Centre for Health Economics and Medicines Evaluation, Bangor University. https://cheme.bangor.ac.uk/documents/transforming-young-lives/CHEME%20transforming%20Young%20Lives%20Full%20Report%20Eng%20WEB%202.pdf

Edwards, R. T., & McIntosh, E. (Eds.). (2019). *Applied health economics for public health practice and research.* Oxford University Press.

Edwards, R. T., Spencer, L. H., Anthony, B. F., & Bryning, L. (2019). *Wellness in work: The economic arguments for investing in the health and wellbeing of the workforce in Wales.* Centre for Health Economics and Medicines Evaluation, Bangor University. https://cheme.bangor.ac.uk/documents/Wellness-in-Work-Report.pdf

Edwards, R. T., Spencer, L. H., Bryning, L., & Anthony, B. F. (2018). *Living well for longer: The economic argument for investing in the health and wellbeing of older people in Wales.* Centre for Health Economics and Medicines Evaluation, Bangor University. https://cheme.bangor.ac.uk/documents/livingwell2018.pdf

Emmel, N., Monaghan, M., Manzano, A., & Greenhalgh, J. (Eds.) (2018). *Doing realist research.* Sage Publications.

Etheridge, B., & Spantig, L. (2020). *The gender gap in mental well-being during the Covid-19 outbreak: Evidence from the UK.* ISER Working Paper Series. Institute for Social and Economic Research. https://www.iser.essex.ac.uk/wp-content/uploads/files/working-papers/iser/2020-08.pdf

Fagerström, C., Borg, C., Balducci, C., Burholt, V., Wenger, C. G., Ferring, D., Weber, G., Holst, G., & Hallberg, I. R. (2007). Life satisfaction and associated factors among people aged 60 years and above in six European countries. *Applied Research in Quality of Life*, 2, 33–50. https://doi.org/10.1007/s11482-007-9028-0

Farmer, P., & Stevenson, D. (2017). *Thriving at work: The Stevenson / Farmer review of mental health and employers*. https://assets.publishing.service.gov.uk/government/uplo ads/system/uploads/attachment_data/file/658145/thriving-at-work-stevenson-farmer-review.pdf

Feder, G., d'Oliveira, A. F. L., Rishal, P., & Johnson, M. (2021). Domestic violence during the pandemic. *BMJ*, 372, n722. https://doi.org/10.1136/bmj.n722

Finch, W. H., & Hernández Finch, M. E. (2020). Poverty and Covid-19: Rates of incidence and deaths in the United States during the first 10 weeks of the pandemic. *Frontiers in Sociology*, 5(47), 1–10. https://doi.org/10.3389/fsoc.2020.00047

Freeman, S., & Eykelbosh, A. (2020). *COVID-19 and outdoor safety: Considerations for use of outdoor recreational spaces*. National Collaborating Centre for Environmental Health. https://ncceh.ca/sites/default/files/COVID-19 Outdoor Safety - April 16 2020.pdf

Fulton, L., & Jupp, B. (2015). *Investing to tackle loneliness: A discussion paper*. Social Finance. https://www.socialfinance.org.uk/assets/documents/investing_to_tackle_lon eliness.pdf

Garrett, H., Margoles, S., Mackay, M., & Nicol, S. (2023). *The cost of poor housing in England by tenure. 2023 briefing paper: Tenure-based analysis*. Building Research Establishment Limited. https://files.bregroup.com/corporate/BRE_cost%20of%20p oor%20housing%20tenure%20analysis%202023.pdf

Garstang, J., Debelle, G., Anand, I., Armstrong, J., Botcher, E., Chaplin, H., Hallett, N., Morgans, C., Price, M., Tan, E. E. H., Tudor, E., & Taylor, J. (2020). Effect of COVID-19 lockdown on child protection medical assessments: A retrospective observational study in Birmingham, UK. *BMJ Open*, 10(9), 1–6. https://doi.org/10.1136/bmjopen-2020-042867

Gascon, M., Triguero-mas, M., Martínez, D., & Dadvand, P. (2015). Mental health benefits of long-term exposure to residential green and blue spaces: A systematic review. *International Journal of Environmental Research and Public Health*, 12, 4354–4379. https://doi.org/10.3390/ijerph120404354

Gibson, J. (2020). Domestic violence during COVID-19: The GP role. *The British Journal of General Practice*, 70(696), 340. https://doi.org/10.3399/bjgp20X710477

Gilmore, A. B., Fabbri, A., Baum, F., Bertscher, A., Bondy, K., Chang, H. J., Demaio, S., Erzse, A., Freudenberg, N., Friel, S., Hofman, K. J., Johns, P., Karim, S. A., Lacy-Nichols, J., de Carvalho C. M. P., Marten, R., McKee, M., Petticrew, M., Robertson, L., . . . Thow, A. M. (2023). Defining and conceptualising the commercial determinants of health. *The Lancet*, 401(10383), 1194–1213. https://doi.org/10.1016/S0140-6736(23)00013-2

Gladwell, V. F., Brown, D. K., Wood, C., Sandercock, G. R., & Barton, J. L. (2013). The great outdoors: How a green exercise environment can benefit all. *Extreme Physiology & Medicine*, 2(3), 1–7. https://doi.org/10.1186/2046-7648-2-3

Gladwell, V. F., Kuoppa, P., Tarvainen, M. P., & Rogerson, M. (2016). A lunchtime walk in nature enhances restoration of autonomic control during night-time sleep: Results from a preliminary study. *International Journal of Environmental Research and Public Health,* 13(3), 280. https://doi.org/10.3390/ijerph13030280

Goods, C., Veen, A., & Barratt, T. (2019). 'Is your gig any good?' Analysing job quality in the Australian platform-based food-delivery sector. *Journal of Industrial Relations,* 61(4), 502–527. https://doi.org/10.1177/0022185618817069

Goulden, C. (2020, 7 February). *UK Poverty 2019/20.* Joseph Rowntree Foundation. https://www.jrf.org.uk/report/uk-poverty-2019-20

Granger, R., Genn, H., & Edwards, R. T. (2022). Health economics of health justice partnerships: A rapid review of the economic returns to society of promoting access to legal advice. *Frontiers in Public Health,* 10, 1009964. https://doi.org/10.3389/fpubh.2022.1009964

Grinde, B., & Patil, G. G. (2009). Biophilia: Does visual contact with nature impact on health and well-being? *International Journal of Environmental Research and Public Health,* 6(9), 2332–2343. https://doi.org/10.3390/ijerph6092332

Grunseit, A. C., Richards, J., Reece, L., Bauman, A., & Merom, D. (2020). Evidence on the reach and impact of the social physical activity phenomenon parkrun: A scoping review. *Preventive Medicine Reports,* 20, 101231. https://doi.org/10.1016/j.pmedr.2020.101231

Gunn, C., Mackus, M., Griffin, C., Munafò, M. R., & Adams, S. (2018). A systematic review of the next day effects of heavy alcohol consumption on cognitive performance. *Addiction,* 113(12), 2182–2193. https://doi.org/10.1111/add.14404

Gwadry-Sridhar, F. H., Manias, E., Zhang, Y., Roy, A., Yu-Isenberg, K., Hughes, D. A., & Nichol, M. B. (2009). A framework for planning and critiquing medication compliance and persistence research using prospective study designs. *Clinical Therapeutics,* 31(2), 421–435. https://doi.org/10.1016/j.clinthera.2009.02.021

Harari, D., Francis-Devine, B., Bolton, P., & Keep, M. (2023). *Rising cost of living in the UK.* Research Briefing. House of Commons Library. https://researchbriefings.files.parliament.uk/documents/CBP-9428/CBP-9428.pdf

Hart, J. T. (1971). The inverse care law. *The Lancet,* 297(7696), 405–412. https://doi.org/10.1016/S0140-6736(71)92410-X

Hartfiel, N., Gittins, H., Morrison, V., Wynne-Jones, S., Dandy, N., & Edwards, R. T. (2023). Social return on investment of nature-based activities for adults with mental wellbeing challenges. *International Journal of Environmental Research and Public Health,* 20(15), 6500. https://doi.org/10.3390/ijerph20156500

Health and Safety Executive. (2021). *Managing drug and alcohol misuse at work.* https://www.hse.gov.uk/alcoholdrugs/

Henseke, G. (2018). Good jobs, good pay, better health? The effects of job quality on health among older European workers. *The European Journal of Health Economics,* 19(1), 59–73. https://doi.org/10.1007/s10198-017-0867-9

Hill, K., & Webber, R. (2022, 12 May). *From pandemic to cost of living crisis: Low-income households in challenging times.* Joseph Rowntree Foundation. https://www.jrf.org.uk/from-pandemic-to-cost-of-living-crisis-low-income-families-in-challenging-times

Hill, S. (2019). *An investigation of economic evaluation methods for public health interventions: Meeting the needs of public health decision-makers* [Doctoral thesis, Newcastle University]. https://theses.ncl.ac.uk/jspui/bitstream/10443/4908/1/Hill%20SR%202019.pdf

Hills, J. (2012, March). *Getting the measure of fuel poverty. Final Report of the Fuel Poverty Review.* Centre for Analysis and Social Exclusion report 72. https://assets.publishing. service.gov.uk/media/5a796f55e5274a2acd18ccde/4662-getting-measure-fuel-pov-final-hills-rpt.pdf

Hinson, S., Bolton, P., & Kennedy, S. (2023, 24 March). *Fuel poverty in the UK.* House of Commons Library. https://commonslibrary.parliament.uk/research-briefings/cbp-8730/

HM Government. (2017a). *Drug strategy 2017.* Home Office [Policy paper]. https://www. gov.uk/government/publications/drug-strategy-2017

HM Government. (2017b). *Industrial strategy. Building a Britain fit for the future* [White paper]. https://assets.publishing.service.gov.uk/media/5a8224cbed915d74e3401f69/ind ustrial-strategy-white-paper-web-ready-version.pdf

HM Government. (2018). *A connected society. A strategy for tackling loneliness—laying the foundations for change.* Department for Digital, Culture, Media and Sport. HM Government. https://assets.publishing.service.gov.uk/government/uploads/system/ uploads/attachment_data/file/936725/6.4882_DCMS_Loneliness_Strategy_web_Up date_V2.pdf

HM Treasury. (2020). *Magenta Book 2020. Supplementary guide: Realist evaluation.* HM Treasury. https://assets.publishing.service.gov.uk/government/uploads/system/ uploads/attachment_data/file/879435/Magenta_Book_supplementary_guide._ Realist_Evaluation.pdf

Hoevenaar-Blom, M. P., Wendel-Vos, G. W., Spijkerman, A. M., Kromhout, D., & Verschuren, W. M. (2011). Cycling and sports, but not walking, are associated with 10-year cardiovascular disease incidence: The MORGEN Study. *European Journal of Preventive Cardiology, 18*(1), 41–47. https://doi.org/10.1097/HJR.0b013e32833bfc87

Holt-Lunstad, J., Smith, T. B., Baker, M., Harris, T., & Stephenson, D. (2015). Loneliness and social isolation as risk factors for mortality: A meta-analytic review. *Perspectives on Psychological Science, 10*(2), 227–237. https://doi.org/10.1177/1745691614568352

Holt-Lunstad, J., Smith, T. B., & Layton, J. B. (2010). Social relationships and mortality risk: A meta-analytic review. *PLoS Medicine, 7*(7), e1000316. https://doi.org/10.1371/ journal.pmed.1000316

Holwerda, T. J., Deeg, D. J., Beekman, A. T., Van Tilburg, T. G., Stek, M. L., Jonker, C., & Schoevers, R. A. (2014). Feelings of loneliness, but not social isolation, predict dementia onset: Results from the Amsterdam Study of the Elderly (AMSTEL). *Journal of Neurology, Neurosurgery & Psychiatry, 85*(2), 135–142. http://https://doi.org/10.1136/ jnnp-2012-302755

House of Commons Education Committee. (2019). *Tackling disadvantage in the early years. Ninth report of session 2017–2019.* House of Commons Education Committee. https:// publications.parliament.uk/pa/cm201719/cmselect/cmeduc/1006/1006.pdf

Hunter, D. (2010). What makes people healthy and what makes people ill? In F. Campbell (Ed.), *The social determinants of health and the role of local government improvement and development agency* (pp. 11–16). IDeA.

Hunter, R. F., Cleland, C., Cleary, A., Droomers, M., Wheeler, B. W., Sinnett, D., Nieuwenhuijsen, M. J., & Braubach, M. (2019). Environmental, health, wellbeing, social and equity effects of urban green space interventions: A meta-narrative evidence synthesis. *Environment International, 130*, 104923. https://doi.org/10.1016/j.env int.2019.104923

Husk, K., Blockley, K., Lovell, R., Bethel, A., Lang, I., Byng, R., & Garside, R. (2019). What approaches to social prescribing work, for whom, and in what circumstances? A realist review. *Health & Social Care in the Community*, **28**(2), 309–324. https://doi. org/10.1111/hsc.12839

Inge, N., Ford, R., & Hogan, J. (2012). *Social return on investment of Ready for Work*. Business in the Community. https://socialvalueuk.org/wp-content/uploads/2016/06/ socialreturn.pdf

Institute for Government. (2022). *Timeline of UK government coronavirus lockdowns and measures, March 2020 to December 2021*. https://www.instituteforgovernment.org.uk/ sites/default/files/2022-12/timeline-coronavirus-lockdown-december-2021.pdf

Institute of Alcohol Studies. (2017). *Splitting the bill: Alcohol's impact on the economy*. https://www.ias.org.uk/uploads/pdf/IAS%20reports/rp23022017.pdf

Institute of Alcohol Studies. (2020). *Alcohol in the workforce*. Alcohol Knowledge Centre Briefing. https://www.ias.org.uk/wp-content/uploads/2020/12/Alcohol-in-the-workpl ace.pdf

International Longevity Centre UK (ILC). (2021, 2 August). *Smoking costs UK economy in excess of £19 billion a year, new report finds*. https://ilcuk.org.uk/smoking-costs-uk-econ omy-in-excess-of-19-billion-a-year-new-report-finds/

Iparraguirre, J. (2017). *The economic contribution of older people in the United Kingdom – An update to 2017*. https://www.ageuk.org.uk/globalassets/age-uk/documents/reports-and- publications/reports-and-briefings/active-communities/the_economic_contribution_ of_older_-people_-update_-to_-2017.pdf

Ireland, N. (2013). *Gardening in mind. Social return on investment (SROI) report*. Social Value UK. https://socialvalueuk.org/report/gardening-in-mind-social-return-on-inv estment-report/

Jephcote, C., Hansell, A. L., Adams, K., & Gulliver, J. (2021). Changes in air quality during COVID-19 'lockdown' in the United Kingdom. *Environmental Pollution*, **272**, 116011. https://doi.org/10.1016/j.envpol.2020.116011

Jin, S., Guo, J., Wheeler, S., Kan, L., & Che, S. (2014). Evaluation of impacts of trees on PM2.5 dispersion in urban streets. *Atmospheric Environment*, **99**, 277–287. https://doi. org/10.1016/j.atmosenv.2014.10.002

Jones, A., Valero-Silva, N., & Lucas, D. (2016). *The effects of 'Secure Warm Modern' homes in Nottingham: Decent Homes impact study*. Nottingham City Homes. http://irep.ntu. ac.uk/28087/

Jones, C., Hartfiel, N., Brocklehurst, P., Lynch, M., & Edwards, R. T. (2020). Social return on investment analysis of the Health Precinct community hub for chronic conditions. *International Journal of Environmental Research and Public Health*, **17**(14), 5249. https://doi.org/10.3390/ijerph17145249

Jones, M. K., Latreille, P. L., Sloane, P. J., & Staneva, A. V. (2013). Work-related health risks in Europe: Are older workers more vulnerable? *Social Science and Medicine*, **88**, 18–29. https://doi.org/10.1016/j.socscimed.2013.03.027

Jones, R., Ashurst, E., Atkey, J., & Duffy, B. (2015). Older people going online: Its value and before-after evaluation of volunteer support. *Journal of Medical Internet Research*, **17**, 1–12. https://doi.org/10.2196/jmir.3943

Joseph Rowntree Foundation. (2021, 13 January). *UK Poverty 2020/21*. https://www.jrf.org. uk/report/uk-poverty-2020-21

Joseph Rowntree Foundation. (2022, 18 January). *UK Poverty 2022: The essential guide to understanding poverty in the UK*. https://www.jrf.org.uk/report/uk-poverty-2022

Kabisch, N., van den Bosch, M., & Lafortezza, R. (2017). The health benefits of nature-based solutions to urbanization challenges for children and the elderly—a systematic review. *Environmental Research*, 159, 362–373. https://doi.org/10.1016/j.env res.2017.08.004

Keenan, C., Miller, S., Hanratty, J., Pigott, T., Hamilton, J., Coughlan, C., Mackie, P., Fitzpatrick, S., & Cowman, J. (2021). Accommodation-based interventions for individuals experiencing, or at risk of experiencing, homelessness. *Campbell Systematic Reviews*, 17(2), e1165. https://doi.org/10.1002/cl2.1165

Kelly, T., Unwin, D., & Finucane, F. (2020). Low-carbohydrate diets in the management of obesity and Type 2 diabetes: A review from clinicians using the approach in practice. *International Journal of Environmental Research and Public Health*, 17(7), 2557. https://doi.org/10.3390/ijerph17072557

Kickbusch, I., Allen, L., & Franz, C. (2016). The commercial determinants of health. *The Lancet Global Health*, 4(12), e895–e896. https://doi.org/10.1016/S2214-109X(16)30217-0

Kinsella, S. (2014). *Older people and social isolation evidence: A review of the evidence*. Wirral Council Business and Public Health Intelligence Team. https://www.wirralinte lligenceservice.org/media/1076/older_people__social_isolation_2015_final.pdf

Kmietowicz, Z. (2020). Covid-19: Highest risk patients are asked to stay at home for 12 weeks. *BMJ*, 368, 1–2. https://doi.org/10.1136/bmj.m1170

Lamu, A. N., Jbaily, A., Verguet, S., Robberstad, B., & Norheim, O. F. (2020). Is cycle network expansion cost-effective? A health economic evaluation of cycling in Oslo. *BMC Public Health*, 20(1869), 1–11. https://doi.org/10.1186/s12889-020-09764-5

Landeiro, F., Leal, J., & Gray, A. M. (2016). The impact of social isolation on delayed hospital discharges of older hip fracture patients and associated costs. *Osteoporosis International*, 27(2), 737–745. https://doi.org/10.1007/s00198-015-3293-9

Langham, S., Wright, A., Kenworthy, J., Grieve, R., & Dunlop, W. C. (2018). Cost-effectiveness of take-home naloxone for the prevention of overdose fatalities among heroin users in the United Kingdom. *Value in Health*, 21(4), 407–415. https://doi.org/10.1016/j.jval.2017.07.014

Lee, A., Sinha, I., Boyce, T., Allen, J., & Goldblatt, P. (2022). *Fuel poverty, cold homes and health inequalities*. Institute of Health Equity. https://www.instituteofhealthequity.org/resources-reports/fuel-poverty-cold-homes-and-health-inequalities-in-the-uk/read-the-report.pdf

Leigh-Hunt, N., Bagguley, D., Bash, K., Turner, V., Turnbull, S., Valtorta, N., & Caan, W. (2017). An overview of systematic reviews on the public health consequences of social isolation and loneliness. *Public Health*, 152, 157–171. https://doi.org/10.1016/j.puhe.2017.07.035

Leitzmann, M. F., Park, Y., Blair, A., Ballard-Barbash, R., Mouw, T., Hollenbeck, A. R., & Schatzkin, A. (2007). Physical activity recommendations and decreased risk of mortality. *Archives of Internal Medicine*, 167(22), 2453–2460. http://doi.org/10.1001/archinte.167.22.2453

Li, Q. (2010). Effect of forest bathing trips on human immune function. *Environmental Health and Preventive Medicine*, 15(1), 9–17. https://doi.org/10.1007/s12 199-008-0068-3

Logan, K. G., Nelson, J. D., & Hastings, A. (2020). Electric and hydrogen buses: Shifting from conventionally fuelled cars in the UK. *Transportation Research Part D: Transport and Environment*, 85, 102350. https://doi.org/10.1016/j.trd.2020.102350

Lynch, M., Spencer, L. H., & Edwards, R. T. (2020). A systematic review exploring the economic valuation of accessing and using green and blue spaces to improve public health. *International Journal of Environmental Research and Public Health*, 17(11), 4142. https://doi.org/10.3390/ijerph17114142

Maas, J., Verheij, R. A., de Vries, S., Spreeuwenberg, P., Schellevis, F. G., & Groenewegen, P. P. (2009). Morbidity is related to a green living environment. *Journal of Epidemiology & Community Health*, 63(12), 967–973. https://doi.org/10.1136/jech.2008.079038

Mackay, L., Egli, V., Booker, L. J., & Prendergast, K. (2019). New Zealand's engagement with the Five Ways to Wellbeing: Evidence from a large cross-sectional survey. *Kōtuitui: New Zealand Journal of Social Sciences Online*, 14(2), 230–244. https://doi.org/10.1080/1177083X.2019.1603165

Marmot, M. (2015). The health gap: The challenge of an unequal world. *The Lancet*, 386(10011), 2442–2444. https://doi.org/10.1016/S0140-6736(15)00150-6

Marmot, M., Allen, J., Boyce, T., Goldblatt, P., & Morrison, J. (2020). *Health equity in England: The Marmot review 10 years on*. Institute of Health Equity. https://www.health.org.uk/publications/reports/the-marmot-review-10-years-on

Marmot, M., Allen, J., Goldblatt, P., Boyce, T., McNeish, D., Grady, M., & Geddes, I. (2010). *Fair society, healthy lives: The Marmot review. Strategic review of health inequalities in England post-2010*. https://www.instituteofhealthequity.org/resources-reports/fair-society-healthy-lives-the-marmot-review

Marmot, M. G., Stansfeld, S., Patel, C., North, F., Head, J., White, I., Brunner, E., Feeney, A., Marmot, M. G., & Smith, G. D. (1991). Health inequalities among British civil servants: The Whitehall II study. *The Lancet*, 337(8754), 1387–1393. https://doi.org/10.1016/0140-6736(91)93068-K

Maslow, A. H. (1943). A theory of human motivation. *Psychological Review*, 50(4), 370–396. https://doi.org/10.1037/h0054346

Maslow, A. H. (2017). *A theory of human motivation*. BN Publishing.

Mason, V., & Roys, M. (2011). *The health costs of cold dwellings*. Building Research Establishment. http://www.somersetintelligence.org.uk/files/Health Costs of Cold Dwellings report.pdf

McCall, H., Adams, N., Mason, D., & Willis, J. (2015). What is chemsex and why does it matter? *BMJ*, 351(h5790). https://doi.org/10.1136/bmj.h5790

McIntosh, T. (2021). parkrun: A panacea for health and wellbeing? *Journal of Research in Nursing*, 26(5), 472–477. https://doi.org/10.1177/17449871211037327

Mental Health Foundation. (2023). *Relationships and community: Statistics*. https://www.mentalhealth.org.uk/statistics/mental-health-statistics-relationships-and-community

Milovanska-Farrington, S. (2021). Education in the times of a pandemic: Parental socioeconomic characteristics and time spent educating children. *Journal of Economic Studies*, 49(4), 716–734. https://doi.org/10.1108/JES-01-2021-0013

Mitchell, R. (2013). Is physical activity in natural environments better for mental health than physical activity in other environments? *Social Science & Medicine*, 91, 130–134. https://doi.org/10.1016/j.socscimed.2012.04.012

Muggleton, N., Parpart, P., Newall, P., Leake, D., Gathergood, J., & Stewart, N. (2021). The association between gambling and financial, social and health outcomes in big financial data. *Nature Human Behaviour*, 5(3), 319–326. https://doi.org/10.1038/s41 562-020-01045-w

National Health Service. (2021, 9 June). *Addiction: What is it?* https://www.nhs.uk/live-well/healthy-body/addiction-what-is-it/

National Health Service. (2022a, 16 September). *What are the health risks of smoking?* https://www.nhs.uk/common-health-questions/lifestyle/what-are-the-health-risks-of-smoking/

National Health Service. (2022b, 10 October). *Using e-cigarettes to stop smoking.* https://www.nhs.uk/live-well/quit-smoking/using-e-cigarettes-to-stop-smoking/

National Health Service Digital. (2020, 5 May). *Statistics on obesity, physical activity and diet, England 2020.* https://digital.nhs.uk/data-and-information/publications/statistical/statistics-on-obesity-physical-activity-and-diet/england-2020

National Health Service Digital. (2021, 18 May). *Statistics on obesity, physical activity and diet, England 2021.* https://digital.nhs.uk/data-and-information/publications/statistical/statistics-on-obesity-physical-activity-and-diet/england-2021

National Health Service Digital. (2022, 3 November). *National Child Measurement Programme, England, 2021/22 school year.* https://digital.nhs.uk/data-and-information/publications/statistical/national-child-measurement-programme/2021-22-school-year

National Health Service England. (2019, 3 September). *Putting health into place.* https://www.england.nhs.uk/publication/putting-health-into-place-executive-summary/

National Health Service England. (2020). *Personalised Care. Social prescribing and community-based support. Summary guide.* NHS Improvement. https://www.engl and.nhs.uk/wp-content/uploads/2020/06/social-prescribing-summary-guide-upda ted-june-20.pdf

National Institute for Health and Care Excellence. (2017). *Air pollution: Outdoor air quality and health* (NG70). https://www.nice.org.uk/guidance/ng70

National Institute for Health and Care Excellence. (2021). *Tobacco: Preventing uptake, promoting quitting and treating dependence* (NG209). https://www.nice.org.uk/guida nce/ng209

Newton, B., Sinclair, A., Tyers, C., & Wilson, T. (2020). *Supporting disadvantaged young people into meaningful work: An initial evidence review to identify what works and inform good practice among practitioners and employers.* IES & Youth Futures Foundation. https://www.voced.edu.au/content/ngv%3A86249

Nicholson, P., Mayho, G., & Sharp, C. (2016). *Alcohol, drugs and the workplace—the role of medical professionals. A briefing from the BMA Occupational Medicine Committee* (2nd ed.). British Medical Association. https://www.bma.org.uk/media/1067/bma_alcohol-and-drugs-in-the-workplace-_oct_2019.pdf

Noltemeyer, A., Bush, K., Patton, J., & Bergen, D. (2012). The relationship among deficiency needs and growth needs: An empirical investigation of Maslow's theory. *Children and Youth Services Review*, 34(9), 1862–1867. https://doi.org/10.1016/j.childyouth.2012.05.021

Nystrand, C., Gebreslassie, M., Ssegonja, R., Feldman, I., & Sampaio, F. (2021). A systematic review of economic evaluations of public health interventions targeting alcohol, tobacco, illicit drug use and problematic gambling: Using a case study to assess transferability. *Health Policy*, 125(1), 54–74. https://doi.org/10.1016/j.health pol.2020.09.002

Office for National Statistics. (2019, 24 July). *Net zero and the different official measures of the UK's greenhouse gas emissions.* https://www.ons.gov.uk/economy/environmentala ccounts/articles/netzeroandthedifferentofficialmeasuresoftheuksgreenhousegasemissi ons/2019-07-24

Office for National Statistics. (2020a, 27 November). *Excess winter mortality in England and Wales: 2019 to 2020 (provisional) and 2018 to 2019 (final).* https://www.ons.gov. uk/peoplepopulationandcommunity/birthsdeathsandmarriages/deaths/bulletins/ excesswintermortalityinenglandandwales/2019to2020provisionaland2018to2019final

Office for National Statistics. (2020b, 9 December). *Drug misuse in England and Wales: Year ending March 2020.* https://www.ons.gov.uk/peoplepopulationandcommunity/crim eandjustice/articles/drugmisuseinenglandandwales/yearendingmarch2020

Office for National Statistics. (2021a, 23 October). *Measures of National Well-being Dashboard.* https://www.ons.gov.uk/peoplepopulationandcommunity/wellbeing/artic les/measuresofnationalwellbeingdashboard/2018-04-25

Office for National Statistics. (2021b, 11 February). *Updated estimates of coronavirus (COVID-19) related deaths by disability status, England: 24 January to 20 November 2020.* https://www.ons.gov.uk/peoplepopulationandcommunity/birthsdeathsandmarria ges/deaths/articles/coronaviruscovid19relateddeathsbydisabilitystatusenglandandwa les/24januaryto20november2020

Office for National Statistics. (2022, 6 December). *Adult smoking habits in the UK: 2021.* https://www.ons.gov.uk/peoplepopulationandcommunity/healthandsocialcare/health andlifeexpectancies/bulletins/adultsmokinghabitsingreatbritain/2021/pdf

Office for National Statistics. (2023, 25 August). *Cost of living insights: Food.* https://www. ons.gov.uk/economy/inflationandpriceindices/articles/costoflivinginsights/food

Oliver, R., Alexander, B., Roe, S., & Wlasny, M. (2019). *The economic and social costs of domestic abuse.* Home Office. https://www.gov.uk/government/publications/the-econo mic-and-social-costs-of-domestic-abuse

Orhan, E. (2022). The effects of the Russia-Ukraine war on global trade. *Journal of International Trade, Logistics and Law,* 8(1), 141–146.

Owen, L., Tierney, R., Rtveladze, K., Pritchard, C., & Nolan, K. (2015). Cost-utility analysis of an internet and computer training intervention to improve independence and mental wellbeing of older people. *The Lancet,* 386, S62. https://doi.org/10.1016/S0140-6736(15)00900-9

Palmer, D. (2022). *Estimating the full costs of obesity: A report for Novo Nordisk.* Frontier Economics. https://www.frontier-economics.com/media/hgwd4e4a/the-full-cost-of-obesity-in-the-uk.pdf

Papathanasopoulou, E., White, M. P., Hattam, C., Lannin, A., Harvey, A., & Spencer, A. (2016). Valuing the health benefits of physical activities in the marine environment and their importance for marine spatial planning. *Marine Policy,* 63, 144–152. https://doi. org/10.1016/j.marpol.2015.10.009

parkrun Group. (2021, 13 August). *UK update—13 August.* https://blog.parkrun.com/uk/ 2021/08/13/uk-update-13-august/

Patterson, R., Webb, E., Millett, C., & Laverty, A. A. (2018). Physical activity accrued as part of public transport use in England. *Journal of Public Health,* 41(2), 222–230. https:// doi.org/10.1093/pubmed/fdy099

Pereira, G., Foster, S., Martin, K., Christian, H., Boruff, B. J., Knuiman, M., & Giles-Corti, B. (2012). The association between neighborhood greenness and cardiovascular disease: an observational study. *BMC Public Health*, **12**, 466. https://doi.org/10.1186/1471-2458-12-466

Polley, M., Whitehouse, J., Elnaschie, S., & Fixsen, A. (2019). *What does successful social prescribing look like? Mapping meaningful outcomes.* University of Westminster. https://42b7de07-529d-4774-b3e1-225090d531bd.filesusr.com/ugd/14f499_5f193389d80c4503a4c800e026189713.pdf

Poole, R., & Huxley, P. (2023). Social prescribing: An inadequate response to the degradation of social care in mental health. *British Journal of Psychiatry Bulletin*, **48**(1), 30–33. https://doi.org/10.1192/bjb.2023.61

Pretty, J., Peacock, J., Hine, R., Sellens, M., South, N., & Griffin, M. (2007). Green exercise in the UK countryside: Effects on health and psychological well-being, and implications for policy and planning. *Journal of Environmental Planning and Management*, **50**(2), 211–231. https://doi.org/10.1080/09640560601156466

Public Health England. (2016, 21 January). *Health matters: Harmful drinking and alcohol dependence.* https://www.gov.uk/government/publications/health-matters-harmful-drinking-and-alcohol-dependence/health-matters-harmful-drinking-and-alcohol-dependence

Public Health England. (2017a, 31 March). *Health matters: Obesity and the food environment.* https://www.gov.uk/government/publications/health-matters-obesity-and-the-food-environment/health-matters-obesity-and-the-food-environment--2

Public Health England. (2017b). *An evidence review of the outcomes that can be expected of drug misuse treatment in England.* https://assets.publishing.service.gov.uk/government/uploads/system/uploads/attachment_data/file/586111/PHE_Evidence_review_of_drug_treatment_outcomes.pdf

Public Health England. (2018a, 7 August). *Creating a logic model for an intervention: Evaluation in health and wellbeing.* https://www.gov.uk/guidance/evaluation-in-health-and-wellbeing-creating-a-logic-model

Public Health England. (2018b, 22 May). *New tool calculates NHS and social care costs of air pollution.* https://www.gov.uk/government/news/new-tool-calculates-nhs-and-social-care-costs-of-air-pollution

Public Health England. (2019a, 23 May). *Health matters: Prevention—a life course approach.* https://www.gov.uk/government/publications/health-matters-life-course-approach-to-prevention/health-matters-prevention-a-life-course-approach

Public Health England. (2019b). *Review of interventions to improve outdoor air quality and public health.* https://www.gov.uk/government/publications/improving-outdoor-air-quality-and-health-review-of-interventions

Public Health England. (2020). *Improving access to greenspace: A new review for 2020.* https://assets.publishing.service.gov.uk/government/uploads/system/uploads/attachment_data/file/904439/Improving_access_to_greenspace_2020_review.pdf

Public Health England. (2021). *Gambling-related harms evidence review: The economic and social cost of harms.* https://assets.publishing.service.gov.uk/government/uploads/system/uploads/attachment_data/file/1022208/Gambling-evidence-review_economic-costs.pdf

Public Health Wales. (2018). *Substance misuse—drugs & alcohol.* https://phw.nhs.wales/topics/substance-misuse-drugs-alcohol/

Quirk, H., Bullas, A., Haake, S., Goyder, E., Graney, M., Wellington, C., Copeland, R., Reece, L., & Stevinson, C. (2021). Exploring the benefits of participation in community-based running and walking events: A cross-sectional survey of parkrun participants. *BMC Public Health*, 21, 1–15. https://doi.org/10.1186/s12889-021-11986-0

Rassafi, A. A., & Vaziri, M. (2005). Sustainable transport indicators: Definition and integration. *International Journal of Environmental Science & Technology*, 2, 83–96. https://doi.org/10.1007/BF03325861

Reece, L. J., Quirk, H., Wellington, C., Haake, S. J., & Wilson, F. (2019). Bright Spots, physical activity investments that work: parkrun; A global initiative striving for healthier and happier communities. *British Journal of Sports Medicine*, 53(6), 326–327. http://dx.doi.org/10.1136/bjsports-2018-100041

Rehfuess, E. A., Booth, A., Brereton, L., Burns, J., Gerhardus, A., Mozygemba, K., Oortwijn, W., Pfadenhauer, L. M., Tummers, M., van der Wilt, G.-J., & Rohwer, A. (2018). Towards a taxonomy of logic models in systematic reviews and health technology assessments: A priori, staged, and iterative approaches. *Research Synthesis Methods*, 9(1), 13–24. https://doi.org/10.1002/jrsm.1254

Rogerson, M., Brown, D. K., Sandercock, G., Wooller, J.-J., & Barton, J. (2016). A comparison of four typical green exercise environments and prediction of psychological health outcomes. *Perspectives in Public Health*, 136(3), 171–180. https://doi.org/10.1177/1757913915589845

Schmuecker, K., & Earwaker, R. (2022, 29 June). *Not heating, eating or meeting bills: Managing a cost of living crisis on a low income.* Joseph Rowntree Foundation. https://www.jrf.org.uk/report/not-heating-eating-or-meeting-bills-managing-cost-living-crisis-low-income

Schoen, V., Caputo, S., & Blythe, C. (2020). Valuing physical and social output: A rapid assessment of a London community garden. *Sustainability (Switzerland)*, 12(13), 15452. https://doi.org/10.3390/su12135452

Sempik, J. (2010). Green care and mental health: Gardening and farming as health and social care. *Mental Health and Social Inclusion*, 14(3), 15–22. https://doi.org/10.5042/mhsi.2010.0440

Sewdas, R., de Wind, A., van der Zwaan, L. G. L., van der Borg, W. E., Steenbeek, R., van der Beek, A. J., & Boot, C. R. L. (2017). Why older workers work beyond the retirement age: A qualitative study. *BMC Public Health*, 17(1), 1–9. https://doi.org/10.1186/s12889-017-4675-z

Shakespeare, T., Ndagire, F., & Seketi, Q. E. (2021). Triple jeopardy: Disabled people and the COVID-19 pandemic. *The Lancet*, 397(10282), 1331–1333. https://doi.org/10.1016/S0140-6736(21)00625-5

Sharman, M. J., Nash, M., & Cleland, V. (2019). Health and broader community benefit of parkrun—an exploratory qualitative study. *Health Promotion Journal of Australia*, 30(2), 163–171. https://doi.org/10.1002/hpja.182

Sharp, C., Macleod, S., Bernardinelli, D., Skipp, A., & Higgins, S. (2015). *Supporting the attainment of disadvantaged pupils. Briefing for school leaders.* Department for Education. https://assets.publishing.service.gov.uk/government/uploads/system/uploads/attachment_data/file/473976/DFE-RS411_Supporting_the_attainment_of_disadvantaged_pupils_-_briefing_for_school_leaders.pdf

Simpson, R. J., Campbell, J. P., Gleeson, M., Krüger, K., Nieman, D. C., Pyne, D. B., Turner, J. E., & Walsh, N. P. (2020). Can exercise affect immune function to increase susceptibility to infection? *Exercise Immunology Review*, 26, 8–22. http://researchonl ine.ljmu.ac.uk/id/eprint/12547/

Skivington, K., Matthews, L., Simpson, S. A., Craig, P., Baird, J., Blazeby, J. M., Boyd, K. A., Craig, N., French, D. P., McIntosh, E., Petticrew, M., Rycroft-Malone, J., White, M., & Moore, L. (2021). A new framework for developing and evaluating complex interventions: Update of Medical Research Council guidance. *BMJ*, 374(2061). https://doi.org/10.1136/bmj.n2061

Smith, M. (2020). Delivering the goods: Executing sustainable transport policy through urban planning in Merseyside (2001–2010). *Planning Perspectives*, 36(3), 515–534. https://doi.org/10.1080/02665433.2020.1813620

Social Value Lab. (2011). *Social return on investment evaluation*. https://www.socialvaluelab. org.uk/wp-content/uploads/2013/05/CraftCafeSROI.pdf

Soga, M., Gaston, K. J., & Yamaura, Y. (2017). Gardening is beneficial for health: A meta-analysis. *Preventative Medicine Reports*, 5, 92–99. https://doi.org/10.1016/ j.pmedr.2016.11.007

Spencer, L. H., Lynch, M., Lawrence, C. L., & Edwards, R. T. (2020). A scoping review of how income affects accessing local green space to engage in outdoor physical activity to improve well-being: Implications for post COVID-19. *International Journal of Environmental Research and Public Health*, 17, 9313. https://doi.org/10.3390/ijerph17249313

Steptoe, A. (2019). Happiness and health. *Annual Review of Public Health*, 40, 339–359. https://doi.org/10.1146/annurev-publhealth-040218-044150

Stevinson, C., & Hickson, M. (2014). Exploring the public health potential of a mass community participation event. *Journal of Public Health (United Kingdom)*, 36(2), 268–274. https://doi.org/10.1093/pubmed/fdt082

Stevinson, C. Wiltshire, G., & Hickson, M. (2015). Facilitating participation in health-enhancing physical activity: A qualitative study of parkrun. *International Journal of Behavioral Medicine*, 22(2), 170–177. https://doi.org/10.1007/s12529-014-9431-5

Stride, A., Fitzgerald, H., Rankin-Wright, A., & Barnes, L. (2020). The en/gendering of volunteering: 'I've pretty much always noticed that the tail runner is always female'. *Sport Management Review*, 23(3), 498–508. https://doi.org/10.1016/j.smr.2019.05.006

Stuart, D. (2016). A chemsex crucible: The context and the controversy. *Journal of Family Planning and Reproductive Health Care*, 42(4), 295–296. https://doi.org/10.1136/jfprhc-2016-101603

Suleman, M., Sonthalia, S., Webb, C., Tinson, A., Kane, M., Bunbury, S., & Bibby, J. (2021). *Unequal pandemic, fairer recovery: The COVID-19 impact inquiry report*. The Health Foundation. https://www.health.org.uk/sites/default/files/upload/publications/ 2021/HEAJ8932-COVID-Impact-210705.pdf

Sustrans. (2021, 15 November). *The Cycle to Work scheme explained*. https://www.sustrans. org.uk/our-blog/get-active/2019/everyday-walking-and-cycling/the-cycle-to-work-sch eme-explained

Swinburn, B., & Egger, G. (2002). Preventive strategies against weight gain and obesity. *Obesity Reviews*, 3(4), 289–301. https://doi.org/10.1046/j.1467-789X.2002.00082.x

Swinburn, B., Kraak, V., Rutter, H., Vandevijvere, S., Lobstein, T., Sacks, G., Gomes, F., March, T., & Magnusson, R. (2015). Strengthening of accountability systems to create healthy food environments and reduce global obesity. *The Lancet*, **385**(9986), 2534–2545. https://doi.org/10.1016/S0140-6736(14)61747-5

Swinburn, B. A., Sacks, G., Hall, K. D., McPherson, K., Finegood, D. T., Moodie, M. L., & Gortmaker, S. L. (2011). The global obesity pandemic: Shaped by global drivers and local environments. *The Lancet*, **378**(9793), 804–814. https://doi.org/10.1016/S0140-6736(11)60813-1

The Health Foundation. (2017, 29 June). *Infographic: What makes us healthy?* https://www.health.org.uk/infographic/infographic-what-makes-us-healthy

The Open University. (2020). *The Open University Business Barometer. Navigating the skills landscape.* https://www5.open.ac.uk/business/sites/www.open.ac.uk.business/files/files/OUBB-Methodology.pdf

Thomas, K. H., Dalili, M. N., López-López, J. A., Keeney, E., Phillippo, D. M., Munafò, M. R., Stevenson, M., Caldwell, D. M., & Welton, N. J. (2021). Smoking cessation medicines and e-cigarettes: A systematic review, network meta-analysis and cost-effectiveness analysis. *Health Technology Assessment*, **25**(59), 1–224. https://doi.org/10.3310/hta25590

Thompson Coon, J., Boddy, K., Stein, K., Whear, R., Barton, J., & Depledge, M. H. (2011). Does participating in physical activity in outdoor natural environments have a greater effect on physical and mental wellbeing than physical activity indoors? A systematic review. *Environmental Science & Technology*, **45**(5), 1761–1772. https://doi.org/10.1021/es102947t

Tinson, A. (2020, 25 July). *Living in poverty was bad for your health long before COVID-19.* The Health Foundation. https://www.health.org.uk/publications/long-reads/living-in-poverty-was-bad-for-your-health-long-before-COVID-19

United Kingdom Government. (2018, 17 December). *Good work plan.* https://www.gov.uk/government/publications/good-work-plan/good-work-plan

United Kingdom Government. (2020). *Staying at home and away from others (social distancing).* https://assets.publishing.service.gov.uk/government/uploads/system/uploads/attachment_data/file/876279/Full_guidance_on_staying_at_home_and_a way_from_others__1_.pdf

United Kingdom Government. (2021a). *Working after state pension age.* https://www.gov.uk/working-retirement-pension-age

United Kingdom Government. (2021b). *From harm to hope: A 10-year drugs plan to cut crime and save lives.* https://assets.publishing.service.gov.uk/government/uploads/system/uploads/attachment_data/file/1079147/From_harm_to_hope_PDF.pdf

United Nations Climate Change Conference UK. (2021). *COP26 explained.* https://ukcop26.org/wp-content/uploads/2021/07/COP26-Explained.pdf

Valtorta, N. K., Kanaan, M., Gilbody, S., Ronzi, S., & Hanratty, B. (2016). Loneliness and social isolation as risk factors for coronary heart disease and stroke: Systematic review and meta-analysis of longitudinal observational studies. *Heart*, **102**(13), 1009–1016. http://dx.doi.org/10.1136/heartjnl-2015-308790

van Soest, D., Tight, M. R., & Rogers, C. D. F. (2020). Exploring the distances people walk to access public transport. *Transport Reviews*, **40**(2), 160–182. https://doi.org/10.1080/01441647.2019.1575491

van Tulleken, C. (2023). Ultra-processed people: *Why do we eat stuff that isn't food . . . and why can't we stop?* Cornerstone Press.

Vardakoulias, O. (2013). *The economic benefits of Ecominds: A case study approach.* NEF Consulting. https://www.mind.org.uk/media-a/4424/the-economic-benefits-of-ecominds-report.pdf

Waste and Resources Action Plan UK. (2019). *WRAP and the circular economy.* http://www.wrap.org.uk/about-us/about/wrap-and-circular-economy

Watson, I., MacKenzie, F., Woodfine, L., & Azam, S. (2019). *Making a difference. Housing and health: A case for investment. Executive summary.* Public Health Wales. https://phw.nhs.wales/files/housing-and-health-reports/a-case-for-investment-executive-summary/

Watt, W., Lawton, R., & Fujiwara, D. (2018). *Revaluing parks and green spaces: Measuring their economic and wellbeing value to individuals.* Fields in Trust. https://fieldsintrust.org/insights/revaluing-parks-and-green-spaces

Weatherly, H. L. A., Neves De Faria, R. I., Van den Berg, B., Sculpher, M. J., O'Neill, P., Nolan, K., Glanville, J., Isojarvi, J., Baragula, E., & Edwards, M. (2017). *Scoping review on social care economic evaluation methods* [Discussion paper]. CHE research paper. Centre for Health Economics, University of York, York. https://eprints.whiterose.ac.uk/135405/1/CHERP150_social_care_evaluation_methods.pdf

Welsh, J., Strazdins, L., Charlesworth, S., Kulik, C. T., & Butterworth, P. (2016). Health or harm? A cohort study of the importance of job quality in extended workforce participation by older adults. *BMC Public Health,* 16(1), 1–14. https://doi.org/10.1186/s12889-016-3478-y

White, M. P., Elliott, L. R., Grellier, J., Economou, T., Bell, S., Bratman, G. N., Cirach, M., Gascon, M., Lima, M. L., Lõhmus, M., Nieuwenhuijsen, M., Ojala, A., Roiko, A., Schultz, P. W., van den Bosch, M., & Fleming, L. E. (2021). Associations between green/blue spaces and mental health across 18 countries. *Scientific Reports,* 11(1), 1–12. https://doi.org/10.1038/s41598-021-87675-0

Williams, C. Y., Townson, A. T., Kapur, M., Ferreira, A. F., Nunn, R., Galante, J., Phillips, V., Gentry, S., & Usher-Smith, J. A. (2021). Interventions to reduce social isolation and loneliness during COVID-19 physical distancing measures: A rapid systematic review. *PLoS One,* 16(2), e0247139. https://doi.org/10.1371/journal.pone.0247139

Wiltshire, G., & Stevinson, C. (2018). Exploring the role of social capital in community-based physical activity: Qualitative insights from parkrun. *Qualitative Research in Sport, Exercise and Health,* 10(1), 47–62. https://doi.org/10.1080/2159676X.2017.1376347

Women's Royal Voluntary Service. (2012). *Loneliness amongst older people and the impact of family connections.* https://www.royalvoluntaryservice.org.uk/Uploads/Documents/How_we_help/loneliness-amongst-older-people-and-the-impact-of-family-connections.pdf

World Health Organization. (2006). *WHO air quality guidelines for particulate matter, ozone, nitrogen dioxide and sulfur dioxide. Global update 2005. Summary of risk assessment.* https://apps.who.int/iris/bitstream/handle/10665/69477/WHO_SDE_PHE_OEH_06.02_eng.pdf

World Health Organization. (2018). *WHO housing and health guidelines.* https://apps.who.int/iris/rest/bitstreams/1161792/retrieve

World Health Organization. (2020, 19 December). *Ambient (outdoor) air quality and health.* https://www.who.int/en/news-room/fact-sheets/detail/ambient-(outdoor)-air-quality-and-health

Younan, D., Tuvblad, C., Li, L., Wu, J., Lurmann, F., Franklin, M., Berhane, K., McConnell, R., Wu, A. H., Baker, L. A., & Chen, J. C. (2016). Environmental determinants of aggression in adolescents: Role of urban neighborhood greenspace. *Journal of the American Academy of Child and Adolescent Psychiatry*, **55**(7), 591–601. https://doi.org/10.1016/j.jaac.2016.05.002

Zapata-Diomedi, B., Gunn, L., Giles-Corti, B., Shiell, A., & Lennert Veerman, J. (2018). A method for the inclusion of physical activity-related health benefits in cost-benefit analysis of built environment initiatives. *Preventive Medicine*, **106**, 224–230. https://doi.org/10.1016/j.ypmed.2017.11.009

Chapter 3

Well-being in the Early Years and Childhood

Lucy Bryning, Bethany F. Anthony,
Nathan Bray, Huw Lloyd-Williams,
Joanna Charles, Lorna Tuersley,
Catherine L. Lawrence, and
Rhiannon T. Edwards

Introduction

In Chapter 2, we examined some of the key cross-cutting themes influencing well-being and well-becoming across the life-course. This current chapter focuses on the start of the life-course: the early years. A well-known proverb states that, 'We do not inherit the Earth from Our Ancestors; we borrow it from our children'. Investment that focuses on the critical window of the first few years of life is likely to provide the most efficient use of public resources, yielding returns over and above other forms of financial investment and investment at other points of the life-course. This chapter explores the economic case for investment in early childhood, helping to ensure that children are as healthy as possible and well-nourished, receive high-quality early-learning opportunities, and are nurtured and protected from harm. This chapter focuses on topics such as adverse childhood experiences (ACEs), maternal mental health, growing up in poverty, housing, preschool experience, early years vaccinations, dental health, and free school meals.

We define 'children' and particularly 'early years' as from birth to seven years of age, as used in reports by the World Health Organization's (WHO's) Commission on Social Determinants of Health (Irwin et al., 2007), Field (2010), Allen (2011a, 2011b), and Marmot and colleagues (2020, 2010). Understanding what supports healthy child development is crucial for protecting early childhood health and well-being, increasing life chances, and improving lifetime outcomes. A child's development and subsequent life chances are influenced by

Lucy Bryning, Bethany F. Anthony, Nathan Bray, Huw Lloyd-Williams, Joanna Charles, Lorna Tuersley, Catherine L. Lawrence, and Rhiannon T. Edwards, *Well-being in the Early Years and Childhood* In: *Health Economics of Well-being and Well-becoming across the Life-course*. Edited by: Rhiannon T. Edwards and Catherine L. Lawrence, Oxford University Press. © Oxford University Press 2024. DOI: 10.1093/9780191919336.003.0003 many factors before birth and throughout childhood, such as the child's environment and experience (Shonkoff & Phillips, 2000; Walker et al., 2011). Field (2010) brought together compelling evidence to show that the first five years of life are the most important for determining life chances. He identified key factors that affect life chances: healthy pregnancy, effective parenting, and access to high-quality childcare. His report argued that the United Kingdom (UK) Government should move funding into the early years, specifically targeting the most deprived children. Around the same time, Allen (2011a, 2011b) reported how intervention in children's earliest years can address or mitigate some of the damaging social problems later in life, which have a substantial cost associated with them. Although both reports focused on the age range from birth to five years, they acknowledged that early years programmes will not be effective in the long term unless they are followed up with high-quality, evidence-based programmes for older children and families who need them.

There is overwhelming evidence from neuroscience research of the impact of the early years environment and experience on a child's brain development (Miguel et al., 2019; Perry, 2002). Figure 3.1 illustrates abnormal brain development following sensory neglect in early childhood (Perry, 2002). The brain image on the left is from a healthy three-year-old child with an average head

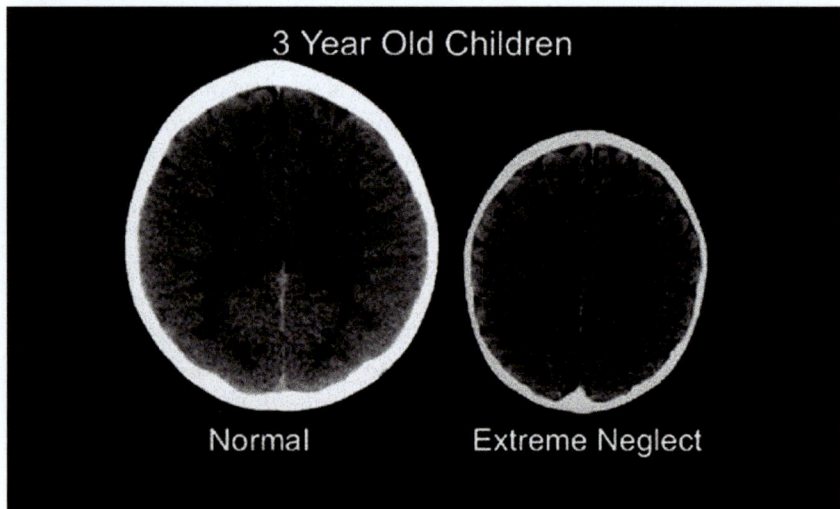

Figure 3.1 Abnormal brain development following sensory neglect in early childhood
Reproduced with permission from Perry, B. D. (2002). Childhood experience and the expression of genetic potential: What childhood neglect tells us about nature and nurture. *Brain and Mind*, 3(1), 79–100. Copyright © 2002 Kluwer Academic Publishers. Published by Springer Nature. All rights reserved.

size. The brain image on the right is from a series of three-year-old children following severe sensory-deprivation neglect in early childhood. The brain image on the right is much smaller than the healthy brain image (on the left) and shows abnormal development of the brain. Healthy brain development is crucial for ensuring that children acquire the social and emotional foundations necessary for learning in school, developing healthy relationships with family and friends, and being ready for the workplace.

The United Nations Children's Fund (UNICEF, 2007) identified six dimensions of child well-being:

1. Material well-being: the percentage of children living in relative income poverty, in households without jobs, and in reported deprivation (in terms of low family affluence, few educational resources, and fewer than ten books in the home).

2. Health and safety: health from birth to age one year (mortality and low birthweight), preventative health services (immunizations), and safety (deaths from accidents and injuries).

3. Educational well-being: school achievement at age fifteen (average achievement in reading and mathematical and science literacy), beyond basics (percentage of children staying in education at age fifteen to nineteen years), and transition to employment (percentage of children aged fifteen to nineteen years not in education, employment, or training (NEET), or expecting to find low-skilled work).

4. Family and peer relationships: family structure (percentage of children in single-parent families or stepfamilies), family relationships (percentage of children eating the main meal with parents more than once per week, percentage of children reporting parents spending time 'just talking' to them), and peer relationships (percentage of children reporting their peers as 'kind and helpful').

5. Behaviours and risks: health behaviours (percentage of children who eat breakfast/fruit daily; are physically active/overweight), risk behaviours (percentage of children who smoke/have been drunk/use cannabis/have sex by fifteen/use condoms and teenage fertility rate), and experience of violence (percentage of children involved in fighting and being bullied).

6. Subjective well-being: health (percentage of children rating their health as 'fair' or 'poor'), school life (percentage of children 'liking school a lot'), and personal well-being (percentage of children rating themselves above the mid-point of a Life Satisfaction Scale and percentage of children reporting negatively about personal well-being).

Measurement Challenges in the Well-being of the Early Years and Childhood

For the health economist, one of the challenges of objectively evaluating interventions, programmes, and policies to promote well-being in the early years is the difficulty in undertaking randomized controlled trials (RCTs) in the community. Another challenge involves isolating the impact or outcomes of one specific intervention in a defined neighbourhood or geographical area when there may be a number of interventions, programmes, or policies in place or initiated during the study period stage, with similar aims to promote well-being in the early years. Health economists have welcomed guidance from the Medical Research Council (MRC) on how to develop and evaluate 'complex interventions', influencing how we identify, measure, and value costs and outcomes (Craig et al., 2008). The update to this guidance pays more attention to roll-out and implementation of complex interventions (Skivington et al., 2021). A key publication in this area is a framework for economic evaluation alongside 'natural experiments' (Deidda et al., 2019). Relevant to this question of the evaluation of large-scale programmes and policies, Carter (2019, p. 721) argued that, 'Projects are ubiquitous throughout the management of public services and the implementation of public policy but implementation processes often remain a "black box"'. This may explain to some extent why, for example, economic evaluation of longer-term follow-up of the Sure Start programme (see Box 3.1) has provided ambiguous findings compounded by programmes varying in implementation, style, intensity, and reach (Carter, 2019).

Where an RCT is possible, another challenge for health economists is the choice of a meaningful outcome measure, often determined by the design of the trial, power calculation, and the age of child participants. For example, in a trial of the Incredible Years Parenting Programme for children at risk of developing conduct disorder, the main outcome measure was the incremental cost per unit of improvement on the intensity score of the Eyberg Child Behaviour Inventory (Eyberg & Ross, 1978). Though this was a logical decision given the nature of the programme and the research in the field of the early years, there was no payer threshold with which to compare the estimated cost of £73 per 1 point improvement on the Eyberg Child Behaviour Inventory (Edwards et al., 2007; Hutchings et al., 2007). The Child Health Utility 9 Dimension (CHU-9D) is a paediatric generic preference-based measure of health-related quality of life suitable for children aged seven to seventeen years. The estimation of preference weights allows for calculation of quality-adjusted life years (QALYs) for use in economic evaluation of paediatric health care interventions (Stevens, 2012).

Maternal Mental Health

Maternal mental health problems can have lifelong implications for both parents and the child (Verbeke et al., 2022). It is estimated that 10 per cent of pregnant women and 13 per cent of postnatal women experience a mental health disorder globally (WHO, 2023). In the UK, the National Institute for Health and Care Excellence (NICE, 2020) guidelines consider the following disorders most relevant for antenatal and postnatal mental health: anxiety, depression, psychosis, bipolar disorder, schizophrenia, eating disorders, drug-use disorders, alcohol-use disorders, and post-traumatic stress disorder (PTSD) following traumatic birth experiences. A systematic review investigating the cost-effectiveness evidence on interventions addressing maternal mental health conditions during and after pregnancy found that relatively few studies have been conducted in this area (Verbeke et al., 2022). The majority of studies were found to be cost-effective which highlights a need for further research to consider the long-term effectiveness and cost-effectiveness of interventions to address methodological challenges related to measuring health outcomes for both parents and the child (Verbeke et al., 2022).

Growing Up in Poverty

In 2021, there were 2.92 million children (aged zero to nineteen years) living in families in relative low income and 2.37 million children (aged zero to nineteen years) in absolute low income in the UK (Department for Work & Pensions, 2022). Relative low income refers to people living in households with income below 60 per cent of the current median income. Absolute low income refers to people living in households with income below 60 per cent of the median income in 2010/2011, adjusted for inflation (UK Parliament, 2023). Prior to the coronavirus disease 2019 (COVID-19) pandemic, nearly a third of children in the UK were growing up and living in poverty (Joseph Rowntree Foundation, 2020). At the extreme, children affected by ACEs face a lifetime trajectory of poverty, ill-health, and intergenerational consequences (Bellis et al., 2015a). As introduced in Chapter 1, ACEs can lead to an elevated risk of experiencing negative health outcomes across the life-course and represent a great cost to society, including public sector services (see Figure 3.2; Bellis et al., 2015a, 2015b).

Children growing up in poorer families are more likely to have poorer physical and mental health outcomes, be less likely to reach development and skills milestones in the early years, have lower educational attainment, and eventually be less likely to be in education, employment, or training between ages sixteen and twenty-four (Pillas et al., 2014; Sidebotham et al., 2014; Wickham et al., 2016). Intergenerationally, children growing up in poorer families are more

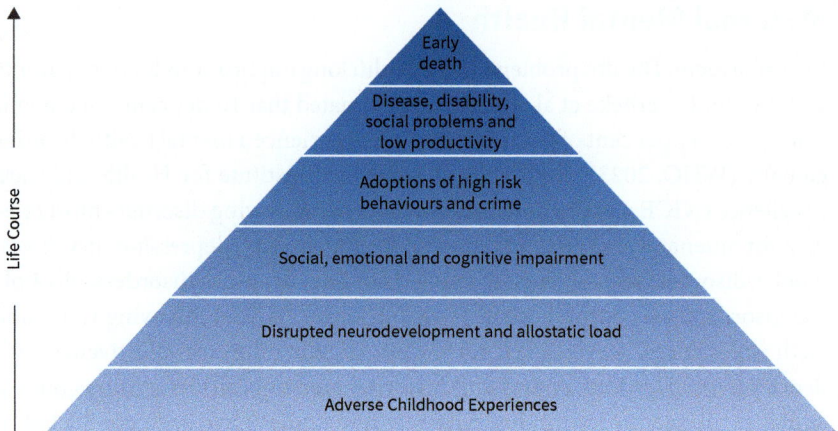

Figure 3.2 Model of ACE impacts across the life-course
Reproduced from Bellis, M. A., Ashton, K., Hughes, K., Ford, K., Bishop, J., & Paranjothy, S. (2015a). *Adverse childhood experiences and their impact on health-harming behaviours in the Welsh adult population*. Public Health Wales. https://www.ljmu.ac.uk/~/media/phi-reports/pdf/2016_01_ adverse_childhood_experiences_and_their_impact_on_health_harming_behaviours_in_the.pdf. Acknowledgment to Public Health Wales NHS Trust. Licence: Creative Commons BY 3.0 IGO.

likely to be living in poverty or unemployed in adulthood and have children who will also be living in poverty (Griggs & Walker, 2008). Work is recognized as one of the main routes out of poverty. There is an economic argument for a continued commitment to the economic regeneration of employment opportunities for the poorest communities across the UK, reducing the number of economically inactive families, some of whom claim long-term sickness benefits intergenerationally as the main source of household income. Transforming young lives and helping children reach their full potential has many wider economic benefits, including improving health and well-being, increasing educational attainment, lifetime earnings and economic productivity, reducing inequalities, and generating substantial savings to the National Health Service (NHS), social care, and social security system.

Pre-pandemic and Pre-cost of Living Crisis—Shifting the Curve

The UK had a significant policy direction and investment in programmes and practice relating to the early years, but this pales into insignificance when compared with what is spent on end of life care when taking a life-course perspective, as shown in Chapter 1, Figure 1.7. In times of mounting austerity it becomes more challenging to argue for investment in childhood, which helps

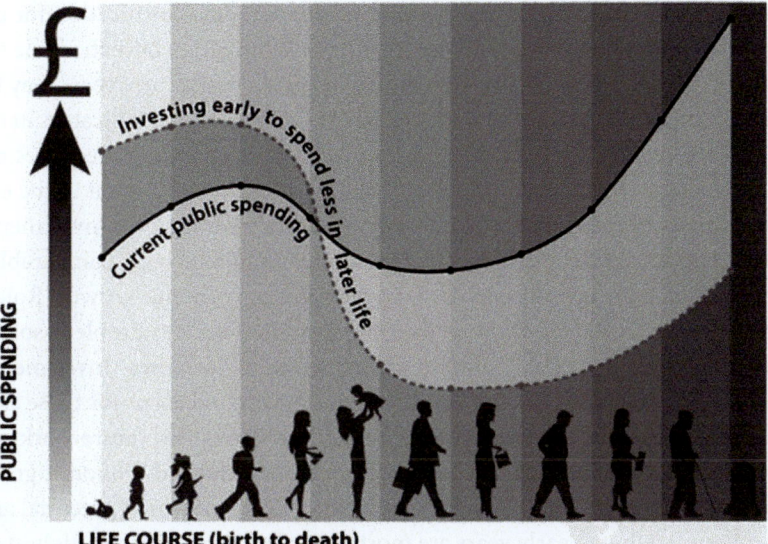

Figure 3.3 Shifting the curve towards prevention and early years investment
Reproduced from Edwards, R. T., Bryning, L., & Lloyd-Williams, H. (2016). *Transforming young lives across Wales: The economic argument for investing in early years.* Centre for Health Economics and Medicines Evaluation, Bangor University. https://cheme.bangor.ac.uk/documents/transforming-young-lives/CHEME%20transforming%20Young%20Lives%20Full%20Report%20Eng%20WEB%202.pdf

shift the curve towards prevention and earlier intervention; but taking a longer-term view, there is a need to shift this curve (see Figure 3.3).

Efficiency and Equity Arguments for Investing in the Early Years

Investing in the early years offers many potential benefits to society and a country's economy. The Organisation for Economic Co-operation and Development (OECD) argues that investing in the early years can provide significant short, medium, and long-term economic returns (OECD, 2011). This investment supports employment opportunities for women and helps educate children, which may interrupt the intergenerational poverty cycle (OECD, 2011; Price Waterhouse Coopers, 2016). From an economist's perspective, there is an efficiency argument for public policy on the early years to redress existing market failures. Societal welfare is lower where there is market failure, that is, resources are not used in their most valued use. Parents, who make decisions on behalf of young children, may not have adequate information upon which to base decisions about, for example, benefits of early preschool childcare

(Suhrcke & Kenkel, 2015). There is also an equity-based justification for governments investing in the early years to allow all children to have the same start in life regardless of family circumstances. Investing in the early years may be a way of reducing disparities in a wide range of socioeconomic indicators in later life across the social gradient—going some way to redressing inequities over the life-course (Suhrcke & Kenkel, 2015). Importantly, investment in the early years can be considered in the same way as European or national investment in wider economic development, as the internal rates of return are comparable or greater than many investments made in the name of economic growth (Rolnick & Grunewald, 2003). In developed economies, skills such as problem-solving, communication, and collaboration are valued in a workforce. Investment in the early years, which aids the development of the foundations for these skills, can lead to better educational attainment and a more skilled future workforce. This investment can contribute to building social capital and economic growth (Karoly & Bigelow, 2005). There is a need to understand which potential areas for investment in the early years are most cost-effective or have the highest rate of return, and a substantial body of evidence developed over the last twenty-five years can help guide a case for early childhood interventions as being an instrument for social change (Suhrcke & Kenkel, 2015).

The Need for Cultural Awareness in Early Years Programmes

Cultural sensitivity is important to consider when designing and implementing early years programmes that aim to improve child well-being. Conti and Heckman (2012) argued that the goal of early childhood programmes is to create a base of productive skills and traits for disadvantaged children from all social, ethnic, and religious groups. This called for 'a move from a policy of redistribution to one of pre-distribution of resources' (Conti & Heckman, 2012, p. 48).

Evidence of Intergenerational Benefits from Early Years Programmes

The Perry Preschool Project was a randomized study developed by American psychologist David Weikart, conducted in the early 1960s, to track the impact of high-quality early childhood education on disadvantaged African-American children from low-income families living in Ypsilanti, Michigan, United States (US). Families were randomly assigned to either the intervention group or the control group. Over a two-year period, children aged between three and four years in the intervention group worked on projects where they planned, exe-cuted, and reviewed tasks collectively in the school classroom and received home visits by teachers to help improve parent-child interactions (Schweinhart et al., 2005). The children were systematically followed through to age forty, with information collected on education, employment, earnings, crime, as well as other outcomes. A number of studies have reported on the rate of return of the intervention. For example, Rolnick and Grunewald (2003) reported a rate of return of 16 per cent to the Perry Preschool Project, and Belfield and col-leagues (2006) reported a 17 per cent rate of return. Heckman and colleagues (2010) estimated that the Perry Preschool Project saved society between $7 and $12 for every $1 invested, mostly due to reduced crime.

In the Perry Preschool Project involving children and siblings of the original participants, the children of participants receiving the intervention had fewer school suspensions, higher levels of education and employment, and lower levels of participation in crime compared with the children of participants in the control condition. The original Perry study has been criticized for having a relatively small sample size and for aspects of the randomization; however, it remains one of the longest follow-up and most influential studies on breaking the cycle of intergenerational poverty (Heckman, 2019). Conti and Heckman (2012) found the impacts were especially pronounced for the children of male participants. These treatment effects were associated with improved childhood home environments. The intergenerational effects arose despite families in the intervention group living in similar or poorer neighbourhoods than the control families. Conti and Heckman also found substantial positive effects of the Perry programme on the siblings of participants who did not directly participate in the program, especially for male siblings.

Methodological Considerations in Economic Evaluation of Childhood Interventions and Policy

Early years interventions can be seen from two distinct but related view-points: 'universal' or 'targeted'. Universal programmes or interventions are aimed at the whole population, while for targeted programmes, the aim is to reduce the inequalities in health by focusing on high-risk disadvantaged groups within the population. Substantial methodological challenges face those under-taking economic evaluations (particularly cost-benefit analysis (CBA) and return on investment (ROI)) of early child development programmes. For ex-ample, a long follow-up period is desirable, the need to discount costs and out-comes at an appropriate discount rate, and differing methods for monetizing benefits with no market price (Karoly & Bigelow, 2005). The evaluation of some early childhood development programmes has been particularly challenging as a result of several components and goals, which we would now define as 'complex interventions' (Skivington et al., 2021; Craig et al., 2008; Karoly & Bigelow, 2005). For example, some early childhood development programmes target high-risk preschool children and have multidisciplinary input from various sectors, including education, health, and social care services. Investing in the early years and child development can mean investing in a range of groups, such as babies and young children directly, women with the potential to become pregnant or who are pregnant, parents and families as a whole, and their wider communities.

Building on the argument above, there is a general need to record spill-over effects in the economic evaluation of public health interventions in the UK (Weatherly et al., 2009). Such positive or negative spill-over effects might relate to younger siblings, parents, offspring (in an intergenerational context), and communities (Karoly & Bigelow, 2005). Investment can be through a range of different one-to-one or group programmes, through multidisciplinary, collaborative practice, developing communities and their assets and changing environments. Investment can be on a universal or targeted basis. Marmot and colleagues (2010) advocated the concept of 'proportionate universalism' whereby actions are universal but with a scale and intensity that reflects, and is proportionate to, the level of disadvantage. Economic returns to investment may well likely be much larger from targeted programmes aimed at the most disadvantaged children and families at high risk (Heckman, 2013; Hutchings et al., 2013; Suhrcke & Kenkel, 2015). Understanding the risk factors, the protective factors, and the factors that promote thriving through life can help determine an appropriate mix of universal programmes for all babies, children, and families, and targeted programmes for families most at risk (Walker et al., 2011).

Evidence of the cost-effectiveness and/or the ROI of early years interventions from one setting may not apply to another. It is difficult to compare the findings of different evaluative studies of the effectiveness of early childhood development programmes, which can vary considerably. Results from targeted programmes cannot be assumed to be transferrable across to universal programmes. In general, there has been a view that more resource-intensive programmes, that is, one-to-one or small groups that adhere with fidelity and are delivered by appropriately trained practitioners tend to be most effective. However, these programmes are delivered at a higher cost than interventions to larger groups of children or families (Karoly & Bigelow, 2005). This is where the need for evidence of the relative cost-effectiveness or value for money is especially relevant. Problems of implementation and translation from one setting to another have been put forward as reasons why programmes seen to be effective in one setting have not proved as effective or cost-effective in large trials in subsequent settings (Suhrcke & Kenkel, 2015).

Most of the evidence of the effectiveness and potential economic returns from investing in early child development has originated from the US, for example, the evaluation of targeted programmes including the Nurse-Family Partnership (Olds et al., 2010), Headstart (Vinovskis, 2005), and the Perry Preschool Project (Schweinhart et al., 2005). Box 3.1 describes the UK-based Sure Start programme of early intervention for children aged up to four years (Cattan et al., 2019, 2021). These early years programmes have been adopted in

Box 3.1 Case study: The Sure Start programme

Sure Start is a programme of early intervention for children aged up to four years. It experienced a rapid roll-out following its launch in 1999 by the UK Government, driven by local partnerships of voluntary groups, parents, and local authorities in some of the most disadvantaged areas of the country. Sure Start projects deliver a wide range of services designed to support children's learning skills, health, and well-being, as well as social and emotional development. In 2004, the 10-Year Strategy for Children called for a children's centre in every community, changing the initiative into a universal service, and at its peak in 2009/2010, Sure Start accounted for £1.8 billion of public spending, a third of overall spending on programmes for children under five years. Since then, following a decade of austerity, funding cuts, and centre closures have meant that funding fell by two-thirds to £600 million in 2017/2018. The services offered by Sure Start vary across the county and over time (Cattan et al., 2019). Interestingly, expansions and cuts to the Sure Start programme and the reshaping of the UK Early Years policy landscape have occurred with a limited evidence base (Cattan et al., 2019). Indeed, the decision to universalize Sure Start Local Programmes occurred before the first impact report by the National Evaluation of Sure Start was published.

In the Evaluation of Children's Centres in England (ECCE) report published in 2016, looking at the overall value for money of children's centre services, most of the value of the benefits derived from improved later labour market outcomes for the children in the families using the services (Gaheer & Paull, 2016). Baby health and parental support services were estimated to provide financial benefits on a per person basis (£2,236 and £5,395, respectively). However, after costs to the state of providing services was taken into account, it was estimated that most services provided a net loss to the UK Government. Some parenting services did provide a net benefit to the UK Government because they were cheaper to provide than baby health services (Bate & Foster, 2017).

The Institute for Fiscal Studies assessed how the Sure Start programme affected children and families, particularly relating to children's hospitalizations (Cattan et al., 2021). For example, at age one, having access to an extra Sure Start centre per 1,000 children under five years increased the probability of hospitalization in the neighbourhood cohort by 10 per cent (i.e. 6,700 additional hospitalizations a year), as families are offered more support to health services, and children are exposed to a variety of infectious diseases. However, at age five, an additional Sure Start centre per 1,000 children prevented around 2,900 hospitalizations a year. For eleven to fifteen-year-olds, over 13,150 hospitalizations were prevented each year due to children developing stronger immune systems, better disease management, safer home environments, and fewer behavioural difficulties (Cattan et al., 2021). The reduction in hospitalizations at age five to eleven years as a result of Sure Start saved the NHS around £5 million per cohort, which is equivalent to 0.4 per cent on average annual spending on Sure Start (Cattan et al., 2019). The programme had significantly larger impacts on boys than on girls across most ages. The programme also had larger benefits for children in deprived areas, at least from age nine onwards. This suggests that a model incorporating universal services with an area-based focus on disadvantaged neighbourhoods can be a promising approach to early years interventions (Cattan et al., 2021). The financial benefits from reducing hospitalizations offset approximately 31 per cent of the cost of Sure Start provision. Cattan and colleagues (2021) believed this figure is likely to underestimate the benefits of Sure Start since the programme may have impacted on other outcomes beyond hospitalizations. Sure Start affects children's health through direct and indirect pathways, such as providing health-related information, improved maternal mental health, and safer parenting practices.

several developed countries, namely Australia, Canada, and France. Evidence of costs and benefits of a range of early years programmes report returns of between $1 and $17 for every $1 invested (Aos et al., 2004; Karoly & Bigelow, 2005; Watson & Tully, 2008). Studies that took a longer time horizon or had a longer follow-up period had a greater ROI or benefit-cost ratio (BCR), as they could consider benefits that occurred later in life (Karoly & Bigelow, 2005). It is difficult to transfer the findings of studies from the US and elsewhere to a UK setting. For example, juvenile detention rates have decreased significantly in recent years in the UK through the use of alternative programmes such as community service, so the rates from the US, with associated savings, are not necessarily applicable to the UK (Penn & Thomas, 2005; Youth Justice Board & Ministry of Justice, 2019, 2020).

The Economic Evidence for Investing in the Early Years and Childhood

The World Bank (2020) highlighted three priority societal objectives to ensure children reach their full potential:

1. Children are as healthy as possible and well-nourished (particularly in the critical window of the first 1,000 days). There is a strong economic case for investing in family planning and pregnancy care, supporting breastfeeding, childhood vaccinations, free school meals, and childhood obesity prevention, with many considered 'best buys' in public health.

2. Children receive good quality early learning opportunities: the ROI of good quality early childhood development is well acknowledged, with learning through play essential in the early years. Good quality childcare and education have many wider economic benefits supporting parents to continue participating in the UK workforce (which was difficult and has changed since the COVID-19 pandemic nationwide lockdowns).

3. Children are nurtured and protected from harm. Cost-effective parenting programmes, preventing childhood accidents, and protection from ACEs can be effective and cost-effective for preventing poor mental and physical health and longer-term adverse economic outcomes.

In the first few months following birth, adequate nutrition is vital to physical and intellectual development. International efforts to reduce malnutrition in developing countries, through the first 1,000 days campaign, have begun to concentrate resources on women during pregnancy and for babies up to the age of two years. It is estimated that every $1 spent on improving nutrition can have as much as a $138 ROI (Hoddinott et al., 2012). In the UK, our focus may not primarily be on nutrition, as it is in aid programmes to low and middle-income countries, but rather on establishing healthy lifestyle choices and reducing the impact of poverty and inequality. This was the case certainly before the COVID-19 pandemic and cost of living crisis, but is more and more the case now too.

Pregnancy

The foundations for thriving are laid down long before birth, with a critical time for investment in pre-conception and early pregnancy. The physical, mental, and emotional health of women while pregnant and in an infant's early years will have a lifelong effect on a child's life chances (Marmot et al., 2010). Promoting good maternal health is crucial in order to provide babies with the best start in life. For example, during pregnancy, factors such as maternal smoking, stress, diet, and alcohol or drug misuse can significantly impact the child's development (Newman, 2002; Nykjaer et al., 2014; Polańska et al., 2015). Concerning maternal nutrition, the universal provision of vitamin supplements is a cost-effective way of promoting good maternal health and healthy pregnancies and child outcomes (NICE, 2015a; Filby et al., 2015).

Until recently there has been a long-term downward trend of teenage pregnancies in the UK. In 2018, conception rates for under eighteen-year-olds in England and Wales declined by 6.1 per cent to 16.8 conceptions per 1,000 women aged fifteen to seventeen years. From 1999 to 2018, conception rates for women under eighteen years have decreased by 62.7 per cent (ONS, 2020). However, in 2021, the number of conceptions for women aged under eighteen years had a small increase from 12,576 in 2020 to 13,131 (ONS, 2023a). Teenagers who have a baby are at a greater risk of social exclusion and poverty because they are less likely to have a good education and well-paid employment (Lyons & Ashton, 2004). They are therefore more likely to suffer poverty and ill health throughout their lives. There is evidence that interventions aimed at promoting planned pregnancy or reducing unwanted teenage pregnancy have a positive ROI. For example, the ROI of a publicly funded family planning programme in the US was found to be $7.09 for every $1 invested (Frost et al., 2014). These family planning programmes, as well as reducing unintended pregnancy, can also help prevent cervical cancer, human immunodeficiency virus (HIV), and other sexually transmitted diseases. In 2010, these government programmes were estimated to have had the effect of avoiding 2.2 million unplanned pregnancies. Evidence from England suggests that for every £1 invested in publicly funded contraception would return £4.64 in savings across the public sector over five years, and £9 per invested £1 over ten years (Public Health England, 2018a). Planned pregnancy significantly affects the life-course with a higher likelihood of positive outcomes for parent and child (Lyons & Ashton, 2004).

Low Birth Weight

Babies born with a low birth weight (under 2,500 grams) are at an increased risk of infant mortality, developmental problems in childhood, and poorer health in later life. Low birth weight affects 6.4 per cent of all UK births (Nuffield Trust, 2023). Babies are often born with a low birth weight because they are preterm births (born before thirty-seven weeks of pregnancy). The risk of low birth weight is related to: smoking while pregnant; substance and alcohol misuse; pregnancy health and nutrition; pregnancy-related complications, and a mother's young age (Nuffield Trust, 2023). Delivery of low birth weight babies entails high direct neonatal treatment costs (Godfrey et al., 2010). Removing exposure to modifiable risk factors and concomitant reduction in low birth weight could prevent 24,000 low birth weight births costing the UK NHS £49 million (Johnson et al., 2016). Low birth weight babies have poorer short and long-term outcomes, such as adverse health consequences, lower educational attainment, and lower lifetime earning outcomes (Currie, 2009; Currie & Moretti, 2007; Jefferis et al., 2002). Stopping smoking is an effective strategy for preventing low birth weight and neonatal mortality (Public Health England, 2015). Chapters 4 and 5 of this book discuss the economic evidence on smoking prevention and cessation programmes both for adolescents and later in the workplace.

Breastfeeding

Breast milk contains essential nutrients, antibodies, hormones, and anti-oxidants that can improve the immune system of the infant (UNICEF, 2021; Victora et al., 2016). A UNICEF UK report proposed that a mid-level policy scenario to increase exclusive breastfeeding rates from 7 per cent to 45 per cent at four months could result in £3.63 million in savings every year due to the reduced prevalence of gastro-intestinal infections in breastfed babies (Renfrew et al., 2012). These savings rise to £17.18 million when considering the savings from avoiding treatment costs from a further three acute diseases in infants (specifically respiratory tract infection, acute otitis media, and necrotizing enterocolitis). Supporting mothers in the UK to continue to exclusively breastfeed up to four months would reduce the incidence of three childhood infectious conditions and save £11 million per annum (Pokhrel et al., 2015).

A systematic search and narrative literature review of economic evaluations of strategies to support or promote breastfeeding found limited published evidence of the cost-effectiveness of strategies to promote breastfeeding (Camacho & Hussain, 2020). Two studies reported that breastfeeding promotion for low birth weight babies in critical care was associated with lower costs and greater health benefits compared with usual care, and likely to be cost-effective. Peer-support for breastfeeding was associated with longer duration of exclusive breastfeeding with costs ranging from £19 to £107 per additional month (Camacho & Hussain, 2020). In a cohort of 313,817 first-time mothers, if 50

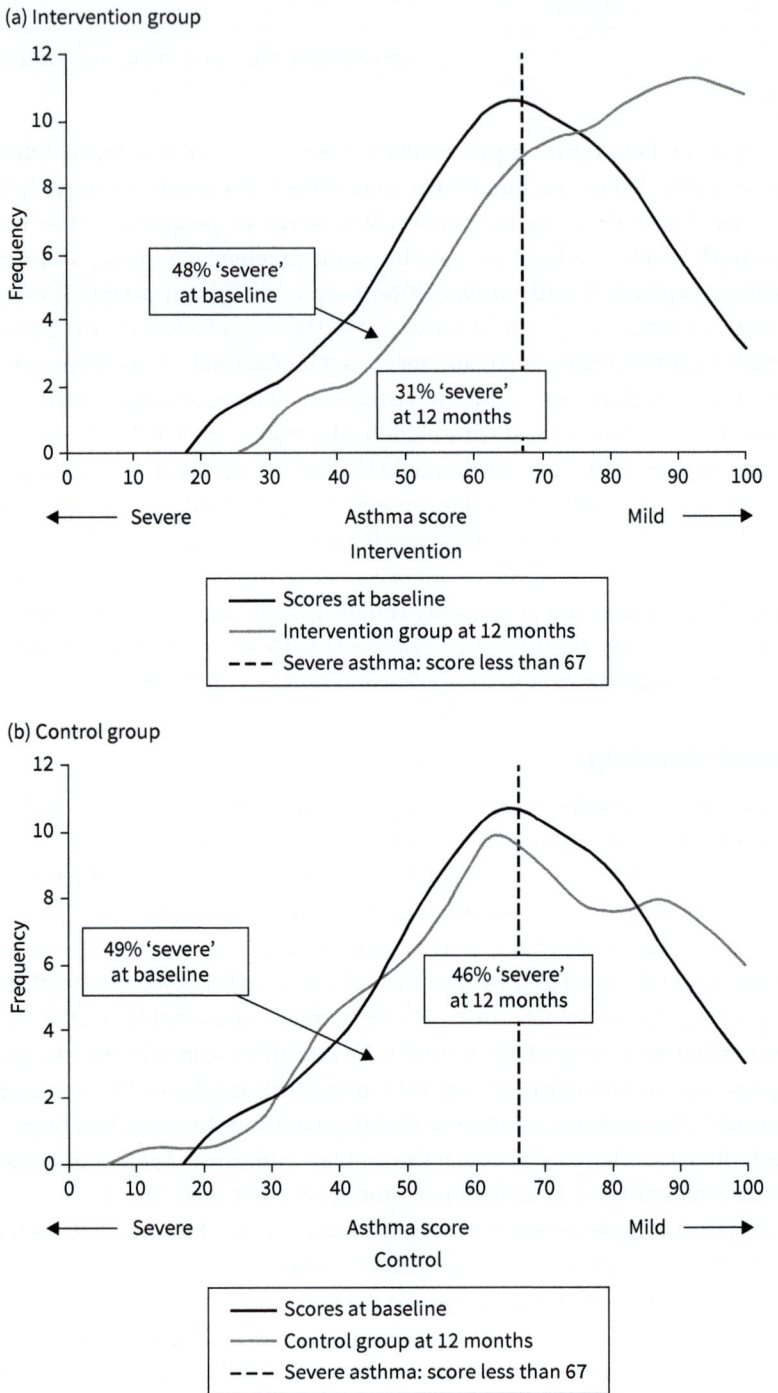

Figure 3.4 Changes in the distribution of asthma scores from baseline to twelve months. All distribution curves are smoothed. Baseline distributions are very similar in the two groups, and the baseline median of both intervention and control groups is 67 (although the proportions are marginally different, as a few scored exactly 67), so the same baseline curve is used in both graphs. From: Edwards, R. T., Neal, R. D., Linck, P., Bruce, N., Mullock, L., Nelhans, N., Pasterfield, D., Russell, D., Russell, I., & Woodfine, L. (2011). Enhancing ventilation in homes of children with asthma: Cost-effectiveness study alongside randomised controlled trial. *British Journal of General Practice*, 61(592), e733–e741. https://doi.org/10.3399/bjgp11X606645

per cent of those who were not currently breastfeeding had been supported to breastfeed for six months across their lifetime, this would result in a total of 371 QALYs gained from a decreased incidence of breast cancer (Pokhrel et al., 2015). Children who were not breastfed were significantly less likely to breast-feed their own babies in later life (Renfrew et al., 2012). Changing social norms through evidence-based interventions that increase rates of breastfeeding may help break this intergenerational cycle.

Housing

Where we grow up can have a significant impact on our life chances. Children who live in more cohesive neighbourhoods, who have stronger family units, and attend better schools tend to maintain a higher economic status later in life (Alexander et al., 2014). As discussed in Chapter 2 of this book, poor housing conditions increase the likelihood of disability and ill-health by up to 25 per cent during childhood and early adulthood (Harker, 2006). Poor housing can place substantial costs on the NHS due to cold, damp homes increasing the risk of cardiovascular, respiratory, and rheumatoid conditions. If the most se-vere hazards were removed from housing in Wales, there would be benefits to the NHS of £95 million a year in saved treatment costs (Nicol et al., 2019). The cost to society of leaving people living in poor housing in Wales is £1 billion a year (Nichol et al., 2019). There are currently few examples of RCTs of housing modification to improve health. The Children's health in asthma: Research to improve status through modifying accommodation (CHARISMA) study, a pragmatic RCT of housing modifications for families of children with moderate and severe asthma ($n = 177$) was undertaken in Wrexham, North Wales. The economic analysis reported that heating and ventilation modifications led to a 14 per cent shift of children from 'severe' to 'moderate' asthma for a total pro-gramme cost of £151,152 to Wrexham Borough Council (Edwards et al., 2011; Woodfine et al., 2011). Figure 3.4 shows that tailored heating and ventilation housing modifications led to a 17 per cent shift of children in the intervention group from 'severe' to 'moderate' asthma, compared with a 3 per cent shift for the control group, at a mean cost of £1,718 per child treated or £12,300 per child shifted from 'severe' to 'moderate' asthma (Edwards et al., 2011).

Preschool Experience

A good preschool experience can lead to better job prospects and higher in-come levels in later life (Paes de Barros & Mendonca, 1999; Goodman & Sianesi, 2005). Children from low socioeconomic backgrounds are more likely to succeed if they receive high-quality preschool education (Melhuish, 2004;

Sylva et al., 2004). Most evidence seems to come from the US, where follow-up studies suggest that every $1 investment in preschool programmes can yield up to $16 in return in adulthood (Schweinhart et al., 2005). *Sesame Street* is an American educational children's television programme that includes puppetry, animation, and sketch comedy. It was first premiered in 1969 and is now shown in more than 150 countries around the world. The aim of this early childhood intervention was to reduce educational deficits experienced by disadvantaged children based on differences in their preschool environment (see Box 3.2; Kearney & Levine, 2019).

Box 3.2 Case study: Sesame Street educational television

Sesame Street is a long-running educational television programme for children which is shown in more than 150 countries around the world. Kearney and Levine (2015) reported that the cost of producing the show in the US was $1 million per show, at a cost of $5 per child. There have been numerous academic studies evaluating the effect of Sesame Street on educational attainment, particularly literacy and numeracy, and school readiness in the early years (Kearney & Levine, 2015; Mares & Pan, 2013; Wright et al., 2001). This produces comparable outcomes to other effective programmes, such as Head Start, but delivered at a fraction of the cost (Kearney & Levine, 2015). Kearney and Levine examined the effects of exposure to Sesame Street on indicators of early school performance, ultimate educational attainment, and labour market outcomes at a cost of around $5 per child per year. They found that children who experienced their preschool years in areas when Sesame Street had the greatest broadcast coverage benefitted the most. This positive outcome was particularly prevalent for boys and Black, non-Hispanic children, and children who grew up in countries with greater economic disadvantage (Kearney & Levine, 2015).

A rapid evidence review of the accessibility and cost-effectiveness of educational television was undertaken during the COVID-19 pandemic (Watson & McIntyre, 2020). The review found that educational television supports academic outcomes in low-income contexts; supports the development of prosocial skills such as sharing, cooperation, and conflict resolution; and promotes positive attitudes towards those with medical conditions. Cost-effectiveness evidence has focused on the role of educational television in low and middle-income countries (Watson et al., 2021).

In the UK, early years education is generally provided to all three and four-year-olds and some eligible two-year-olds. The main aims of early years education are to provide high-quality stimulating learning and improve children's outcomes, helping to close the poverty-related attainment gap; to ensure that children develop well by improving the health and well-being of both child and parent, and to support parents into work, study, or training. There are some differences in how education provision is offered across the UK. The statutory duty lies with local authorities to provide nursery education from the age of three onwards, and at least ten hours a week for thirty-eight weeks is provided by the state. The actual number of hours varies between local authorities. The cost to local authorities in Wales for disadvantaged children enrolled in Flying Start Initiatives was found to be £11.32 per hour (National Assembly for Wales, 2014). From September 2022, Welsh Government is investing £26 million to expand Flying Start to deliver funded part-time childcare to more two-year-olds during 2023/2024 and 2024/2025. The initiative also includes support packages to enhance parenting skills in supporting child development, care, and well-being (Welsh Government, 2022). In England, all three and four-year-olds, and eligible disadvantaged two-year-olds, are entitled to 570 hours of government-funded education and childcare (UK Government, 2022a). These hours are usually taken as fifteen hours a week over thirty-eight weeks of the year. Children with eligible working parents are entitled to an additional 570 hours, typically taken as thirty hours a week over thirty-eight weeks of the year. The hourly funding rate is £4.88 for three to four-year-olds and £5.56 for two-year-olds (Education & Skills Funding Agency, 2021). In Scotland, funded early learning and childcare is available to all three to four-year-olds and eligible two-year-olds. From August 2021, the entitlement increased to 1,140 hours a year (thirty hours a week during term-time). The Scottish Government (2022) has increased investment by £567 million by 2021/2022. In Northern Ireland, Sure Start Services support parents with children aged under four years old living in disadvantaged areas. In 2020/2021, there were 37,376 children aged up to three years registered on one of thirty-eight Sure Start projects across Northern Ireland (Department of Education, 2021).

Early Years Vaccinations

In this section on vaccinations, we begin our focus on routine vaccinations prior to the COVID-19 pandemic. Vaccinations in the early years significantly reduce disease, disability, death, and inequity worldwide (Andre et al., 2008). Compared with other common public health interventions, vaccinations are considered a good investment and are generally highly cost-effective (Chabot et al., 2004; Public Health England, 2018a). However, with the rapid expansion of available vaccines in recent years the costs to governments and other payers for vaccines, and the associated delivery programmes, have been increasing as recommended schedules have become increasingly multifaceted (Atchison & Hassounah, 2015; Crocker-Buque et al., 2019). Evidence from the US showed that for every $1 invested in the measles, mumps, and rubella (MMR; German measles) vaccine, there was $26 in benefits to society (Zhou et al., 2004).

In the UK, though not a current practice, it has been estimated that the childhood flu vaccine could be cost-effective across the whole population with a cost per QALY of £251, dramatically below the NICE threshold of £20,000 used for decisions about new medicines and services (Pitman et al., 2013). Paediatric vaccination would appear to be a highly cost-effective intervention that directly protects those targeted for vaccination, with indirect protection extending to both the very young and the elderly through increased herd immunity (Pitman et al., 2013). NICE has published a routine immunization schedule for children aged between eight weeks old to fourteen years old (NICE, 2023). Since 2012, the uptake of nearly all preschool vaccinations in England has declined, meaning that NHS England has failed to meet performance standards set by the Department of Health and Social Care (DHSC; Bamber et al., 2019). The impact of the COVID-19 pandemic and series of national lockdowns on early vaccination has been documented by Public Health England (2021) and NHS Digital (2022). In 2021 to 2022, no vaccination met the 95 per cent target set by WHO for children aged up to five years. For example, MMR1 coverage at twenty-four months was 90.3 per cent in 2020/2021 and fell to 89.2 per cent in 2021/2022 (NHS Digital, 2022). It has been recommended that General Practitioners (GPs) continue offering routine immunizations and reschedule missed immunizations so that vaccine coverage does not drop further (Public Health England, 2021).

Dental Health

Tooth decay continues to be the primary cause of hospital admissions among children aged between six and ten years, with rates for children and young people living in the most deprived communities being nearly 3.5 times that of those living in the most affluent communities (British Dental Journal (BDJ) Team, 2023; Information Services Division, 2016; Royal College of Surgeons, 2015). In 2016, the cost of tooth extractions was £50.5 million among children aged between zero and nineteen years (Public Health England, 2017a). A number of historical cohort and modelling studies have shown that population-level programmes to improve child dental hygiene can be cost saving. For example, Anopa and colleagues (2015) reported that the ChildSmile programme in Scotland generated substantial cost-savings in avoided dental extractions, fillings, and potential treatments for decay. Population standardized analysis by deprivation groups showed that the largest decrease in modelled costs was for the most deprived cohort of children (Anopa et al., 2015). Pine and colleagues (2020) reported that the Dental RECUR study, a single low-cost, low-intensity intervention, was successful in significantly reducing the risk of recurrence of dental caries in children. The intervention involved training in, and implementation of, a motivational interviewing-informed brief intervention which provided opportunities for dental nurses to facilitate behaviour change. This proactive talking intervention improved the oral health of children at risk of developing caries and was found to have a very moderate cost (£6.47) (Ezeofor et al., 2022; Pine et al., 2020). The intervention was effective in providing better health-related quality of life gains and the QALYs gained for the prevention of reoccurrence of dental caries was higher in the intervention arm by 0.023 QALYs (Ezeofor et al., 2022).

Public Health England (2017a) estimated that the ROI for target fluoride varnish programmes was £2.29 for every £1 spent after five years, increasing to £2.74 after ten years. These interventions can result in an extra 3,049 school days gained per 5,000 children. A systematic review of economic evaluations of primary caries prevention in two- to five-year-old preschool children found variation across studies around the types of caries prevention examined, the effectiveness measures used, how costs and outcomes were reported, and the study perspective, making it difficult for comparisons to be made (Anopa et al., 2020).

Children Living with Disability

The Family Resources Survey 2018/2019 estimated that 8 per cent of children in the UK have a disability (Department for Work and Pensions, 2020a). Disability is associated with living in poverty due to a variety of factors including lack of access to employment for parents with additional caring roles and additional costs of living as a result of a household having a child with a disability. Once extra-cost disability benefits (e.g. Disability Living Allowance and Personal Independence Payment) are discounted, nearly half of all individuals living in poverty live in a household where someone is disabled (Joseph Rowntree Foundation, 2020). Over one-fifth of all children with a disability have mobility limitations (Department for Work and Pensions, 2020b). In relation specifically to the early years, an evidence synthesis of powered mobility interventions for very young children with mobility limitations suggested that additional support for mobility-related issues could have multiple benefits (Bray et al., 2020). Self-directed mobility in early childhood results in a major step-change in children's engagement with the world and thus in their perceptual, cognitive, social, and physical development. As this is usually attained through rolling, crawling, and bottom-shuffling, children with mobility limitations have less self-directed movement and thus fewer opportunities to explore the world around them (Barton et al., 2015; Morris et al., 2014, 2015; Tatla et al., 2013). Children with mobility limitations are also at a greater risk of secondary disabilities in terms of motor, cognitive, and social abilities related to daily tasks; other life skills such as general independence and autonomy; and participation in daily life across home, education, and leisure (Livingstone & Field, 2014; Uchiyama et al., 2008). Such secondary disabilities are thought to be negatively related to a child's long-term health, development, and social integration through the life-course. Not only can this impact on their access to education and the workplace in later life, but there is also a negative impact on parental physical and mental health, productivity, and on wider society (Bray et al., 2020).

The provision of early powered mobility to provide 'movement for movement's sake' and directional mobility as appropriate could prevent these secondary disabilities by enabling self-directed mobility and exploration, and subsequent developmental benefits (Bray et al., 2020). Provision of a powered wheelchair to a young child has been estimated to cost less than £10,000, taking into account the equipment, staffing, and costs of adaptations to the home. Provision of ride-on toys for the experience of movement for movement's sake could be provided at an even lower cost (Bray et al., 2020). However, provision of powered mobility to children aged up to five years through the NHS is limited and has been estimated at 400 children per year in England, with further provision though the third sector including ride-on toys to a further 225 children (Bray et al., 2020). A review of current evidence found no studies on cost-effectiveness of such powered mobility aids for very young children (Bray et al., 2020). The third sector plays a major part in the provision of powered mobility for disabled children. For example, the charity Whiz Kids supply vital mobility equipment across the UK and support young wheelchair users through skills training, clubs, and employability.

Parenting Programmes and Conduct Disorder

Conduct disorder is a psychological disorder diagnosed in childhood or adolescence presenting as persistent antisocial and aggressive behaviour. Conduct disorder is one of the most common mental and behavioural problems affecting children and young people, occurring in 6 per cent of school-aged children (NICE, 2013a, 2013b). It is twice as prevalent in males than in females (Coghill, 2013; Polanczyk et al., 2015). Parenting programmes, when delivered well, can be effective and cost-effective in preventing and reducing the long-term effect of conduct disorder in children, with potential savings across multiple sectors (Edwards et al., 2007, 2016; Hutchings et al., 2007; Knapp et al., 2011). A systematic review found that despite economic studies of parenting programmes tending to focus on short-term outcomes, many studies found evidence of economic benefits including savings to the economy (Duncan et al., 2017). Parenting interventions could save the NHS £2,500 per family over twenty-five years and could save the criminal justice system over £145,000 per person over the life-course (Duncan et al., 2017).

Children with conduct disorder cost the public sector ten times more than children with no conduct disorder (Knapp et al., 2011). It is estimated that preventing conduct disorder in the most serious of cases could provide lifetime savings of around £150,000 per case (Friedli & Parsonage, 2007). This is where it seems necessary to take a very wide societal perspective in future economic evaluations of interventions to support families living with children affected by conduct disorder. There are potential savings to the judicial system of early intervention (Parsonage, 2009).

Attention Deficit-Hyperactivity Disorder

Attention deficit-hyperactivity disorder (ADHD) is one of the most common neurodevelopmental disorders in childhood, prevalent in around 5 per cent of children worldwide (Thomas et al., 2015). In the UK, the prevalence of ADHD in children aged three to seventeen years is 1.8 per cent in males and 0.4 per cent in females (McKechnie et al., 2023). There are three different subtypes of ADHD: the inattentive subtype (which accounts for 20 per cent to 30 per cent of cases); the hyperactive-impulsive subtype (which accounts for 15 per cent of cases), and the combined subtype (which accounts for 50 per cent to 75 per cent of cases; NICE, 2022). ADHD can be treated using medicine and/or therapy (e.g. psychoeducation, behaviour therapy, parent training and education programmes, and social skills training; NHS, 2021). Although there are evidence-based national guidelines for ADHD in the UK, the condition is under-identified, under-diagnosed, and under-treated (Young et al., 2021). This leaves people who are seeking help with inconsistent and inaccessible services, often with lengthy waiting lists (Crenna-Jennings & Hutchinson, 2018). As a result, some individuals and families seek out costly private diagnosis and treatment (Vibert, 2018).

ADHD is associated with a number of adverse outcomes which can persist into adult life, even after symptoms of the condition have resolved. For example, a negative impact on educational attainment might have implications for future employment and earnings prospects. The societal financial impact of ADHD in Europe has been estimated to cost up to €14,483 per child with ADHD, with high direct costs of psychological support and pharmacotherapy, coupled with the indirect costs of productivity losses from caregiver lost wages and productivity (as cited in Sampaio et al., 2021). In the UK, cost estimates per case of ADHD have been estimated at around £102,135 per case due to additional costs of health care, additional educational support provision, and a projection of lifetime earnings lost (Khong, 2014). When considering the prevalence of ADHD in the UK, this equates to a total long-term cost of ADHD for each one-year cohort of children of £1,070 million.

Economic evaluations of interventions to treat ADHD have largely focused on pharmacotherapy treatments. There is evidence to support the cost-effectiveness of these treatment when compared with no treatment (Wu et al., 2012). The wider impacts, including potential negative adverse effects of medication, are not always considered and there remains uncertainty about the longer-term effects of ADHD medication (Sampaio et al., 2021). Research evaluating behavioural and psychosocial interventions to manage ADHD have highlighted benefits to child outcomes including cognitive gains, improved social functioning, behaviour and language development, and improvements in daily living skills (Sampaio et al., 2021). However, few studies have included an economic evaluation of non-pharmacotherapy options for ADHD management (Sampaio et al., 2021). There have been some attempts to measure economic returns from programmes delivered within primary schools. Estimates range widely, for example, returns of £1.96 for every £1 invested for group Multimodal Therapy for children with ADHD (Social Research Unit, 2013a) to returns of nearly £27 for every £1 invested for the Good Behaviour Game (Social Research Unit, 2013b).

Troubled Families

Troubled families are characterized by there being no adult in the family in employment, children not being in school, and family members being involved in crime and antisocial behaviour. Troubled families cause problems to the community around them, putting high costs on the public sector (Ministry of Housing, Communities and Local Government, & The Rt Hon Lord Pickles, 2015). Between 2015 and 2020, the UK Government invested £920 million into the Troubled Families Programme to support interventions for 400,000 families with complex needs across the UK (Ministry of Housing, Communities and Local Government, 2019). A keyworker or lead worker considers the problems experienced by the family as a whole and works with family members in a persistent and assertive way towards an agreed improvement plan. A CBA analysis of a cohort of 124,000 families that joined the programme between 2017/2018 found that for every £1 invested in the programme, there was a return of £2.28 of economic benefits (Ministry of Housing, Communities and Local Government, 2019). Supporting troubled families effectively requires joined-up services that consider the whole family unit.

Early interventions targeting disadvantaged high-risk communities, such as the Sure Start and Flying Start programmes, have become part of the UK Government's nationwide strategy. However, the UK Government did not specify effective and cost-effective interventions, resulting in service providers delivering widely differing services, with some delivering evidence-based programmes and others developing their own (Belsky et al., 2006). Subsequently, the evaluation of nationwide strategies in this area is currently unclear. Early evaluation within a cost-benefit framework concluded that by the time children had reached the age of five years, the Sure Start Local Programme had already delivered benefits to the public purse valued between £279 and £557 per eligible child (coming from a reduction in workless households), which is 6 per cent to 12 per cent of the total cost of the programme (Meadows, 2011). A follow-up paper found similar findings (Gaheer & Paull, 2016). Cattan and colleagues (2019) focused on the return to spending on the Sure Start programme in terms of reduced hospitalizations, specifically for infections and injury. Cattan and colleagues reported a CBA using 2018/2019 prices using a discount rate of 3.5 per cent with a life-course time horizon. They found the total financial benefit from averted costs, obtained by adding together the direct health care costs, indirect costs throughout childhood and long-term costs, amounted to £65 million. Of this, £5 million was attributed to direct cost savings to the NHS from fewer hospitalizations at ages five to eleven years. Most of the total averted cost was attributable to the lifetime costs of traumatic brain injury. This was compared with the estimated cost of providing an additional Sure Start centre per 1,000 children to a representative cohort, which was calculated at £1,055 million. The financial benefits from reducing hospitalizations offset 6 per cent of the cost of Sure Start provision (with direct savings from the reduction in hospitalizations at ages five to eleven years coming to 0.4 per cent of spending on Sure Start). This is comparable to the findings of Meadows (2011) for the National Evaluation of Sure Start. Cattan and colleagues (2019) found no evidence that the Sure Start programme impacted on the prevalence of child obesity at age five or maternal mental health. A clear prospective evaluation was not instigated, arguably crucial to such a large-scale public spending programme.

Care Experienced Children

There are slight differences in the definitions of the terms 'looked after children', 'children in care', and 'care experienced children' used across the UK nations (National Society for the Prevention of Cruelty to Children (NSPCC), 2023). Generally, looked after children or children in care include children living with foster parents, living in a residential children's home, or living in residential settings such as schools or secure units (NSPCC, 2023). In the UK, since 2010, the number of looked after children has risen every year. In 2018/2019, there were 102,000 looked after children (NSPCC, 2021). During the COVID-19 pandemic, there were fewer children starting to be looked after, a higher proportion of children needing care due to family stress or dysfunction, fewer placement moves, fewer children leaving care, and changes in the accommodation of young people leaving care (UK Government, 2022b; Welsh Government, 2021). Looked after children at a high risk of being mistreated are more likely to suffer from emotional and behavioural difficulties and have poorer mental health and educational outcomes than the general population (Wilkinson & Bowyer, 2017). The total estimated annual costs for providing support and services to meet the needs of children and families during reunification is £56 million (Holmes, 2014). In 2015, the average cost per year for each child returning to care from their home was £61,614, whereas the average annual cost of supporting a child to return home was £5,627 (Wilkins & Farmer, 2015).

Adverse Childhood Experiences

As described in Chapter 1, at the extreme, children facing ACEs face a lifetime trajectory of poverty, ill-health, and intergenerational consequences (Bellis et al., 2015a). ACEs include the following: experiencing stressful events in childhood, such as domestic violence; experiencing physical, sexual, or verbal abuse; experiencing physical or emotional neglect; having a family member who has a mental health issue or experiences substance misuse; and losing a parent through divorce, separation, or death. A well-defined set of ACEs linked to poor outcomes has been identified and refined as a tool for measuring childhood adversity and its impact on population health (Bellis et al., 2015b). ACEs lead to an elevated risk of experiencing negative health outcomes across the life-course and represent a great cost to society, including public sector services (Bellis et al., 2015a, 2015b). ACEs are clustered around, but not exclusive to, families from lower socioeconomic backgrounds (Björkenstam et al., 2013). Box 3.3 outlines the costs to some sectors of some of the individual outcomes associated with ACEs.

Box 3.3 The costs to some sectors of some of the individual outcomes associated with ACEs

- Early sex and unplanned teenage pregnancy: the total cost of unplanned pregnancies and sexually transmitted infections in the UK between 2015 and 2025 has been estimated to be £259.012 billion (Family Planning Association, 2015; UK Parliament, 2016).

- Child sexual abuse: the annual cost of child sexual abuse in the UK was £3.2 billion in 2012/2013 (Saied-Tessier, 2014). The financial and non-financial (monetized) costs relating to all children who began to experience contact sexual abuse, or who continued to experience contact sexual abuse, in England and Wales in the year ending March 2019 was estimated to be at least £10.1 billion (Home Office, 2021).

- Smoking: the mean incremental lifetime cost of smoking in maltreated children in the UK was estimated to be £528 per maltreated child (Conti et al., 2017).

- Binge drinking: the average discounted lifetime cost of alcohol abuse per victim of child maltreatment was estimated to be £537 (Conti et al., 2017).

- Drug abuse: in 2014, it was estimated that the overall annual cost of drug misuse was £15.4 billion, comprising of £13.9 billion for drug-related crime and £0.5 billion for NHS medical costs (National Treatment Agency for Substance Misuse, 2014). Every £1 spent on drugs treatment saves society £2.50 in reduced NHS and social care costs and reduced crime (National Treatment Agency for Substance Misuse, 2014).

- Crime: it was estimated that the total costs of crime in England and Wales in 2015/2016 was £50 billion for crimes against individuals and £9 billion for crimes against businesses (Heeks et al., 2018).

- Poor diet: in 2006/2007, poor diet-related ill-health cost the NHS £5.8 billion (Scarborough et al., 2011). The UK-wide NHS costs attributable to overweight and obesity are projected to reach £9.7 billion by 2050, with wider costs to society estimated to reach £49.9 billion per year (Public Health England, 2017b).

- In the UK, the lifetime attributable cost of cancer for those with more than four ACEs was £13,791, while the attributable cost of depression for those with four or more ACEs was £42,453 (Lloyd-Williams, 2023).

Youth Crime

There are links between aggression, hyperactivity, concentration problems, and impulsivity in early childhood, and later risk-taking and subsequent violent behaviour in adolescence (Hawkins et al., 1998). Family characteristics such as poor parenting skills, family size, home discord, child maltreatment, and anti-social parents are risk factors linked to juvenile delinquency (Wasserman & Seracini, 2001). Eighty per cent of prolific adult offenders committed a crime as children. In 2018, Black children were four times more likely than White children to be arrested (Youth Justice Board & Ministry of Justice, 2019, 2020). Being arrested is typically the first interaction a child has with the justice system. Ethnic disproportionality is evident at other stages of the youth justice system (Youth Justice Board & Ministry of Justice, 2020, 2022). The cost of late intervention to the UK economy is estimated to be £17 billion a year. To tackle this issue, the UK Government is investing £300 million between 2022 and 2025 to support councils across England and Wales in preventing youth offending at an earlier stage and stopping children from committing more serious offences (Ministry of Justice, Youth Justice Board for England & Wales et al., 2022). The Dartington Service Design Lab (previously the Dartington Social Research Unit) has adapted some evidence from the US to a UK context, listing the benefits, costs, and risks of a range of programmes (see https://www.dartington.org.uk). For example, the Good Behaviour Game is a universal classroom-based intervention aimed at children aged six to eight years. It seeks to reduce aggressive behaviour in order to prevent problem behaviours in middle childhood through to early adulthood. For every £1 invested, the Good Behaviour Game intervention yielded £27 in avoided costs to society as a result of crime (Social Research Unit, 2013b).

Provision of Free School Meals

In England and Wales, children aged four to sixteen years are eligible for free school meals if they live in a household which receives income-related benefits (e.g. universal credit) and has an annual income of less than £7,400 after tax (not including welfare payments; British Broadcasting Corporation (BBC), 2022). In Scotland, the income cap is set at £7,920, and in Northern Ireland, this is set as £14,000 (BBC, 2022). During the COVID-19 pandemic, footballer Marcus Rashford called on ministers to review the free school meals system and to offer a guaranteed 'meal a day' to pupils from low-income families. Rashford called on the UK Government to lower the threshold for free school meals eligibility so that a further 1.7 million children from low-income families on universal credit could claim school meal support. Prior to the pandemic, two in five children (1.6 million) in England living below the poverty line were not entitled to free school meals (UK Government, 2021). In Wales, there is a commitment to meet the rise in demand for free school meals resulting from the COVID-19 pandemic and to extend entitlement for free school meals. Younger children are more likely to be living in relative income poverty and, in taking this action, an additional 196,000 children will become eligible to take up the offer of a free school meal in Wales (Miles, 2021).

Due to rising global food prices, many families have experienced a rise in the cost of their weekly food shop, resulting in increased demand on food banks. Food and non-alcoholic drinks inflation was at 19.1 per cent in March 2023 (ONS, 2023b). Food bank networks reported increased demand and falling food donations in the first half of 2022 (Gorb, 2022). Between August 2019 and August 2022, social tenants, those with a disability or health condition were most likely to need a referral to food banks. More referrals were also given to single people and single people with children compared to couples with or without children (Citizens Advice, 2023). Families with children have also been using uniform banks (Newlands, 2022).

The Cost-effectiveness of Childhood Obesity Interventions

Establishing healthy eating practices early in life, such as a healthy breakfast, can yield educational attainment benefits (Littlecott et al., 2016). Nearly a third of children aged two to fifteen years are overweight or obese, and younger generations are becoming obese at earlier ages and staying obese for longer (UK Government, 2017). Obesity rates are highest in the poorest communities. The overall cost of obesity to the wider society is £27 billion and this figure is rising (Public Health England, 2017b). The UK-wide NHS costs attributable to people being overweight and obese are projected to reach £9.7 billion by 2050, with wider costs to society estimated to reach £49.9 billion per year. During the COVID-19 pandemic, people with obesity were at a higher risk of dying from COVID-19 compared with people without obesity. This is partly due to the link between obesity and other health conditions such as cardiovascular diseases, diabetes, and asthma, which can lead to worse COVID-19 outcomes and an increase in risk of death in general (ONS, 2022).

NICE (2015b) has published guidance on the prevention of obesity in children and adults with the aim to: 1) reduce the rising prevalence of obesity and diseases associated with it; 2) increase the effectiveness of interventions to prevent people becoming overweight and obese; and 3) improve the care provided to children and adults at risk of becoming overweight and obese. The guidance highlights that there is currently little evidence of the cost-effectiveness of interventions. This is due to a lack of outcome measures that are amenable to health economics evaluations; the use of crude measures such as average weight loss rather than response rates, and short follow-up data collection time-points. The development of the CHU-9D instrument for children over the age of seven years will help with this issue going forward (Stevens, 2012). NICE (2015b) has called for clinical research to obtain more information from quality of life questionnaires throughout the intervention and follow-up periods to help assess any clinical improvement to the individual.

The West Midlands ActiVe lifestyle and healthy Eating in School children (WAVES) cluster RCT was undertaken in fifty-four schools across the West Midlands (Canaway et al., 2019). The trial involved a twelve-month intervention aimed to increase physical activity by thirty minutes per day and encourage healthy eating. At thirty months, the total adjusted incremental mean cost of the intervention was £155 per child and the incremental mean QALYs gained was 0.006. The incremental cost-effectiveness was £26,815 per QALY and using a standard willingness to pay (WTP) threshold of £30,000 per QALY, there was a 52 per cent chance that the intervention was cost-effective. Canaway and colleagues (2019) highlighted that although the results of this economic evaluation appeared to show the WAVES intervention to be a potentially cost-effective use of public resources, there were high levels of uncertainty, as shown by the low probability of cost-effectiveness at varying threshold levels of WTP. In terms of implementation science, the WAVES study provided evidence that schools can play an important role in addressing childhood obesity and that the upstream determinants of obesity, as well as the wider social, physical, and family environment, need to be considered (Canaway et al., 2019).

The Daily Mile programme was designed to increase physical activity levels by encouraging children to walk or run around school grounds for fifteen minutes a day. It has been adopted by schools worldwide and endorsed as a solution to tackle obesity, despite no current robust evidence of its benefits. Breheny and colleagues (2020) conducted a cluster RCT in forty schools to determine the clinical and cost-effectiveness of The Daily Mile programme. They found the programme to be highly cost-effective in girls (£2,492 per QALY), but not in boys, and overall to have a 76 per cent chance of cost-effectiveness for the whole sample, at the commonly applied UK threshold of £20,000 per QALY.

Both these large school-based trials take a public sector perspective and use the CHU-9D instrument as a source of QALY weights. It is interesting that they generate such different estimates of a cost per QALY. The Daily Mile programme had a small but non-significant effect on body mass index z-score (BMIz), and had a greater effect in girls (Breheny et al., 2020). In the WAVES programme, which had a higher cost per QALY estimate, the researchers argued this was due to uncertainty (Canaway et al., 2019). Further research is needed to explore obesity prevention within schools as part of a whole system approach to obesity prevention.

Promoting Music and Arts

There has been some adaptation of the South American El Sistema programme encouraging music in schools to the UK. El Sistema is the national music education programme of Venezuela, which aims to give young children from disadvantaged backgrounds a better start in life through music. The five fundamental principles of El Sistema are: 1) social transformation through the pursuit of musical excellence; 2) the focus is the orchestra or choral experience; 3) the ensembles meet multiple times every week over extended periods; 4) programmes are free and are not selective in admission; and 5) every music school is linked at the urban, regional, and national levels, forming a cohesive network of services and opportunities for students across the county (Govias, 2011). This type of music intervention in schools has been explored in England (through the In Harmony programme and more recently, The Nucleo Project), in Scotland (through the Big Noise programme), and in Wales (through the Codi'r To programme; Scottish Government Social Research, 2011; Wilson, 2013; Winrow & Edwards, 2018). Evaluations of all of these programmes have uncovered 'added value', meaning that the interventions offer benefits for a wider range of stakeholders than expected. In the case of the El Sistema programmes, the community has benefitted enormously and has helped integrate both young children and families.

The Codi'r To project was a music-based intervention pilot that brought the El Sistema teaching method to schools in deprived areas in North Wales. Its adaptation in Wales has proved to have a positive social return on investment (SROI) ratio. Research by the Centre for Health Economics and Medicines Evaluation (CHEME) at Bangor University found the Codi'r To project generated an ROI of between £4.59 and £8.95 for every £1 spent on the project, and improved pupil confidence, pupil relationships, family relationships, and classroom behaviour (Winrow & Edwards, 2018). In Scotland, the Big Noise project generated £9 for every £1 spent and improved team-working, communication, and leadership; increased resilience, happiness, and sense of belonging and fulfilment, and gave respite and protection for vulnerable children (Harkins & Moore, 2019).

Playgrounds and Public Spaces

As discussed in Chapter 2, neighbourhoods, or where we live, contribute to our lifetime health and opportunities. Play provision provides an important context in which children can counter the effects of poverty and deprivation. Where the home environment is poor or there is a restricted range of stimuli, play services and spaces offer variety and even comfort. Good play provision can offer a welcoming space where children can meet on a more equal basis. For this reason, play provision can be the starting point for tackling social exclusion, engaging with marginalized families and communities, and working to build their capacity to improve their social, environmental, and economic circumstances (Dobson et al., 2019; Hill-Tout et al., 1991).

A pilot study in England assessed the cost-effectiveness of a playground intervention (Pre-schoolers in the Playground) involving 164 children aged between eighteen months and four years who were allocated to either six thirty-minute sessions per week for thirty weeks or usual practice (Barber et al., 2015). Results demonstrated improvement in health-related quality of life in parents by 0.058 QALYs at an additional cost of £1,173 per participant, generating an incremental cost-effectiveness ratio (ICER) of £20,215, which is considered borderline cost-effective (Barber et al., 2015). Findings from the pilot study suggested that a full RCT is feasible but that the intervention requires some modification, such as running the intervention during the summer term only as attendance during other seasons was low (Barber et al., 2015).

Childhood Accidents

Unintentional injuries (i.e. accidents) in and around the home are a leading cause of preventable death for children under five years and are a major cause of ill-health and serious disability (Public Health England, 2018b). See Box 3.4 for a case study on the Keeping Children Safe programme, which evaluated the effectiveness and cost-effectiveness of home safety interventions (Kendrick et al., 2017). In England, on average per year, fifty children under the age of five have died due to an unintentional injury, 370,000 children attended accident and emergency (A&E) departments, and 40,000 children were admitted to hospital as an emergency (Public Health England, 2018b). The economic cost to health and social care services is estimated at £36 million a year for emergency hospital admissions alone (de Sousa, 2017). The lifetime social care cost for just one child who suffers a severe traumatic brain injury at age three years is £1.19 million (de Sousa, 2017). Accidental injuries are a feature of inequalities, with children from poorer backgrounds

Box 3.4 Case study: The Keeping Children Safe programme

The Keeping Children Safe programme provided evidence of the effectiveness and cost-effectiveness of home safety interventions (Kendrick et al., 2017). The programme comprised multicentre case-control studies assessing risk and protective factors, a study measuring quality of life and injury costs, national surveys of children's centres, interviews with children's centre staff and parents, a systematic review of barriers to, and facilitators of, prevention, and systematic overviews, meta-analyses and decision analyses of home safety interventions. Kendrick and colleagues (2017) developed evidence-based resources for preventing thermal injuries, falls, and scalds in children. They found that providing these resources to children's centres increased their injury prevention activity and some parental safety behaviours. They found a significant association with modifiable risk factors for falls from furniture and on stairs, poisoning, and scalds in children aged up to four years. They developed an injury prevention briefing (IPB) intervention, which combined evidence of the effectiveness of fire safety interventions with best practice from those who had experience of running injury prevention programmes. Key messages in the IPB were: the importance of smoke alarm use and maintenance; having a family fire escape plan; identifying potential causes of house fires; the safe storage of matches and lighters, and having a bedtime fire safety routine. In the IPB with support (IPB+) group, children's centres were provided with IPB (immediately before the start of the twelve-month intervention period) and a facilitation package to support implementation of the IPB. The researchers found that the IPB for children's centres intervention was less costly and marginally more effective than usual care. The IPB+ intervention was more costly and marginally more effective than usual care (Kendrick et al., 2017).

As part of the Keeping Children Safe programme, Kendrick and colleagues (2017) examined the NHS, child and family costs of falls, poisonings, and scalds in children aged under two years. Mean NHS costs ranged from £2,588 to £2,989 across injury mechanisms for children admitted for up to two days, from £719 to £1,011 for children admitted for up to one day, and from £97 to £178 for children attending an emergency department but not admitted. Scalds incurred the highest NHS costs for admissions for up to one day and for emergency department attendances. Mean costs to families ranged from £99 to £399 across injury mechanisms for those admitted for up to two days, from £38 to £200 for those admitted for up to one day, and from £18 to £68 for those attending an emergency department but not admitted. Family costs were highest for scalds for admissions for up to one day and for falls from furniture for emergency department attendances. Family costs mainly consisted of the costs of informal child care and the costs of taking time off work (Kendrick et al., 2017).

being three times more likely to be admitted to hospital and five times more likely to die as a result of an accident than children from less deprived families (Royal Society for the Prevention of Accidents (ROSPA), 2013; White et al., 2000).

The NHS spends £131 million per year on emergency hospital admissions related to childhood accidents (Tyrrell & Prasad, 2021). Five in every 1,000 children under four years are injured by burns and scalds each year in England (Baker et al., 2016). Scald injuries place a considerable burden on health care services, with the individual lifetime cost for treating a severe scald estimated to be £250,000 (Phillips et al., 2011). The cost of treating serious bathwater scalds ranges from £25,226 to £71,902. Investing in injury prevention could produce savings further down the line. Thermostatic mixer valves can control water temperature for bathing, washing and hand-washing. Phillips and colleagues (2011) evaluated the cost-effectiveness of introducing bath thermostatic mixer valves in social housing. Unit costs associated with installation were £13.68. The cost of an avoided bath water scald ranged from net savings to the public purse of £1,887 to £75,520, and at baseline produced a net saving of over £3 million. This study demonstrated that installing thermostatic mixers would save £1.41 for every £1 spent (Phillips et al., 2011). Interventions designed by ROSPA are reported to have reduced accidents and saved money, reducing accidents by 20 per cent to 30 per cent in the target population/area. The ROI ranges between three times to ten times the initial investment (ROSPA, 2012).

A Generation at Risk from Lost Learning

In their editorial, Margaret Whitehead and colleagues argued that, 'Covid-19 does not strike at random—mortality is much higher in elderly people, poorer groups, and ethnic minorities, and its economic effect is also unevenly distributed across the population. . . . Without concerted preventive action worse off families and communities will be disproportionately affected, increasing health inequalities in the UK and globally' (Whitehead et al., 2021, p. 1). One in six children and young people reported experiencing mental health problems at the start of the pandemic, exacerbated as their lives were 'put on hold' due to national lockdowns, with implications for their long-term health and wellbecoming (NHS Digital, 2020). Nearly half of parents (47 per cent) reported that their child experienced more social and emotional difficulties in February 2021 than a year earlier, while around one in six parents reported fewer challenges (Cattan et al., 2023). For children, the pandemic has impacted on their education, training, and future earning potential (Bambra et al., 2020; Hefferon et al., 2021). The Institute for Fiscal Studies estimated that missing half a year of school could mean losing £40,000 in lifetime earnings, with negative effects concentrated among children from disadvantaged backgrounds (Sibieta, 2021). The National Tutoring Programme was launched in November 2020 to help pupils across the country to catch-up on missed time in school, providing access to one-to-one or small group teaching with specialist tutors (Department for Education, 2022).

Summary

This chapter highlights the concept that investment in the early years should be viewed as part of wider economic investment policy (Edwards et al., 2016). Intervention in the earliest years of childhood can address or mitigate the damaging social problems later in life, which has substantial costs to society. A third of children in the UK are growing up in poverty, a figure that will have risen following the impacts of the COVID-19 pandemic. Transforming young lives and helping children reach their full potential has many wider economic benefits, including improving health and well-being; increasing educational attainment, lifetime earnings, and economic productivity; reducing inequalities; and generating substantial savings to the NHS, social care, and social security system. This chapter explores the economic case for investing in the early years and childhood, helping to ensure that children are as healthy as possible and well-nourished, receive good quality early learning opportunities, and are nurtured and protected from harm.

Based on international evidence, investment that focuses on the critical window of the first few years of life is argued to provide the most efficient use of public resources. In many cases, yielding returns over and above other forms of financial investment and investment at other points of the life-course. UK higher education institutions continue to make a significant contribution to the international evidence of the effectiveness and cost-effectiveness of programmes and practice relating to early years. There is an economic argument for disinvestment in programmes without a strong evidence-base, and re-investment in programmes, both universal and targeted, with a strong evidence-base of effectiveness and cost-effectiveness. What is unlikely to work is, in the interest of keeping costs down, delivering watered-down versions of evidence-based programmes in an attempt to bring their key principles into current practice.

Curiosity Questions

- Are universal or targeted interventions, programmes, and policies most cost-effective within an early years or school context or environment?

- What evidence is there that interventions that are cost-effective in the short run in terms of promoting well-being in the early years have a lasting impact into adolescence?

- Public sector agencies, including local councils, wanting to invest in the early years would benefit from true valuations of the financial, economic, environmental, and social value of community assets that already exist in the UK, such as playgrounds and public spaces. How could this be achieved?

- How can the short and long-term returns to the economy of the early care and education sector as a source of employment and wider economic driver across the UK best be integrated into systems level thinking about population well-being and well-becoming?

- How can the sharing of data across sectors be used to both improve statutory services and be used in health economics research?

- How can the cost-effectiveness of more 'joined-up' services that better consider the whole family, rather than just the individual child, best be evaluated?

References

Alexander, K., Entwisle, D., & Olson, L. (2014). *The long shadow: Family background, disadvantaged urban youth, and the transition to adulthood*. Russell Sage Foundation.

Allen, G. (2011a). *Early intervention: The next steps. An independent report to Her Majesty's Government*. HM Government. https://assets.publishing.service.gov.uk/government/uploads/system/uploads/attachment_data/file/284086/early-intervention-next-steps2.pdf

Allen, G. (2011b). *Early intervention: Smart investment, massive savings. The second independent report to Her Majesty's Government*. UK Government. https://assets.publishing.service.gov.uk/government/uploads/system/uploads/attachment_data/file/61012/earlyintervention-smartinvestment.pdf

Andre, F. E., Booy, R., Bock, H. L., Clemens, J., Datta, S. K., John, T. J., Lee, B. W., Lolekha, S., Peltola, H., Ruff, T. A., Santosham, M., & Schmitt, H. J. (2008). Vaccination greatly reduces disease, disability, death and inequity worldwide. *Bulletin of the World Health Organization*, 86, 140–146. https://doi.org/10.2471/BLT.07.040089

Anopa, Y., Macpherson, L., & McIntosh, E. (2020). Systematic review of economic evaluations of primary caries prevention in 2-to 5-year-old preschool children. *Value in Health*, 23(8), 1109–1118. https://doi.org/10.1016/j.jval.2020.04.1823

Anopa, Y., McMahon, A. D., Conway, D. I., Ball, G. E., McIntosh, E., & Macpherson, L. M. (2015). Improving child oral health: Cost analysis of a national nursery toothbrushing programme. *PLoS One*, **10**(8), e0136211. https://doi.org/10.1371/journal.pone.0136211

Aos, S., Lieb, R., Mayfield, J., Miller, M., & Pennucci, A. (2004). *Benefits and costs of prevention and early intervention programs for youth*. Washington State Institute for Public Policy. https://www.wsipp.wa.gov/ReportFile/882

Atchison, C. J., & Hassounah, S. (2015). The UK immunisation schedule: Changes to vaccine policy and practice in 2013/14. *JRSM Open*, **6**(4), 1–7. https://doi.org/10.1177/2054270415577762

Baker, R., Tata, L. J., Kendrick, D., Burch, T., Kennedy, M., & Orton, E. (2016). Differing patterns in thermal injury incidence and hospitalisations among 0–4 year old children from England. *Burns*, **42**(7), 1609–1616. https://doi.org/10.1016/j.burns.2016.05.007

Bambra, C., Munford, L., Alexandros, A., Barr, B., Brown, H., Davies, H., Konstantinos, D., Mason, K., Pickett, K., Taylor, C., Taylor-Robinson, D., & Wickham, S. (2020). *COVID-19 and the Northern Powerhouse: Tackling inequalities for UK health and productivity*. Northern Health Science Alliance. https://www.thenhsa.co.uk/app/uplo ads/2020/11/NP-COVID-REPORT-101120-.pdf

Bamber, F., Burke, M., Chambers, M., Jobling, S., Taylor, A., & McDougall, A. (2019, 25 October). *Investigation into pre-school vaccinations*. Report by the Comptroller and Auditor General. Department of Health and Social Care. National Audit Office. https:// publications.parliament.uk/pa/cm201919/cmselect/cmhealth/correspondence/NAO-vaccinations-report-2019-10-25.pdf

Barber, S. E., Akhtar, S., Jackson, C., Bingham, D. D., Hewitt, C., Routen, A., Richardson, G., Ainsworth, H., Moore, H. J., Summerbell, C. D., Pickett, K. E., O'Malley, C., Brierley, S., & Wright, J. (2015). Preschoolers in the playground: A pilot cluster randomised controlled trial of a physical activity intervention for children aged 18 months to 4 years. *Public Health Research*, **3**(5), 1–242. https://doi.org/10.3310/phr03050

Barton, E. E., Reichow, B., Schnitz, A., Smith, I. C., & Sherlock, D. (2015). A systematic review of sensory-based treatments for children with disabilities. *Research in Developmental Disabilities*, **37**, 64–80. https://doi.org/10.1016/j.ridd.2014.11.006

Bate, A., & Foster, D. (2017, 9 June). *Sure Start (England)* [Briefing paper]. House of Commons Library. https://researchbriefings.files.parliament.uk/documents/CBP-7257/CBP-7257.pdf

Belfield, C. R., Nores, M., Barnett, S., & Schweinhart, L. (2006). The High/Scope Perry Preschool Program cost–benefit analysis using data from the age-40 followup. *Journal of Human Resources*, **41**(1), 162–190. https://doi.org/10.3368/jhr.XLI.1.162

Bellis, M. A., Ashton, K., Hughes, K., Ford, K., Bishop, J., & Paranjothy, S. (2015a). *Adverse childhood experiences and their impact on health-harming behaviours in the Welsh adult population*. Public Health Wales. https://www.ljmu.ac.uk/~/media/phi-reports/pdf/2016_01_adverse_childhood_experiences_and_their_impact_on_health_harming_be haviours_in_the.pdf

Bellis, M. A., Hughes, K., Leckenby, N., Hardcastle, K. A., Perkins, C., & Lowey, H. (2015b). Measuring mortality and the burden of adult disease associated with adverse childhood experiences in England: a national survey. *Journal of Public Health*, **37**(3), 445–454. https://doi.org/10.1093/pubmed/fdu065

Belsky, J., Melhuish, E., Barnes, J., Leyland, A. H., & Romaniuk, H. (2006). Effects of Sure Start local programmes on children and families: Early findings from a quasi-experimental, cross sectional study. *BMJ*, **332**(7556), 1476. https://doi.org/10.1136/bmj.38853.451748.2F

Björkenstam, E., Hjern, A., Mittendorfer-Rutz, E., Vinnerljung, B., Hallqvist, J., & Ljung, R. (2013). Multi-exposure and clustering of adverse childhood experiences, socioeconomic differences and psychotropic medication in young adults. *PLoS One*, **8**(1), e53551. https://doi.org/10.1371/journal.pone.0053551

Bray, N., Kolehmainen, N., McAnuff, J., Tanner, L., Tuersley, L., Beyer, F., Grayston, A., Wilson, D., Edwards, R. T., Noyes, J., & Craig, D. (2020). Powered mobility interventions for very young children with mobility limitations to aid participation and positive development: The EMPoWER evidence synthesis. *Health Technology Assessment*, **24**(50), 1. https://doi.org/10.3310/hta24500

Breheny, K., Passmore, S., Adab, P., Martin, J., Hemming, K., Lancashire, E. R., & Frew, E. (2020). Effectiveness and cost-effectiveness of The Daily Mile on childhood weight outcomes and wellbeing: A cluster randomised controlled trial. *International Journal of Obesity*, **44**(4), 812–822. https://doi.org/10.1038/s41366-019-0511-0

British Broadcasting Corporation (BBC). (2022, 11 October). *Free school meals: How many children can claim them?* https://www.bbc.co.uk/news/54693906

British Dental Journal Team. (2023). Tooth decay remains top reason for child hospital admissions. *BDJ Team*, **10**, 6. https://doi.org/10.1038/s41407-023-1798-1

Camacho, E. M., & Hussain, H. (2020). Cost-effectiveness evidence for strategies to promote or support breastfeeding: A systematic search and narrative literature review. *BMC Pregnancy and Childbirth*, **20**(1), 1–8. https://doi.org/10.1186/s12884-020-03460-3

Canaway, A., Frew, E., Lancashire, E., Pallan, M., Hemming, K., & Adab, P. (on behalf of WAVES Trial Investigators). (2019). Economic evaluation of a childhood obesity prevention programme for children: Results from the WAVES cluster randomised controlled trial conducted in schools. *PLoS One*, **14**(7), e0219500. https://doi.org/10.1371/journal.pone.0219500

Carter, P. (2019). Time tactics: Project managing policy implementation in a network. *Time & Society*, **28**(2), 721–742. https://doi.org/10.1177/0961463X16682517

Cattan, S., Conti, G., Farquharson, C., & Ginja, R. (2019). *The health effects of Sure Start.* The Institute for Fiscal Studies. https://discovery.ucl.ac.uk/id/eprint/10117437/1/Cattan_Conti_etal_IFS_2019_The%20health%20effects%20of%20Sure%20Start%20-%20Final%20Report.pdf

Cattan, S., Conti, G., Farquharson, C., Ginja, R., & Pecher, M. (2021). *The health effects of universal early childhood interventions: Evidence from Sure Start* (IZA Discussion Papers, No. 14868). Institute of Labor Economics (IZA), Bonn. https://www.econstor.eu/bitstream/10419/250529/1/dp14868.pdf

Cattan, S., Farquharson, C., Krutikova, S., McKendrick, A., & Sevilla, A. (2023). *How did parents' experiences in the labour market shape children's social and emotional development during the pandemic?* The Institute for Fiscal Studies. https://ifs.org.uk/sites/default/files/2023-07/Final-Parents-experience-of-labour-market-IFS-Report.pdf

Chabot, I., Goetghebeur, M. M., & Grégoire, J. P. (2004). The societal value of universal childhood vaccination. *Vaccine*, **22**(15–16), 1992–2005. https://doi.org/10.1016/j.vacc ine.2003.10.027

Citizens Advice. (2023, 15 June). *CA cost of living data dashboard*. Flourish. https://public. flourish.studio/story/1634399/

Coghill, D. (2013). Editorial: Do clinical services need to take conduct disorder more seriously? *Journal of Child Psychology and Psychiatry*, **54**(9), 921–923. https://doi.org/ 10.1111/jcpp.12135

Conti, G., & Heckman, J. J. (2012). *The economics of child well-being* [Working paper 18466]. National Bureau of Economic Research. https://doi.org/10.3386/w18466

Conti, G., Morris, S., Melnychuk, M., & Pizzo, E. (2017). *The economic costs of child maltreatment in the UK: A preliminary study*. NSPCC and University College London. https://learning.nspcc.org.uk/media/1094/economic-cost-child-maltreatment-united-kingdom-preliminary-study.pdf

Craig, P., Dieppe, P., Macintyre, S., Michie, S., Nazareth, I., & Petticrew, M. (2008). Developing and evaluating complex interventions: The new Medical Research Council guidance. *BMJ*, **337**(a1655), 1–6. https://doi.org/10.1136/bmj.a1655

Crenna-Jennings, W., & Hutchinson, J. (2018). *Access to children and young people's mental health services—2018*. Education Policy Institute. https://dera.ioe.ac.uk/id/eprint/ 32275/1/EPI_Access-to-CAMHS-2018.pdf

Crocker-Buque, T., Mohan, K., Ramsay, M., Edelstein, M., & Mounier-Jack, S. (2019). What is the cost of delivering routine vaccinations at GP practices in England? A comparative time-driven activity-based costing analysis. *Human Vaccines & Immunotherapeutics*, **15**(12), 3016–3023. https://doi.org/10.1080/21645515.2019.1619403

Currie, J. (2009). Healthy, wealthy, and wise: Socioeconomic status, poor health in childhood, and human capital development. *Journal of Economic Literature*, **47**(1), 87–122. https:// doi.org/10.1257/jel.47.1.87

Currie, J., & Moretti, E., (2007). Biology as destiny? Short- and long-run determinants of intergenerational transmission of birth weight. *Journal of Labor Economics*, **25**(2), 231–264. http://dx.doi.org/10.1086/511377

de Sousa, E. (2017, 28 February). *Preventing accidents in children under five*. UK Health Security Agency. UK Government. https://ukhsa.blog.gov.uk/2017/02/28/preventing-accidents-in-children-under-five/

Deidda, M., Geue, C., Kreif, N., Dundas, R., & McIntosh, E. (2019). A framework for conducting economic evaluations alongside natural experiments. *Social Science & Medicine*, **220**, 353–361. https://doi.org/10.1016/j.socscimed.2018.11.032

Department for Education. (2021, 18 November). *Sure Start report card 2020/21*. https:// www.education-ni.gov.uk/publications/sure-start-report-card-202021

Department for Education. (2022, 11 January). *How the National Tutoring Programme is helping young people catch up on education they missed because of Covid-19*. UK Government. https://educationhub.blog.gov.uk/2022/01/11/how-the-national-tutoring-programme-is-helping-young-people-catch-up-on-education-they-missed-because-of-covid-19/

Department for Work and Pensions. (2020a, 26 March). *Family Resources Survey: Financial year 2018/19*. UK Government. https://www.gov.uk/government/statistics/family-resources-survey-financial-year-201819

Department for Work and Pensions (2020b, 26 March). *Households below average income: An analysis of the UK income distribution: 1994/95–2018/19*. UK Government. https://www.gov.uk/government/statistics/households-below-average-income-199495-to-201819

Department for Work & Pensions. (2022, 31 March). *Children in low income families: local area statistics, financial year ending 2021*. UK Government. https://www.gov.uk/government/statistics/children-in-low-income-families-local-area-statistics-2014-to-2021/children-in-low-income-families-local-area-statistics-financial-year-ending-2021

Dobson, J., Harris, C., Eadson, W., & Gore, T. (2019). *Space to thrive: A rapid evidence review of the benefits of parks and green spaces for people and communities*. The National Lottery Heritage Fund and The National Lottery Community Fund. https://shura.shu.ac.uk/25904/1/space-to-thrive-2019-evidence-review.pdf

Duncan, K. M., MacGillivray, S., & Renfrew, M. J. (2017). Costs and savings of parenting interventions: Results of a systematic review. *Child: Care, Health and Development*, **43**(6), 797–811. https://doi.org/10.1111/cch.12473

Education & Skills Funding Agency. (2021, 25 November). *Early years funded entitlement cost changes forecasts, England: Spending round 2021 to 2022*. UK Government. https://www.gov.uk/government/publications/early-years-funding-2021-2022/early-years-funded-entitlement-cost-changes-forecasts-england-spending-round-2021-to-2022

Edwards, R. T., Bryning, L., & Lloyd-Williams, H. (2016). *Transforming young lives across Wales: The economic argument for investing in early years*. Centre for Health Economics and Medicines Evaluation, Bangor University. https://cheme.bangor.ac.uk/documents/transforming-young-lives/CHEME%20transforming%20Young%20Lives%20Full%20Report%20Eng%20WEB%202.pdf

Edwards, R. T., Céilleachair, A., Bywater, T., Hughes, D. A., & Hutchings, J. (2007). Parenting programme for parents of children at risk of developing conduct disorder: Cost effectiveness analysis. *BMJ*, **334**(7595), 682. https://doi.org/10.1136/bmj.39126.699421.55

Edwards, R. T., Jones, C., Berry, V., Charles, J., Linck, P., Bywater, T., & Hutchings, J. (2016). Incredible Years parenting programme: Cost-effectiveness and implementation. *Journal of Children's Services*, **11**(1), 54–72. https://doi.org/10.1108/JCS-02-2015-0005

Edwards, R. T., Neal, R. D., Linck, P., Bruce, N., Mullock, L., Nelhans, N., Pasterfield, D., Russell, D., Russell, I., & Woodfine, L. (2011). Enhancing ventilation in homes of children with asthma: Cost-effectiveness study alongside randomised controlled trial. *British Journal of General Practice*, **61**(592), e733–e741. https://doi.org/10.3399/bjgp11X606645

Eyberg, S. M., & Ross, A. W. (1978). Assessment of child behavior problems: The validation of a new inventory. *Journal of Clinical Child & Adolescent Psychology*, **7**(2), 113–116. https://doi.org/10.1080/15374417809532835

Ezeofor, V., Edwards, R. T., Burnside, G., Adair, P., & Pine, C. M. (2022). Cost-effectiveness analysis of the dental RECUR pragmatic randomized controlled trial: Evaluating a goal-oriented talking intervention to prevent reoccurrence of dental caries in children. *Applied Health Economics and Health Policy*, **20**(3), 431–445. https://doi.org/10.1007/s40258-022-00720-5

Family Planning Association. (2015). *Unprotected nation: An update on the financial and economic impacts of restricted contraceptive and sexual health services*. https://www.fpa.org.uk/unprotected-nation-cuts-to-sexual-health-services-cost-uk-%C2%AC136-billion/

Field, F. (2010). *The foundation years: preventing poor children becoming poor adults. The report of the Independent Review on Poverty and Life Chances.* Cabinet Office, HM Government. https://dera.ioe.ac.uk/id/eprint/11472/1/ffreport.pdf

Filby, A., Wood, H., Jenks, M., Taylor, M., Burley, V., Barbier, M., & Giunta, G. (2015). *Examining the cost-effectiveness of moving the Healthy Start Vitamin Programme from a targeted to a universal offering: Cost-effectiveness systematic review.* York Health Economics Consortium. https://www.nice.org.uk/Media/Default/About/what-we-do/NICE-guidance/NICE-guidelines/healthy-start-cost-effectiveness-review.pdf

Friedli, L., & Parsonage, M. (2007). Building an economic case for mental health promotion: Part I. *Journal of Public Mental Health, 6*(3), 14–23. https://doi.org/10.1108/17465729200700017

Frost, J. J., Sonfield, A., Zolna, M. R., & Finer, L. B. (2014). Return on investment: A fuller assessment of the benefits and cost savings of the US publicly funded family planning program. *The Milbank Quarterly, 92*(4), 696–749. https://doi.org/10.1111/1468-0009.12080

Gaheer, S., & Paull, G. (2016). *The value for money of children's centre services. Evaluation of Children's Centres in England (ECCE) Strand 5. Research report.* Department for Education. UK Government. https://assets.publishing.service.gov.uk/government/uploads/system/uploads/attachment_data/file/534942/ECCE_Strand_5_Value_for_Money_Analysis_Main_Report.pdf

Godfrey, C., Pickett, K.E., Parrott, S., Mdege, N., & Eapen, D., (2010). *Estimating the costs to the NHS of smoking in pregnancy for pregnant women and infants.* Public Health Research Consortium, University of York. https://www.phrc.online/assets/uploads/files/PHRC_A3_06_Exec_Summary.pdf

Goodman, A., & Sianesi, B. (2005). Early education and children's outcomes: How long do the impacts last? *Fiscal Studies, 26*(4), 513–548. https://doi.org/10.1111/j.1475-5890.2005.00022.x

Gorb, A. (2022, 18 October). *Food bank demand and the rising cost of living.* House of Commons Library. UK Parliament. https://commonslibrary.parliament.uk/food-bank-demand-and-the-rising-cost-of-living/

Govias, J. A. (2011). The five fundamentals of El Sistema. *Canadian Music Educator, 53*(1), 21–23.

Griggs, J., & Walker, R. (2008). *The costs of child poverty for individuals and society: Literature Review.* Joseph Rowntree Foundation. https://www.jrf.org.uk/sites/default/files/jrf/migrated/files/2301-child-poverty-costs.pdf

Harker, L. (2006). *Chance of a lifetime: The impact of bad housing on children's lives.* Shelter. https://england.shelter.org.uk/professional_resources/policy_and_research/policy_library/policy_library_folder/chance_of_a_lifetime_-_the_impact_of_bad_housing_on_childrens_lives

Harkins, C., & Moore, K. (2019). *People change lives: Consolidating five years of evaluation learning from Sistema Scotland's Big Noise centres in Stirling, Glasgow & Aberdeen.* Glasgow Centre for Population Health. https://www.makeabignoise.org.uk/files/3415/5231/4056/People_change_lives_March_2019_FINAL.pdf

Hawkins, J. D., Herrenkohl, T. L., Farrington, D. P., Brewer, D., Catalano, R. F., & Harachi, T. W. (1998). A review of predictors of youth violence. In R. Loeber & D. P. Farrington (Eds.), *Serious and violent juvenile offenders: Risk factors and successful interventions* (pp. 106–146). Sage Publications.

Heckman, J. J. (2013). *Invest in early childhood development: Reduce deficits, strengthen the economy.* The Heckman Equation. https://heckmanequation.org/wp-content/uploads/2013/07/F_HeckmanDeficitPieceCUSTOM-Generic_052714-3.pdf

Heckman, J. J. (2019). *Early childhood education strengthens families and can break the cycle of poverty.* The Heckman Equation. https://heckmanequation.org/www/assets/2019/05/F_Heckman_PerryMidlife_OnePager_050819.pdf

Heckman, J. J., Moon, S. H., Pinto, R., Savelyev, P. A., & Yavitz, A. (2010). The rate of return to the HighScope Perry Preschool Program. *Journal of Public Economics*, **94**(1–2), 114–128. https://doi.org/10.1016/j.jpubeco.2009.11.001

Heeks, M., Reed, S., Tafsiri, M., & Prince, S. (2018). *The economic and social costs of crime.* Home Office. UK Government. https://www.gov.uk/government/publications/the-economic-and-social-costs-of-crime

Hefferon, C., Taylor, C., Bennett, D., Falconer, C., Campbell, M., Williams, J. G., Schwartz, D., Kipping, R., & Taylor-Robinson, D. (2021). Priorities for the child public health response to the COVID-19 pandemic recovery in England. *Archives of Disease in Childhood*, **106**(6), 533–538. http://dx.doi.org/10.1136/archdischild-2020-320214

Hill-Tout, J., Doyle, A., & Allen, D., (1991). Challenging behaviour service, South Glamorgan. In D. Allen, R. Banks, & S. Staite (Eds.), *Meeting the challenge. Some UK perspectives on community services for people with learning disabilities and challenging behaviour* (pp. 40–44). King's Fund.

Hoddinott, J., Rosegrant, M., & Torero, M. (2012, 30 March). *Hunger and malnutrition.* 2012 Global Copenhagen Consensus. https://copenhagenconsensus.com/sites/default/files/Hunger+and+Malnutrition.pdf

Holmes, L., (2014). *Supporting children and families returning home from care: Counting the costs.* NSPCC. Centre for Child and Family Research, Loughborough University.

Home Office. (2021, 13 December). *The economic and social cost of contact child sexual abuse.* UK Government. https://www.gov.uk/government/publications/the-economic-and-social-cost-of-contact-child-sexual-abuse/the-economic-and-social-cost-of-contact-child-sexual-abuse

Hutchings, H. A., Evans, A., Barnes, P., Demmler, J., Heaven, M., Hyatt, M. A., James-Ellison, M., Lyons, R. A., Maddocks, A., Paranjothy, S., Rodgers, S. E., & Dunstan, F. (2013). Do children who move home and school frequently have poorer educational outcomes in their early years at school? An anonymised cohort study. *PLoS One*, **8**(8), e70601. https://doi.org/10.1371/journal.pone.0070601

Hutchings, J., Bywater, T., Daley, D., Gardner, F., Whitaker, C., Jones, K., Eames, C., & Edwards, R. T. (2007). Parenting intervention in Sure Start services for children at risk of developing conduct disorder: Pragmatic randomised controlled trial. *BMJ*, **334**(7595), 678. https://doi.org/10.1136/bmj.39126.620799.55

Information Services Division. (2016). *Childhood admissions summary data, 2011/12–2015/16.* Edinburgh (Scotland): Information Services Division.

Irwin, L. G., Siddiqui, A., & Hertzman, C. (2007). *Early child development: A powerful equalizer.* World Health Organization. https://apps.who.int/iris/bitstream/handle/10665/69729/a91213.pdf

Jefferis, B. J., Power, C., & Hertzman, C. (2002). Birth weight, childhood socioeconomic environment, and cognitive development in the 1958 British birth cohort study. *BMJ*, **325**(7359), 305. https://doi.org/10.1136/bmj.325.7359.305

Johnson, C. D., Jones, S., & Paranjothy, S. (2016). Reducing low birth weight: Prioritizing action to address modifiable risk factors. *Journal of Public Health*, **39**(1), 122–131. https://doi.org/10.1093/pubmed/fdv212

Joseph Rowntree Foundation (2020). *UK poverty 2019/20*. https://www.jrf.org.uk/uk-poverty-2019-20

Karoly, L. A., & Bigelow, J. H. (2005). *The economics of investing in universal preschool education in California*. Rand Corporation. https://www.rand.org/content/dam/rand/pubs/monographs/2005/RAND_MG349.pdf

Kearney, M. S., & Levine, P. B. (2015). *Early childhood education by MOOC: Lessons from Sesame Street* [Working paper 21229]. National Bureau of Economic Research Working Paper Series. https://www.nber.org/system/files/working_papers/w21229/w21229.pdf

Kearney, M. S., & Levine, P. B. (2019). Early childhood education by television: Lessons from Sesame Street. *American Economic Journal: Applied Economics*, **11**(1), 318–50. https://www.doi.org/10.1257/app.20170300

Kendrick, D., Ablewhite, J., Achana, F., Benford, P., Clacy, R., Coffey, F., Cooper, N., Coupland, C., Deave, T., Goodenough, T., Hawkins, A., Hayes, M., Hindmarch, P., Hubbard, S., Kay, B., Kumar, A., Majsak-Newman, G., McColl, E., McDaid, L., … Zou, K. (2017). Keeping children safe: A multicentre programme of research to increase the evidence base for preventing unintentional injuries in the home in the under-fives. *Programme Grants for Applied Research*, **5**(14). https://doi.org/10.3310/pgfar05140

Khong, B. (2014). *The lifetime costs of attention deficit hyperactivity disorder (ADHD)*. [Masters dissertation, London School of Economics and Political Science]. Centre for Mental Health. https://www.centreformentalhealth.org.uk/wp-content/uploads/2018/11/costs_of_ADHD.pdf

Knapp, M., King, D., Healey, A., & Thomas, C. (2011). Economic outcomes in adulthood and their associations with antisocial conduct, attention deficit and anxiety problems in childhood. *Journal of Mental Health Policy and Economics*, **14**(3), 137–147. http://eprints.lse.ac.uk/id/eprint/38200

Littlecott, H. J., Moore, G. F., Moore, L., Lyons, R. A., & Murphy, S. (2016). Association between breakfast consumption and educational outcomes in 9–11-year-old children. *Public Health Nutrition*, **19**(9), 1575–1582. https://doi.org/10.1017/S1368980015002669

Livingstone, R., & Field, D. (2014). Systematic review of power mobility outcomes for infants, children and adolescents with mobility limitations. *Clinical Rehabilitation*, **28**(10), 954–964. https://doi.org/10.1177/0269215514531262

Lloyd-Williams, H. (2023). *Movin' on up? The economics of adverse childhood experiences (ACEs) in terms of health care costs and social mobility*. [Doctoral thesis, Bangor University]. Bangor University Research Portal. https://research.bangor.ac.uk/portal/files/54250031/2023Lloyd_WilliamsPhD.pdf

Lyons, M., & Ashton, J. R. (2004). Contraception, fertility and abortion services. In A. Stevens, J. Raftery, J. Mant, & S. Simpson (Eds.), *Health care needs assessment: The epidemiologically based needs assessment reviews* (2nd ed., pp. 631–676). Radcliffe Publishing.

Mares, M. L., & Pan, Z. (2013). Effects of Sesame Street: A meta-analysis of children's learning in 15 countries. *Journal of Applied Developmental Psychology*, 34(3), 140–151. https://doi.org/10.1016/j.appdev.2013.01.001

Marmot, M., Allen, J., Boyce, T., Goldblatt, P., & Morrison, J. (2020). *Health equity in England: The Marmot review 10 years on*. Institute of Health Equity. https://www.health.org.uk/publications/reports/the-marmot-review-10-years-on

Marmot, M., Allen, J., Goldblatt, P., Boyce, T., McNeish, D., Grady, M., & Geddes, I. (2010). *Fair society, healthy lives: The Marmot review. Strategic review of health inequalities in England post-2010*. https://www.instituteofhealthequity.org/resources-reports/fair-society-healthy-lives-the-marmot-review

McKechnie, D. G., O'Nions, E., Dunsmuir, S., & Petersen, I. (2023). Attention-deficit hyperactivity disorder diagnoses and prescriptions in UK primary care, 2000–2018: Population-based cohort study. *BJPsych Open*, 9(4), e121. https://doi.org/10.1192/bjo.2023.512

Meadows, P. (2011). *National evaluation of Sure Start local programmes: An economic perspective*. Research Report DFE-RR073. Department for Education. https://assets.publishing.service.gov.uk/government/uploads/system/uploads/attachment_data/file/182194/DFE-RR073.pdf

Melhuish, E. C. (2004). *A literature review of the impact of early years provision on young children, with emphasis given to children from disadvantaged backgrounds*. Institute for the Study of Children, Families & Social Issues. National Audit Office. http://media.nao.org.uk/uploads/2004/02/268_literaturereview.pdf

Miguel, P. M., Pereira, L. O., Silveira, P. P., & Meaney, M. J. (2019). Early environmental influences on the development of children's brain structure and function. *Developmental Medicine & Child Neurology*, 61(10), 1127–1133. https://doi.org/10.1111/dmcn.14182

Miles, J. (2021, 17 December). *Written statement: Extending free school meal entitlement to all primary school children*. Welsh Government. https://gov.wales/written-statement-extending-free-school-meal-entitlement-all-primary-school-children

Ministry of Housing, Communities and Local Government. (2019). *Building resilient families: Third annual report of the Troubled Families Programme 2018–19*. https://assets.publishing.service.gov.uk/government/uploads/system/uploads/attachment_data/file/790402/Troubled_Families_Programme_annual_report_2018-19.pdf

Ministry of Housing, Communities and Local Government, & The Rt Hon Lord Pickles. (2015). *Policy paper. 2010 to 2015 government policy: Support for families*. UK Government. https://www.gov.uk/government/publications/2010-to-2015-government-policy-support-for-families

Ministry of Justice, Youth Justice Board for England & Wales, Fraser, K., Raab, D., & Atkins, V. (2022, 20 May). *£300 million to cut youth crime and make streets safer* [Press release]. https://www.gov.uk/government/news/300-million-to-cut-youth-crime-and-make-streets-safer

Morris, C., Janssens, A., Allard, A., Thompson Coon, J., Shilling, V., Tomlinson, R., Williams, J., Fellowes, A., Rogers, M., Allen, K., Beresford, B., Green, G., Jenkinson, C., Tennant, A., & Logan, S. (2014). Informing the NHS Outcomes Framework: What outcomes of NHS care should be measured for children with neurodisability? *Health Services and Delivery Research*, 2(15), 1–224. https://doi.org/10.3310/hsdr02150

Morris, C., Simkiss, D., Busk, M., Morris, M., Allard, A., Denness, J., Janssens, A., Stimson, A., Coghill, J., Robinson, K., Fenton, M., & Cowan, K. (2015). Setting research priorities to improve the health of children and young people with neurodisability: A British Academy of Childhood Disability-James Lind Alliance Research Priority Setting Partnership. *BMJ Open*, 5(1), e006233. https://doi.org/10.1136/bmjopen-2014-006233

National Assembly for Wales. (2014). *Flying Start. Research note.* https://dera.ioe.ac.uk/23963/1/rn14-005-English.pdf

National Health Service. (2021, 24 December). *Treatment. Attention deficit hyperactivity disorder (ADHD).* https://www.nhs.uk/conditions/attention-deficit-hyperactivity-disorder-adhd/treatment/

National Health Service Digital. (2020, 22 October). *Mental health of children and young people in England, 2020: Wave 1 follow up to the 2017 survey.* https://digital.nhs.uk/data-and-information/publications/statistical/mental-health-of-children-and-young-people-in-england/2020-wave-1-follow-up

National Health Service Digital. (2022, 29 September). *Childhood vaccination coverage statistics—England, 2021–22.* https://digital.nhs.uk/data-and-information/publications/statistical/nhs-immunisation-statistics/2021-22

National Institute for Health and Care Excellence. (2013a). *Antisocial behaviour and conduct disorders in children and young people: Recognition and management* (CG158). https://www.nice.org.uk/guidance/cg158

National Institute for Health and Care Excellence. (2013b). *Antisocial behaviour and conduct disorders in children and young people: Costing report* (CG158). https://www.nice.org.uk/guidance/cg158

National Institute for Health and Care Excellence. (2015a). *Healthy start vitamins: Special report on cost effectiveness* (ECD5). https://www.nice.org.uk/corporate/ecd5

National Institute for Health and Care Excellence. (2015b). *Obesity prevention. Clinical guideline* (CG43). https://www.nice.org.uk/guidance/cg43/

National Institute for Health and Care Excellence. (2020). *Antenatal and postnatal mental health: Clinical management and service guidance* (CG192). https://www.nice.org.uk/guidance/cg192

National Institute for Health and Care Excellence. (2022, November). *Attentive deficit hyperactivity disorder: How common is it?* https://cks.nice.org.uk/topics/attention-deficit-hyperactivity-disorder/background-information/prevalence/

National Institute for Health and Care Excellence. (2023, June). *Immunizations—childhood: What is the routine immunization schedule?* https://cks.nice.org.uk/topics/immunizations-childhood/background-information/the-routine-childhood-immunization-schedule/

National Society for the Prevention of Cruelty to Children. (2021). *Statistics briefing: Looked after children.* https://learning.nspcc.org.uk/media/1622/statistics-briefing-looked-after-children.pdf

National Society for the Prevention of Cruelty to Children. (2023, 17 May). *Looked after children.* https://learning.nspcc.org.uk/children-and-families-at-risk/looked-after-children

National Treatment Agency for Substance Misuse. (2014). *Alcohol and drugs prevention, treatment and recovery: Why invest?* Public Health England. https://app.box.com/s/p52mrjh78yryshd9smogm350s7ouggll

Newlands, R. (2022, 25 September). *Glasgow school uniform bank makes plea ahead of winter.* Glasgow Times. https://www.glasgowtimes.co.uk/news/scottish-news/22639028.glasgow-school-uniform-bank-makes-plea-ahead-winter/

Newman, T. (2002). *Promoting resilience: A review of effective strategies for child care services—summary*. Barnardo's. https://nursingacademy.com/wp-content/uploads/2020/01/promotingresiliencenewman.pdf

Nicol, S., Garrett, H., Woodfine, L., Watkins, G., & Woodham, A. (2019). *The full cost of poor housing in Wales*. Building Research Establishment Ltd. Public Health Wales. Welsh Government. https://phw.nhs.wales/news/the-cost-of-poor-housing-in-wales/the-full-cost-of-poor-housing-in-wales/

Nuffield Trust. (2023, 17 August). *Low birth weight*. https://www.nuffieldtrust.org.uk/resource/low-birth-weight

Nykjaer, C., Alwan, N. A., Greenwood, D. C., Simpson, N. A., Hay, A. W., White, K. L., & Cade, J. E. (2014). Maternal alcohol intake prior to and during pregnancy and risk of adverse birth outcomes: Evidence from a British cohort. *Journal of Epidemiology and Community Health*, **68**(6), 542–549. http://dx.doi.org/10.1136/jech-2013-202934

Office for National Statistics. (2020, 4 March). *Conceptions in England and Wales: 2018*. https://www.ons.gov.uk/peoplepopulationandcommunity/birthsdeathsandmarriages/conceptionandfertilityrates/bulletins/conceptionstatistics/2018#teenage-conceptions

Office for National Statistics. (2022, 14 October). *Obesity and mortality during the coronavirus (COVID-19) pandemic, England: 24 January 2020 to August 2022*. https://www.ons.gov.uk/peoplepopulationandcommunity/birthsdeathsandmarriages/deaths/articles/obesityandmortalityduringthecoronaviruscovid19pandemicengland24january2020to30august2022/24january2020to30august2022/pdf

Office for National Statistics. (2023a, 30 March). *Conceptions in England and Wales: 2021*. https://www.ons.gov.uk/peoplepopulationandcommunity/birthsdeathsandmarriages/conceptionandfertilityrates/bulletins/conceptionstatistics/2021

Office for National Statistics. (2023b, 20 September). *CPI annual rate 01: Food and non-alcohol beverages 2015=100*. https://www.ons.gov.uk/economy/inflationandpriceindices/timeseries/d7g8/mm23

Olds, D. L., Kitzman, H. J., Cole, R. E., Hanks, C. A., Arcoleo, K. J., Anson, E. A., Luckey, D. W., Knudtson, M. D., Henderson, C. R., Bondy, J., & Stevenson, A. J. (2010). Enduring effects of prenatal and infancy home visiting by nurses on maternal life course and government spending: Follow-up of a randomized trial among children at age 12 years. *Archives of Pediatrics & Adolescent Medicine*, **164**(5), 419–424. https://doi.org/10.1001/archpediatrics.2010.49

Organisation for Economic Co-operation and Development. (2011). *Investing in high-quality early childhood education and care (ECEC)*. https://www.oecd.org/education/school/48980282.pdf

Paes de Barros, R., & Mendonca, R. (1999). *Costs and benefits of preschool education in Brazil*. Institute of Applied Economic Research.

Penn, J. V., & Thomas, C. (2005). Practice parameter for the assessment and treatment of youth in juvenile detention and correctional facilities. *Journal of the American Academy of Child & Adolescent Psychiatry*, **44**(10), 1085–1098. https://doi.org/10.1097/01.chi.0000175325.14481.21

Perry, B. D. (2002). Childhood experience and the expression of genetic potential: What childhood neglect tells us about nature and nurture. *Brain and Mind*, **3**(1), 79–100. https://doi.org/10.1023/A:1016557824657

Phillips, C. J., Humphreys, I., Kendrick, D., Stewart, J., Hayes, M., Nish, L., Stone, D., Coupland, C., & Towner, E. (2011). Preventing bath water scalds: A cost-effectiveness analysis of introducing bath thermostatic mixer valves in social housing. *Injury Prevention*, 17(4), 238–243. http://dx.https://doi.org/10.1136/ip.2010.031393

Pillas, D., Marmot, M., Naicker, K., Goldblatt, P., Morrison, J., & Pikhart, H. (2014). Social inequalities in early childhood health and development: A European-wide systematic review. *Pediatric Research*, 76(5), 418–424. https://doi.org/10.1038/pr.2014.122

Pine, C. M., Adair, P. M., Burnside, G., Brennan, L., Sutton, L., Edwards, R. T., Ezeofor, V., Albadri, S., Curnow, M. M., Deery, C., Hosey, M. T., Willis-Lake, J., Lynn, J., Parry, J., & Wong, F. S. L. (2020). Dental RECUR randomized trial to prevent caries recurrence in children. *Journal of Dental Research*, 99(2), 168–174. https://doi.org/10.1177/00220 34519886808

Pitman, R. J., Nagy, L. D., & Sculpher, M. J. (2013). Cost-effectiveness of childhood influenza vaccination in England and Wales: Results from a dynamic transmission model. *Vaccine*, 31(6), 927–942. https://doi.org/10.1016/j.vaccine.2012.12.010

Pokhrel, S., Quigley, M. A., Fox-Rushby, J., McCormick, F., Williams, A., Trueman, P., Dodds, R., & Renfrew, M. J. (2015). Potential economic impacts from improving breastfeeding rates in the UK. *Archives of Disease in Childhood*, 100(4), 334–340. https://doi.org/10.1136/archdischild-2014-306701

Polanczyk, G. V., Salum, G. A., Sugaya, L. S., Caye, A., & Rohde, L. A. (2015). Annual research review: A meta-analysis of the worldwide prevalence of mental disorders in children and adolescents. *Journal of Child Psychology and Psychiatry*, 56(3), 345–365. https://doi.org/10.1111/jcpp.12381

Polańska, K., Jurewicz, J., & Hanke, W. (2015). Smoking and alcohol drinking during pregnancy as the risk factors for poor child neurodevelopment—a review of epidemiological studies. *International Journal of Occupational Medicine and Environmental Health*, 28(3), 419. http://dx.doi.org/10.13075/ijomeh.1896.00424

Price Waterhouse Coopers. (2016). *International Women's Day: PwC Women in Work Index*. https://www.pwc.co.uk/economic-services/assets/PwC-Women-in-Work-2016-FINAL-3.pdf

Public Health England. (2015). *Healthy child programme: Rapid review to update evidence*. https://www.gov.uk/government/publications/healthy-child-programme-rapid-review-to-update-evidence

Public Health England. (2017a, 14 June). *Health matters: Child dental health*. https://www.gov.uk/government/publications/health-matters-child-dental-health/health-matters-child-dental-health

Public Health England. (2017b). *Guidance: Health matters: Obesity and the food environment*. https://www.gov.uk/government/publications/health-matters-obesity-and-the-food-environment

Public Health England. (2018a). *Contraception: Economic analysis estimation of the return on investment (ROI) for publicly funded contraception in England*. https://assets.publish ing.service.gov.uk/government/uploads/system/uploads/attachment_data/file/730292/contraception_return_on_investment_report.pdf

Public Health England. (2018b). *Reducing unintentional injuries in and around the home among children under five years*. https://assets.publishing.service.gov.uk/government/

uploads/system/uploads/attachment_data/file/696646/Unintentional_injuries_under_fives_in_home.pdf

Public Health England. (2021). Impact of COVID-19 on routine childhood immunisations: Early vaccine coverage data to June 2021 in England. https://assets.pub lishing.service.gov.uk/government/uploads/system/uploads/attachment_data/file/1010 976/hpr1421_chldhd-vc.pdf

Renfrew, M. J., Pokhrel, S., Quigley, M., McCormick, F., Fox-Rushby, J., Dodds, R., Duffy, S., Trueman, P., & Williams, A. (2012). *Preventing disease and saving resources: The potential contribution of increasing breastfeeding rates in the UK.* https://www.unicef.org.uk/wp-content/uploads/sites/2/2012/11/Preventing_disea se_saving_resources.pdf

Rolnick, A., & Grunewald, R. (2003). Early childhood development: Economic development with a high public return. *The Region, 17*(4), 6–12.

Royal College of Surgeons. (2015). *The state of children's oral health in England.* https:// www.rcseng.ac.uk/-/media/files/rcs/about-rcs/government-relations-consultation/ childrens-oral-health-report-final.pdf

Royal Society for the Prevention of Accidents. (2012). *The big book of accident prevention.* https://www.rospa.com/rospaweb/docs/advice-services/public-health/big-book.pdf

Royal Society for the Prevention of Accidents. (2013). *Delivering accident prevention at local level in the new public health system Part 1: Context.* Public Health England. https:// www.rospa.com/rospaweb/docs/advice-services/public-health/delivering-accident-pre vention-context.pdf

Saied-Tessier, A. (2014). *Estimating the costs of child sexual abuse in the UK.* NSPCC. https:// library.nspcc.org.uk/heritagescripts/hapi.dll/search2

Parsonage, M. (2009). *The chance of a lifetime. Preventing early conduct problems and reducing crime.* Sainsbury Centre for Mental Health. https://www.researchgate.net/publ ication/308383127_The_chance_of_a_lifetime_preventing_early_conduct_problems_ and_reducing_crime

Sampaio, F., Feldman, I., Lavelle, T. A., & Skokauskas, N. (2021). The cost-effectiveness of treatments for attention deficit-hyperactivity disorder and autism spectrum disorder in children and adolescents: A systematic review. *European Child & Adolescent Psychiatry, 31*(11), 1655–1670. https://doi.org/10.1007/s00787-021-01748-z

Scarborough, P., Bhatnagar, P., Wickramasinghe, K. K., Allender, S., Foster, C., & Rayner, M. (2011). The economic burden of ill health due to diet, physical inactivity, smoking, alcohol and obesity in the UK: An update to 2006–07 NHS costs. *Journal of Public Health, 33*(4), 527–535. https://doi.org/10.1093/pubmed/fdr033

Schweinhart, L. J., Montie, J., Xiang, Z., Barnett, W. S., Belfield, C. R., & Nores, M. (2005). *The High/Scope Perry preschool study through age 40. Summary, conclusions, and frequently asked questions.* High/Scope Press. https://nieer.org/wp-content/uploads/ 2014/09/specialsummary_rev2011_02_2.pdf

Scottish Government. (2022). *Early education and care.* https://www.gov.scot/policies/early-education-and-care/early-learning-and-childcare/

Scottish Government Social Research. (2011). *Evaluation of Big Noise, Sistema Scotland.* https://www.makeabignoise.org.uk/files/5514/9749/1161/0114922.pdf

Shonkoff, J. P., & Phillips, D. A. (Eds.). (2000). *From neurons to neighborhoods: The science of early childhood development.* National Academies Press.

Sibieta, L. (2021, 1 February). *The crisis in lost learning calls for a massive national policy response*. Institute for Fiscal Studies. https://www.ifs.org.uk/publications/15291

Sidebotham, P., Fraser, J., Covington, T., Freemantle, J., Petrou, S., Pulikottil-Jacob, R., Cutler, T., & Ellis, C. (2014). Understanding why children die in high-income countries. *The Lancet*, 384(9946), 915–927. https://doi.org/10.1016/S0140-6736(14)60581-X

Skivington, K., Matthews, L., Simpson, S. A., Craig, P., Baird, J., Blazeby, J. M., Boyd, K. A., Craig, N., French, D. P., McIntosh, E., Petticrew, M., Rycroft-Malone, J., White, M., & Moore, L. (2021). A new framework for developing and evaluating complex interventions: Update of Medical Research Council guidance. *BMJ*, 374(2061). http://dx.doi.org/10.1136/bmj.n206

Social Research Unit. (2013a). *Family Nurse Partnership*. The Social Research Unit at Dartington. https://archive.dartington.org.uk/projects/family_nurse_partnership__3

Social Research Unit. (2013b). *Investing in children*. The Social Research Unit at Dartington. http://investinginchildren.eu

Stevens, K. (2012). Valuation of the child health utility 9D index. *Pharmacoeconomics*, 30(8), 729–747. https://doi.org/10.2165/11599120-000000000-00000

Suhrcke, M., & Kenkel, D. (2015). Social determinants of health: Early childhood development and education. In D. McDaid, F. Sassi, & S. Merkur (Eds.), *Promoting health, preventing disease* (pp. 237–258). Open University Press.

Sylva, K., Melhuish, E. C., Sammons, P., Siraj-Blatchford, I., & Taggart, B. (2004). *The Effective Provision of Pre-School Education (EPPE) Project: Findings from pre-school to end of key stage 1*. SureStart/DfES. https://dera.ioe.ac.uk/18189/2/SSU-SF-2004-01.pdf

Tatla, S. K., Sauve, K., Virji-Babul, N., Holsti, L., Butler, C., & Van Der Loos, H. F. M. (2013). Evidence for outcomes of motivational rehabilitation interventions for children and adolescents with cerebral palsy: An American Academy for Cerebral Palsy and Developmental Medicine systematic review. *Developmental Medicine & Child Neurology*, 55(7), 593–601. https://doi.org/10.1111/dmcn.12147

Thomas, R., Sanders, S., Doust, J., Beller, E., & Glasziou, P. (2015). Prevalence of attention-deficit/hyperactivity disorder: A systematic review and meta-analysis. *Pediatrics*, 135(4), e994–e1001. https://doi.org/10.1542/peds.2014-3482

Tyrrell, E., & Prasad, V. (2021). Risk and prevention of unintentional injuries in children and young people with attention-deficit/hyperactivity disorder. *Paediatrics and Child Health*, 31(10), 371–375. https://doi.org/10.1016/j.paed.2021.07.001

Uchiyama, I., Anderson, D. I., Campos, J. J., Witherington, D., Frankel, C. B., Lejeune, L., & Barbu-Roth, M. (2008). Locomotor experience affects self and emotion. *Developmental Psychology*, 44(5), 1225. https://doi.org/10.1037/a0013224

United Kingdom Government. (2017, 20 January). *Childhood obesity: A plan for action*. https://www.gov.uk/government/publications/childhood-obesity-a-plan-for-action/childhood-obesity-a-plan-for-action

United Kingdom Government. (2021, 30 March). *Free school meals: Autumn term*. https://explore-education-statistics.service.gov.uk/find-statistics/free-school-meals-autumn-term/2020-21-autumn-term

United Kingdom Government. (2022a, 30 June). *Education provision: Childcare under 5 years of age*. https://explore-education-statistics.service.gov.uk/find-statistics/education-provision-children-under-5

United Kingdom Government. (2022b, 27 July). *Children's social care 2022: Recovering from the COVID-19 pandemic.* https://www.gov.uk/government/publications/childrens-soc ial-care-2022-recovering-from-the-covid-19-pandemic/childrens-social-care-2022-rec overing-from-the-covid-19-pandemic

United Kingdom Parliament. (2016, 22 January). *Written evidence submitted by the sexual health charity, FPA (CSR0030).* https://committees.parliament.uk/writtenevidence/ 63263/html/

United Kingdom Parliament. (2023, 6 April). *Poverty in the UK: Statistics.* House of Commons Library. https://commonslibrary.parliament.uk/research-briefings/sn07096/

United Nations Children's Fund. (2007). *An overview of child well-being in rich countries: A comprehensive assessment of the lives and well-being of children and adolescents in the economically advanced nations.* https://www.unicef-irc.org/publications/pdf/rc7_eng.pdf

United Nations Children's Fund. (2021, 31 July). *Breastmilk is the best protection for babies against infections during COVID-19, says UNICEF.* https://www.unicef.org/thailand/ press-releases/breastmilk-best-protection-babies-against-infections-during-covid-19- says-unicef

Verbeke, E., Bogaerts, A., Nuyts, T., Crombag, N., & Luyten, J. (2022). Cost-effectiveness of mental health interventions during and after pregnancy: A systematic review. *Birth,* **49**(3), 364–402. https://doi.org/10.1111/birt.12623

Vibert, S. (2018). *Your attention please: The social and economic impact of ADHD.* Demos. https://demos.co.uk/wp-content/uploads/2018/02/Your-Attention-Please-the-social- and-economic-impact-of-ADHD-.pdf

Victora, C. G., Bahl, R., Barros, A. J., França, G. V., Horton, S., Krasevec, J., Murch, S., Sankar, M. J., Walker, N., & Rollins, N. C. (for The Lancet Breastfeeding Series Group). (2016). Breastfeeding in the 21st century: Epidemiology, mechanisms, and lifelong effect. *The Lancet,* **387**(10017), 475–490. https://doi.org/10.1016/ S0140-6736(15)01024-7

Vinovskis, M. A. (2005). *The birth of Head Start: Preschool education policies in the Kennedy and Johnson Administrations.* University of Chicago Press.

Walker, S. P., Wachs, T. D., Grantham-McGregor, S., Black, M. M., Nelson, C. A., Huffman, S. L., Baker-Henningham, H., Chang, S. M., Hamadani, J. D., Lozoff, B. Gardner, J. M. M., Powell, C. A., Rahman, A., & Richter, L. (2011). Inequality in early childhood: Risk and protective factors for early child development. *The Lancet,* **378**(9799), 1325–1338. https://doi.org/10.1016/S0140-6736(11)60555-2

Wasserman, G. A., & Seracini, A. G. (2001). Family risk factors and interventions. In R. Loeber & D. P. Farrington (Eds.), *Child delinquents: Development, intervention, and service needs* (pp. 165–189). Sage Publications.

Watson, J., Hennessy, S., & Vignoles, A. (2021). The relationship between educational television and mathematics capability in Tanzania. *British Journal of Educational Technology,* **52**(2), 638–658. https://doi.org/10.1111/bjet.13047

Watson. J., & McIntyre, N. (2020). *Educational television: A rapid evidence review.* EdTech Hub. https://docs.edtechhub.org/lib/BVXSZ7G4/download/D8HI7KPH/Educatio nal%20Television_A%20Rapid%20Evidence%20Review_Final.pdf

Watson, J., & Tully, L. (2008). *Prevention and early intervention update—trends in recent research. Literature review.* NSW Department of Community Services. https://www.facs. nsw.gov.au/__data/assets/pdf_file/0015/321603/research_earlyintervention.pdf

Weatherly, H., Drummond, M., Claxton, K., Cookson, R., Ferguson, B., Godfrey, C., Rice, N., Sculpher, M., & Sowden, A. (2009). Methods for assessing the cost-effectiveness of public health interventions: Key challenges and recommendations. *Health Policy*, 93(2-3), 85–92. https://doi.org/10.1016/j.healthpol.2009.07.012

Welsh Government. (2021, 4 November). *Experimental statistics: Children looked after by local authorities, 2020–21.* Statistics for Wales. https://gov.wales/sites/default/files/statist ics-and-research/2021-11/children-looked-after-local-authorities-april-2020-march-2021-experimental-statistics-396.pdf

Welsh Government. (2022, 18 November). *Phased expansion of early years provision.* https://gov.wales/phased-expansion-early-years-provision

White, D., Raeside, R., & Barker, D. (2000). *Road accidents and children living in disadvantaged areas: A literature review.* The Scottish Government. http://docs.scie-socialcareonline.org.uk/fulltext/roadacci.pdf

Whitehead, M., Taylor-Robinson, D., & Barr, B. (2021). Poverty, health, and covid-19. *BMJ*, 372(376). https://doi.org/10.1136/bmj.n376

Wickham, S., Anwar, E., Barr, B., Law, C., & Taylor-Robinson, D. (2016). Poverty and child health in the UK: Using evidence for action. *Archives of Disease in Childhood*, 101(8), 759–766. http://dx.doi.org/10.1136/archdischild-2014-306746

Wilkins, M., & Farmer, E. (2015). *Reunification: An evidence-informed framework for return home practice.* NSPCC. https://proceduresonline.com/trixcms/media/1868/reunificat ion-practice-framework-guidance-3.pdf

Wilkinson, J., & Bowyer, S. (2017). *The impacts of abuse and neglect on children; and comparison of different placement options.* Department for Education. https://assets.pub lishing.service.gov.uk/government/uploads/system/uploads/attachment_data/file/602 148/Childhood_neglect_and_abuse_comparing_placement_options.pdf

Wilson, K. (2013). *The orchestra, the community and cultural value.* Institute for Cultural Capital. https://iccliverpool.ac.uk/wp-content/uploads/2014/05/IHLRN-interim-rep ort-KW-July-2013.pdf

Winrow, E., & Edwards, R. T. (2018). *Social return on investment of Sistema Cymru—Codi'r To.* Centre for Health Economics and Medicines Evaluation, Bangor University. https:// cheme.bangor.ac.uk/documents/Codi'r%20To%20(English)%20.pdf

Woodfine, L., Neal, R. D., Bruce, N., Edwards, R. T., Linck, P., Mullock, L., Nelhans, N., Pasterfield, D., Russell, D., & Russell, I. (2011). Enhancing ventilation in homes of children with asthma: Pragmatic randomised controlled trial. *British Journal of General Practice*, 61(592), e724–e732. https://doi.org/10.3399/bjgp11X606636

World Bank. (2020). *Investing in the early years during COVID-19.* World Bank. https:// openknowledge.worldbank.org/handle/10986/33647

World Health Organization. (2023). *Maternal mental health.* https://www.who.int/teams/ mental-health-and-substance-use/promotion-prevention/maternal-mental-health

Wright, J. C., Huston, A. C., Scantlin, R., & Kotler, J. (2001). The early window project: Sesame Street prepares children for school. In S. Fisch & R. Truglio (Eds.), *'G' is for growing: Thirty years of research on Sesame Street* (pp. 97–114). Lawrence Erlbaum Associates, Inc.

Wu, E. Q., Hodgkins, P., Ben-Hamadi, R., Setyawan, J., Xie, J., Sikirica, V., Du, E. X., Yan, S. Y., & Erder, M. H. (2012). Cost effectiveness of pharmacotherapies for attention-deficit hyperactivity disorder. *CNS Drugs*, 26(7), 581–600. https://doi.org/10.2165/ 11633900-000000000-00000

Young, S., Asherson, P., Lloyd, T., Absoud, M., Arif, M., Colley, W. A., Cortese, S., Cubbin, S., Doyle, N., Morua, S. D., Ferreira-Lay, P., Gudjonsson, G., Ivens, V., Jarvis, C., Lewis, A., Mason, P., Newlove-Delgado, T., Pitts, M., Read, H., . . . Skirrow, C. (2021). Failure of healthcare provision for attention-deficit/hyperactivity disorder in the United Kingdom: A consensus statement. *Frontiers in Psychiatry*, **12**, 649399. https://doi.org/10.3389/fpsyt.2021.649399

Youth Justice Board & Ministry of Justice. (2019). *Youth justice statistics 2017/18: England and Wales*. Ministry of Justice. https://assets.publishing.service.gov.uk/government/uploads/system/uploads/attachment_data/file/774866/youth_justice_statistics_bulletin_2017_2018.pdf

Youth Justice Board & Ministry of Justice. (2020). *Youth justice statistics 2018/19: England and Wales*. Ministry of Justice. https://assets.publishing.service.gov.uk/government/uploads/system/uploads/attachment_data/file/862078/youth-justice-statistics-bulletin-march-2019.pdf

Youth Justice Board & Ministry of Justice. (2022). *Youth justice statistics 2020/21: England and Wales*. Ministry of Justice. https://assets.publishing.service.gov.uk/government/uploads/system/uploads/attachment_data/file/1054236/Youth_Justice_Statistics_2020-21.pdf

Zhou, F., Reef, S., Massoudi, M., Yusuf, H. R., Bardenheier, B., & Zimmerman, L. (2004). An economic analysis of the current universal 2-dose measles-mumps-rubella vaccination program in the United States. *The Journal of Infectious Diseases*, **189**(S1), S131–S145. https://doi.org/10.1086/378987

Chapter 4

The Well-being and Well-becoming of Adolescents and Young Adults

Alexander Torbuck, Eira Winrow, Huw Lloyd-Williams, Catherine L. Lawrence, and Rhiannon T. Edwards

Introduction

In Chapter 3, we focused on the health benefits and some evidence of the economic benefits of investing in the early years. In this chapter, we focus on the well-being and well-becoming of adolescents and young adults. The World Health Organization (WHO; 2023) defines 'adolescents' as individuals aged between ten and nineteen years, while the Office for National Statistics (ONS; 2021) defines 'young people' as individuals aged between sixteen and twenty-four years. This chapter is relevant to individuals spanning these age groups. The transition from adolescence to young adulthood involves biological and psychological development and maturation. There are a number of models of the determinants of well-being at various stages of life. This chapter is structured around the following domains of adolescent well-being proposed by Ross and colleagues (2020):

- good health and optimum nutrition;
- connectedness, positive values, and contribution to society;
- safety and a supportive environment;
- learning, competence, education, skills, and employability; and
- agency and resilience.

Table 4.1 expands on these domains by highlighting the subdomains and requirements necessary that underpin the adolescent well-being framework proposed by Ross and colleagues (2020).

Alexander Torbuck, Eira Winrow, Huw Lloyd-Williams, Catherine L. Lawrence, and Rhiannon T. Edwards, *The Well-being and Well-becoming of Adolescents and Young Adults* In: *Health Economics of Well-being and Well-becoming across the Life-course*. Edited by: Rhiannon T. Edwards, and Catherine L. Lawrence, Oxford University Press. © Oxford University Press 2024. DOI: 10.1093/9780191919336.003.0004

Table 4.1 The five domains of adolescent well-being that underpin the adolescent well-being framework

No.	Domain	Subdomains	Requirements include	Type of well-being
1.	Good health and optimum nutrition	• Physical health and capacities. • Mental health and capacities. • Optimal nutritional status and diet.	• Information, care, and services; access to valid and relevant information and affordable age-appropriate, high-quality, welcoming health services, care, and support, including for self-care. • Healthy environment such as: safe water supply, hygiene, sanitation and without undue danger of injury in the home, safe roads, management of toxic substances in the home and community, access to safe greenspaces, and no air pollution, skills to navigate the environment safely. • Physical activity: access to opportunities for adequate physical activity. • Diet: Has access to local, culturally acceptable, adequate, diversified, balanced, and healthy diet commensurate to the individual's characteristics and requirements, to protect from all forms of malnutrition.	Physical Nutritional Emotional Sociocultural
2.	Connectedness, positive values, and contribution to society	• Connectedness: being part of positive social and cultural networks and having positive, meaningful relationships with others, including family, peers, and, where relevant, teachers and employers. • Valued and respected by others and accepted as part of the community. • Attitudes: responsible, caring, and has respect for others. Has a sense of ethics, integrity, and morality.	• Connectedness: has access to opportunities to become part of positive social and cultural networks and to develop positive, meaningful relationships with others, including family, peers, and, where relevant, teachers and employers. • Valued: has access to opportunities to be involved in decision-making and having their opinions taken seriously, with increasing spaces to influence and engage with their environment commensurate with their evolving capacities and stage of development.	Emotional Sociocultural

- Interpersonal skills: has empathy, friendship skills, and sensitivity.
- Activity: socially, culturally, and civically active.
- Change and development: equipped to contribute to change and development in their own lives and/or in their communities.

- Attitudes: has access to opportunities to develop personal responsibility, caring and respect for others, and a sense of ethics, integrity, and morality.
- Interpersonal skills: has access to opportunities to develop empathy, friendship skills, and sensitivity.
- Activity: has access to opportunities to be socially, culturally, and civically active that are appropriate to their evolving capacities and stages of development.
- Change and development: has access to opportunities to develop the skills to be equipped to contribute to change and development in their own lives and/or in their communities.

3. Safety and a supportive environment

- Safety: emotional and physical safety.
- Material conditions in the physical environment are met.
- Equity: treated fairly and have an equal chance in life.
- Equality: equal distribution of power, resources, rights, and opportunities for all.
- Non-discrimination.
- Privacy.
- Responsive: enriching the opportunities available to the adolescent.

- Safety: has protection from all forms of violence and from exploitative commercial interests in families, communities, among peers and in schools, and the social and virtual environment.
- Material conditions: the adolescent's rights to food and nutrition, water, housing, heating, clothing, and physical security are met.
- Equity: there is a supportive legal framework and policies and equitable access to valid and relevant information, products, and high-quality services.
- Equality: positive social norms, including gender norms, to ensure equal rights and opportunities for all adolescents.
- Non-discrimination: is free to practise personal, cultural, and spiritual beliefs and to express their identity in a non-discriminatory environment and have the liberty to access objective, factual information and services without being exposed to judgemental attitudes.

Physical
Emotional
Sociocultural

(continued)

Table 4.1 Continued

No.	Domain	Subdomains	Requirements include	Type of well-being
			• Privacy: their personal information, views, interpretations, fears, and decisions, including those stored online, are not shared or disclosed without the adolescent's permission. • Responsive: has access to a wide range of safe and stimulating opportunities for leisure or personal development.	
4.	Learning, competence, education, skills, and employability	• Learning: has the commitment to, and motivation for, continual learning. • Education. • Resources, life skills, and competencies: has the necessary cognitive, social, creative, and emotional resources; skills (life/decision-making) and competencies to thrive, including knowing their rights and how to claim them; and how to plan and make choices. • Skills: acquisition of technical, vocational, business, and creative skills to be able to take advantage of current or future economic, cultural, and social opportunities. • Employability. • Confidence that they can do things well.	• Learning: receives support to develop the commitment to, and motivation for, continual learning. • Education: has access to formal education until age sixteen and opportunities for learning through formal or non-formal education or training and beyond. • Resources, life skills, and competencies: has opportunities to develop the resources, skills (life/decision-making), and competencies to thrive. • Skills: has opportunities to develop relevant technical, vocational, business, and creative skills. • Employability: is given the opportunities to participate in non-exploitative and sustainable livelihoods and/or entrepreneurship appropriate for their age and stage of development. • Confidence: is given the necessary encouragement and opportunities to develop self-confidence and is empowered to feel that they can do things well.	Emotional Cognitive

| 5. | Agency and resilience | • Agency: has self-esteem, a sense of agency and of being empowered to make meaningful choices and to influence their social, political, and material environment; and has the capacity for self-expression and self-direction appropriate to their evolving capacities and stage of development.
• Identity: feels comfortable in their own self and with their identity(s), including their physical, cultural, social, sexual, and gender identity.
• Purpose: has a sense of purpose, desire to succeed and optimism about the future.
• Resilience: equipped to handle adversities both now and in the future, in a way that is appropriate to their evolving capacities and stage of development.
• Fulfilment: feels that they are fulfilling their potential now and that they will be able to do so in the future. | • Agency: has opportunities to develop self-esteem, a sense of agency, the ability to make meaningful choices and to influence their social, political, and material environment, for self-expression and self-direction.
• Identity: has the safe space to develop clarity and comfort in their own self and their identity(s), including their physical, cultural, social, sexual, and gender identity.
• Purpose: has opportunities to develop a sense of purpose, desire to succeed, and optimism about the future.
• Resilience: has opportunities to develop the ability to handle adversities both now and in the future, in a way that is appropriate to their evolving capacities and stage of development
• Fulfilment: has opportunities to fulfil their potential now and to be able to do so in the future. | Emotional
Cognitive |

Adapted from Ross, D. A., Hinton, R., Melles-Brewer, M., Engel, D., Zeck, W., Fagan, L., Herat, J., Phaladi, G., Imbago-Jácome, D., Anyona, P., Sanchez, A., Damji, N., Terki, F., Baltag, V., Patton, G., Silverman, A., Fogstad, H., Banerjee, A., & Mohan, A. (2020). Adolescent well-being: A definition and conceptual framework. *Journal of Adolescent Health*, 67(4), 472–476. Copyright © 2020 with permission from Elsevier.

Health behaviours

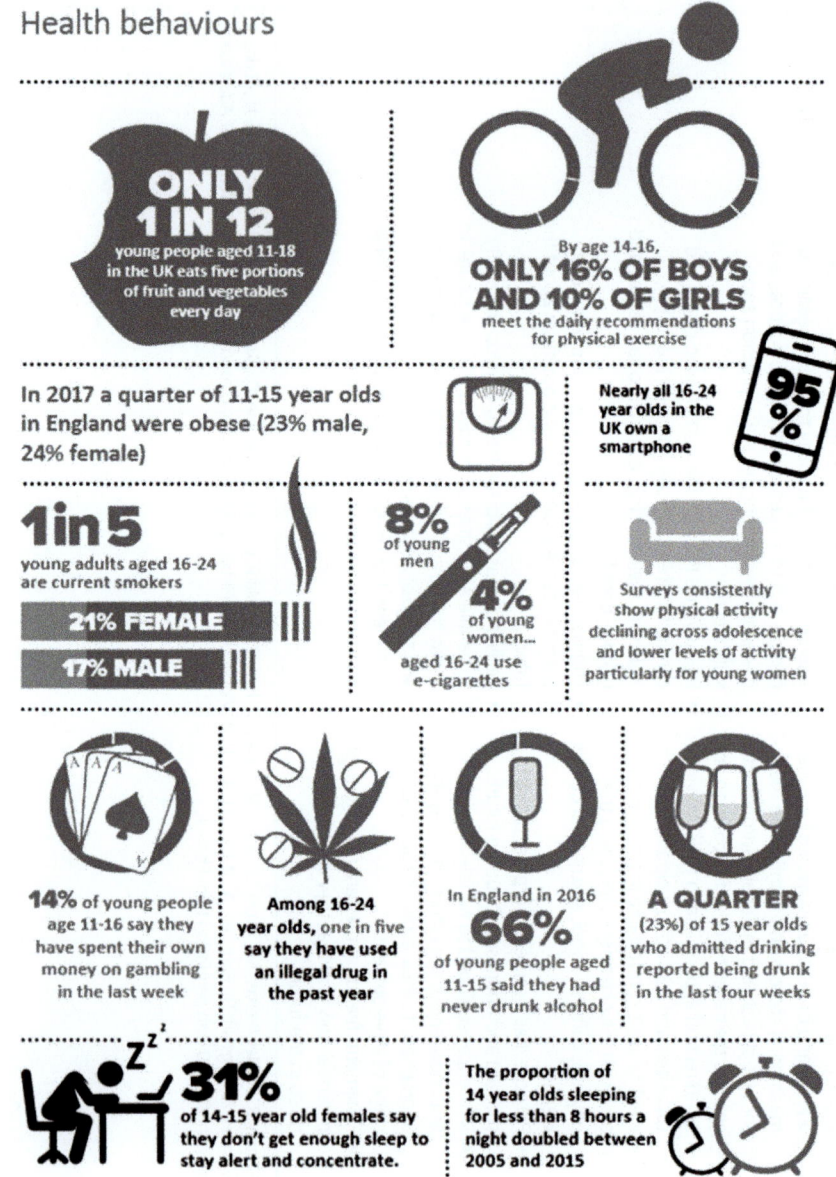

Figure 4.1 Health behaviours in young people
Reproduced from Hagell, A., & Shah, R. (2019). *Highlights: Key data on young people 2019*. Association for Young People's Health. https://www.active-together.org/files/68190/ayph-kdyp2 019-fullversion.pdf. Copyright © AYPH 2019 with permission.

There are over 11.8 million young people aged between ten and twenty-four years in the United Kingdom (UK) (Clark, 2023a, 2023b, 2023c, 2023d). Investing in the health and well-being of adolescents and young people is important because life-long lifestyle and health behaviours, such as diet and exercise habits, are established during this life-stage (see Figure 4.1). These health behaviours can affect health outcomes, including cancer, heart disease, and type 2 diabetes, right through the life-course (Hagell & Shah, 2019). There is a wider economic argument for understanding health behaviour in young people and the wider determinants at play as the consequences of poor health can have both a short-term and long-term cost. However, the role of prevention and early intervention during this life-stage is not a visibly major policy priority at present despite growing evidence that intervening during adolescence can prevent health issues from developing (Hagell & Rigby, 2015).

Good Health and Good Nutrition

The mortality rate for young people has fallen since the 1990s. The most common causes of death in young people include accidents, suicide, and cancer (Hagell & Shah, 2019; ONS, 2022a). In this section we consider the mental health, physical health, and sexual health of young people, and draw on systematic review evidence and cost-effectiveness evidence where relevant.

Mental health

Prior to the coronavirus disease 2019 (COVID-19) pandemic, young people were known to be regular users of health care services, with half of Year 10 pupils (aged fourteen to fifteen) reporting that they have visited their general practitioner (GP) in the last three months for mental health and/or physical health reasons (Hagell & Shah, 2019). Despite at least 10 per cent of adolescents experiencing mental health problems, only eighteen in 1,000 were seen by Child and Adolescent Mental Health Services (CAMHS) (Hagell & Shah, 2019). CAMHS is a National Health Service (NHS) provision that assesses and treats young people with emotional, behavioural, or mental health difficulties. Prior to the COVID-19 pandemic, many health services were failing to meet their waiting time targets. During the pandemic, many NHS Trusts experienced a significant demand for specialist CAMHS and saw a rise in the number of high-risk and urgent case referrals. In 2021, the Department of Health and Social Care pledged to invest an additional £2.3 billion a year into CAMHS by 2023/2024. This funding could provide an additional 345,000 children and young people with timely access to mental health support through the NHS (UK Parliament, 2021).

Deaths registered as suicide have fallen overall since the early 2000s (Hagell & Shah, 2019). There were fears that suicide rates would increase amongst adolescents during the COVID-19 pandemic; however, despite reported increases in anxiety and distress, this does not seem to have been the case (Appleby et al., 2021). Although there was an increase in the rate of deaths registered as suicide in 2021, the increase was due to a low number of deaths by suicide registered in 2020 because of the disruption to coroners' inquests caused by the COVID-19 pandemic (ONS, 2022b). The 2021 suicide rate was similar to the pre-pandemic rates in 2018 and 2019. Females aged twenty-four years or under have seen the largest increase in suicide rate since 1981, when ONS records began (ONS, 2022b).

The transition from CAMHS to adult mental health services (AMHS) can be challenging for young people (Broad et al., 2017; Mulvale et al., 2016). One of the reasons for this is the different philosophies between CAMHS and AMHS. In a systematic review of the different philosophies and their influence on the transition between services, Mulvale and colleagues (2016) described the philosophy of CAMHS as being centred around the family unit, whereas AMHS considers young people as autonomous adults, with a shift away from family involvement to give the young person privacy. In a thematic synthesis of youth experiences of transition from CAMHS to AMHS, Broad and colleagues (2017) found that the transition can be a turbulent time. This is a time when concurrent life transitions coincide with an institutionalized transition system. Making adult services more youth-friendly, responsive to individual needs, clarifying referral pathways, and promoting self-referral where possible could prevent young people from disengaging from services and returning in the future in crisis (Broad et al., 2017; Paul et al., 2015).

Physical health

The adolescent years can be a time of good health as individuals experience rapid physical, cognitive, and psychosocial development (WHO, 2021a). However, nearly a quarter of eleven to fifteen-year-olds have a long-term illness or disability and a tenth of ten to twenty-four-year-olds have a disability that impacts on their daily functioning (Hagell & Shah, 2019). For example, the most common age range for diagnosis of type 1 diabetes is eleven to fourteen years and the most common age range for diagnosis of asthma is sixteen to twenty years. Since health outcomes for adolescents with long-term health conditions are worse during the transition between child and adult services, there is a need for 'systems level' research or service evaluation about this transition period, and specifically design and evaluation of appropriate transition services (Hagell & Shah, 2019).

In a systematic review of reviews exploring the cost-effectiveness of physical activity interventions, four out of the eighteen reviews included in the systematic review focused on the target population of children and adolescents (Abu-Omar et al., 2017). Three of the reviews examined school-based physical activity interventions (Laine et al., 2014; Lehnert et al., 2012; Wu et al., 2011). Laine and colleagues (2014) and Wu and colleagues (2011) found some evidence for the cost-effectiveness of interventions (e.g. health education and improving opportunities for walking and cycling), but advised caution on generalizing the results due to the limited number of population-level studies. The review by Lehnert and colleagues (2012) found that most community interventions were cost-effective, but school-based interventions were not cost-effective (e.g. active commuting). Lewis and colleagues (2010) explored physical activity interventions in the family, home, school, and community settings. The intervention environment was found to have an important role to play in increasing physical activity levels. This review found evidence of cost-effectiveness for some interventions (e.g. dance classes and walking school bus programmes), but not for others (e.g. free swimming classes). Some interventions were found to be cost-effective only for a particular group of children (e.g. curriculum-based interventions to promote healthy diet and physical activity in girls only) (Lewis et al., 2010). From a public health perspective, further work is needed to identify which type of school-based physical activity interventions are cost-effective (Abu-Omar et al., 2017). For example, multi-component interventions that do not require the hiring of additional staff were found to be particularly cost-effective in this review (e.g. Wu et al., 2011). Another important methodological issue for researchers to consider relates to the curvilinear relationship between physical activity level and health benefits: the more active a person is prior to a physical activity intervention, the smaller the health gains experienced after undertaking the intervention (Warburton & Bredin, 2016). This curvilinear relationship should be taken into account when evaluating the cost-effectiveness of physical activity interventions (Abu-Omar et al., 2017).

Sexual health and adolescent pregnancy rates

In the UK, the average age of first heterosexual intercourse is sixteen years (Hagell & Shah, 2019). In 2021 there was no specific guidance on services to support adolescent sexual health in the UK, though the National Institute for Health and Care Excellence (NICE) impact statement and quality standards are available relating to sexual health services in general with a focus on human immunodeficiency virus (HIV) and contraceptive services (NICE, 2019a). The majority of adolescent pregnancies in England are unplanned and half result in abortion (Nuffield Trust, 2021). In the UK, conception rates in the under-eighteens were at a record level of forty-six per 1,000 women in 1999 (Department of Health, 2010). Since then, the rate has fallen by more than half to nineteen conceptions per 1,000 women. This reduction has been attributed to changes in social interaction as adolescents spend less time in physical contact with others and more time on digital media (British Pregnancy Advisory Service, 2018). However, the proportion of repeat pregnancies is still relatively high and accounts for between 12 per cent and 25 per cent of total teenage pregnancies (Public Health England, 2018). Adolescent pregnancy is associated with poorer outcomes for the parents and the children. For example, teenage mothers are more likely to be early school leavers, be a single parent, live in poverty, and have a higher risk of mental health problems than older mothers (Nuffield Trust, 2021). Babies born to teenage mothers have a 60 per cent higher risk of infant mortality, are more likely to have accidents, and more likely to experience behaviour problems than babies born to older mothers (Nuffield Trust, 2021). For repeat pregnancies, where an adolescent who gives birth to two babies within two years, there is an increased risk of premature birth, low birth weight, and child mortality (Conroy, 2016). Twenty per cent of pregnant young women under the age of twenty-five are smokers at their booking appointment and 25 per cent are overweight or obese in early pregnancy (Hagell & Shah, 2019). These are known risk factors for the future health of mothers and their babies.

A systematic review of the effectiveness and cost-effectiveness of interventions to reduce repeat unintended teenage pregnancies identified twelve randomized controlled trials (RCTs), four quasi-RCTs, ten qualitative studies, and fifty-three other quantitative studies published between 1996 and 2012 (Aslam et al., 2017; Whitaker et al., 2016). The review found no evidence for effectiveness of condom use, contraceptive use or rates of unprotected sex, or use of birth control. Repeat conceptions tended to occur in conditions where there was poverty, low expectations and aspirations, and few life opportunities. Motivators for repeat pregnancies included to replace loss or to please a partner (Aslam et al., 2017; Whitaker et al., 2016).

Whole-school and social marketing interventions are promising approaches to addressing unintended teenage pregnancy and promoting adolescent sexual health; however, such interventions have not yet been rigorously trialled in the UK. Ponsford and colleagues (2022a) assessed the feasibility and acceptability of Positive Choices, a whole-school social marketing intervention to promote sexual health among secondary school students across six schools in south-east England. The intervention consisted of a student needs survey; a student/staff-led school health promotion council; a classroom curriculum for Year 9 students (aged thirteen to fourteen); whole-school student-led social marketing activities; parent information; and a review of local and school-based sexual health services. All six schools were successfully randomized and response rates to the survey were above 80 per cent at baseline and follow-up. A full phase-III RCT of Positive Choices is currently underway across fifty schools in England. Economic and process evaluations are due to be conducted in 2024 (Ponsford et al., 2022b).

Smoking

Addictive behavioural patterns can start in adolescence. NICE (2014) has produced guidance on the cost-effectiveness of preventing the uptake of tobacco use in adolescence. This evidence review found mass media campaigns and age restrictions on the sale of tobacco to be cost-effective and raising the legal age of smoking to be cost-saving. A cost-effectiveness modelling analysis for both mass media and point-of-sale interventions were found both to be cost-effective. Limitations of the modelling analyses included uncertainty about how many young people were prevented from taking up smoking and how long the effect of the interventions lasted (NICE, 2014).

E-cigarettes, known as vapes, produce an aerosol by heating a liquid that usually contains nicotine, flavourings, and other chemicals (e.g. propylene glycol and vegetable glycerine; NHS, 2022). As vapes do not burn tobacco or produce tar or carbon monoxide, they are thought to be safer than smoking cigarettes, although the long-term risks of vaping are currently unclear (NHS, 2022). In the UK, vapes can be sold to anyone over the age of eighteen years and there are a range of restrictions in place to prevent their uptake and use in those below this age (Office for Health Improvement and Disparities, 2023). Although vapes are more effective than nicotine replacement therapy in supporting people to stop smoking (Hartmann-Boyce et al., 2022), they are not risk free, particularly for younger users and those who have never smoked (Office for Health Improvement and Disparities, 2022a). In 2022, 6 per cent of people aged eleven to eighteen years in England occasionally or regularly smoked cigarettes (an increase from 4.1 per cent in 2021), and 8.6 per cent of people in this age group vaped (an increase from 4 per cent in 2021). Although there has been a rise in vaping in young people, it remains predominantly limited to current or former smokers, and is mainly experimental in nature. The increase in vaping among young people is thought to be attributed to the introduction of disposable vape products. In 2022, 52 per cent of young people who vape used disposable vape products, compared with 7.8 per cent in 2021 (Office for Health Improvement and Disparities, 2022a). Despite the higher long-term costs associated with disposable vapes, they offer the advantage of not requiring any upfront investment in equipment and are relatively cheap to purchase. The 'Khan review: Making smoking obsolete' is an independent review commissioned by the Department of Health and Social Care (Office for Health Improvement and Disparities, 2022b). It provides recommendations for the UK Government to meet its smokefree 2030 ambition. Relating to young people, the review recommends taking measures to close a loophole that allows the distribution of free samples of vapes to children; restricting packaging images and descriptions so that vapes are not appealing to children, and commissioning a review on vape flavourings (Office for Health Improvement and Disparities, 2022b).

Obesity and physical exercise interventions

Obesity is defined as abnormal or excessive fat accumulation that presents a risk to health. A body mass index (BMI) over 25 is considered overweight, and over 30 is obese (WHO, 2021b). Obesity rates have nearly tripled since 1975, with over 390 million children and adolescents aged five to nineteen years considered to be overweight or obese in 2016 worldwide (WHO, 2021c). Up to 79 per cent of teenagers who are obese are likely to go on to be obese as adults (NICE, 2013). This can lead to health problems in adulthood such as type 2 diabetes, heart disease, and certain cancers. Being overweight also impacts on mental health and well-being, including lower self-esteem, poor health-related quality of life, and can lead to depression (NICE, 2013).

It is well-documented that children who are obese are likely to have obese parents (Lanigan et al., 2019). Obesity that runs in families can be due to environmental factors (e.g. poor eating habits learned during childhood), relational and behavioural factors (e.g. poor boundary setting), and genetic traits inherited from parents (NICE, 2015). Interventions are most effective and cost-effective if they involve the whole household or family and can be maintained over time. NICE (2022a) guidance for planning lifestyle weight management services for children and young people called for family-based, multi-component lifestyle weight management services to be available as part of a community-wide, multi-agency approach to promoting a healthy weight and preventing and managing obesity. The guidance suggested that lifestyle weight management programmes should focus on diet and healthy eating habits; physical activity; reducing the amount of time spent being sedentary; and strategies for changing the behaviour of the child or young person and all close family members. Core components, developed with the input of a multidisciplinary team should also include, for example, behaviour-change techniques to increase motivation and confidence in the ability to change, and positive parenting skills training, including problem-solving skills, to support changes in behaviour (NICE, 2022a).

NICE (2009a, updated in 2018) modelled four types of exercise interventions for children and young people: walking buses, free swimming, dance classes, and community sports programmes. Of these, only walking buses demonstrated cost-effectiveness due to the regularity of participation. The difficulties of designing and evaluating school-based programmes to promote regular physical activity are demonstrated by the Girls Active study, a cluster RCT involving fifty-six schools in the UK (Harrington et al., 2018; Charles et al., 2019). The aim of the Girls Active intervention was to increase physical activity in Key Stage 3 adolescent girls (aged eleven to fourteen years), as levels of physical activity often decline during these years. The main effectiveness and cost consequence results showed that compared with usual practice, Girls Active was not effective in terms of accelerometer measured moderate to vigorous-intensity physical activity (Charles et al., 2019; Harrington et al., 2018). Harrington and colleagues (2018) suggested that differences in subgroups may mean the Girls Active intervention has potential in certain types of pupils or schools. Costs ranged from £1,054 (£2 per pupil, per school year) to £3,498 (£7 per pupil, per school year), depending on how the intervention was implemented. Charles and colleagues (2019) highlighted the difficulty in balancing quantity and quality of data capture in community-based trials and alternative methods of data collection that would better suit the school environment.

In another cluster RCT assessing the effectiveness and cost-effectiveness of a school-based programme to increase moderate to vigorous-intensity physical activity among adolescents, GoActive, Corder and colleagues (2020) found that it was no more effective than standard school practice at preventing declines in adolescent physical activity. The GoActive intervention aimed to increase physical activity through increased peer support, self-efficacy, self-esteem, and friendship quality, and was implemented in tutor groups using a student-led tiered-leadership system. At a cost of £13 per student, compared with standard school practice, GoActive was not cost-effective (Corder et al., 2020). All adolescents became less physically active over time, with no difference in physical activity between intervention and control groups. The researchers described low implementation fidelity and the relatively affluent and ethnically homogeneous study sample as methodological limitations of the trial (Corder et al., 2020).

In contrast, there is some evidence that interventions to reduce obesity in young people can be cost-effective (Borde et al., 2017; Love et al., 2019). Zanganeh and colleagues (2019) undertook a systematic review of economic evaluations, appraising the methods used, assessing the quality of the economic evaluations, and summarizing cost-effectiveness. Thirty-nine economic evaluation studies were reviewed and quality assessed. Almost all the studies had been undertaken in Western countries and methods were found to vary by country, setting, and type of intervention. The majority, particularly 'behavioural and policy' preventative interventions, were cost-effective, even cost-saving. An example of this type of intervention is removing television advertising of high-fat and/or high-sugar food and beverages during children's peak viewing times (Magnus et al., 2009). Some behavioural interventions were multi-component, including modification of the environment and policies. Only four interventions were found to be not cost-effective, for example, the walking school bus intervention, which had a high cost of delivery and low participant rates (Moodie et al., 2009). This systematic review demonstrates that economic evaluation of obesity interventions is an expanding area of research. Of interest is the relative cost-effectiveness of system level changes versus, for example, school or community-level interventions. However, methodological heterogeneity makes evidence synthesis challenging. Whilst upstream interventions show promise, an expanded and consistent approach to evaluate cost-effectiveness is needed to capture health and non-health costs and consequences (Zanganeh et al., 2019).

Returning to school-based interventions, evidence of the cost-effectiveness of school-based physical exercise interventions to tackle obesity and sedentary behaviour amongst adolescents is mixed. There are interesting questions for researchers to consider when designing interventions. For example, what constitutes a meaningful change in physical activity behaviour per week, month, or year? And at what follow-up time-point should activity levels be measured? This issue of 'drop-off' is addressed by social return on investment (SROI) methods. It is very challenging to apply a meaningful lifetime approach to evaluation of costs and outcomes in such studies in a modelling context as is advocated by NICE in the valuation of new medicines and other health technologies. A number of longitudinal studies show that physical activity levels in childhood predict similar physical activity behaviour in the future (Tammelin et al., 2003; Telama et al., 2005). Frech (2012) found that psychosocial resources, social support, and family of origin characteristics during adolescence exert a persistent, though generally not cumulative, influence on healthy behaviour trajectories through young adulthood. Building on the above study, another study from the United States (US) explored how peer disadvantage impacts life-course obesity differently by individual identities in terms of ethnicity, socioeconomic status, and gender (Polos et al., 2021). In this study, Polos and colleagues (2021) used cohort data from the National Longitudinal Study of Adolescent to Adult Health and took a life-course approach. They found that among Black men from lower-income households in adolescence, there was a strong negative relationship between adolescent peer economic disadvantage and adult obesity that strengthened over time. In contrast, they found that among Black women across adolescent household income levels, there was a strong positive relationship between adolescent peer economic disadvantage and obesity that emerged as women leave high school and that this endures into mid-adulthood. Among non-Black women, a more modest positive relationship was found between peer disadvantage and obesity. Among non-Black men, no relationship was found (Polos et al., 2021). These heterogeneous effects highlight social life-course determinants of adult health and inequities, and the importance of using intersectional and quasi-experimental approaches jointly (Polos et al., 2021).

Inequalities in Health Outcomes

In 2021, there were 2.92 million children (aged zero to nineteen) living in families in relative low income, and 2.37 million children in absolute low income across the UK. Nineteen per cent of children aged under sixteen years were in low income families and 15 per cent were in absolute low income families (Department for Work & Pensions, 2022). Young people living in poor areas are more likely to experience physical, mental, and sexual health difficulties, be obese, and be involved in a serious road traffic accident (Hagell & Shah, 2019). Marginalized groups of young people include: care experience children; young carers; those from ethnic minorities; those with learning disabilities; young people who identify as lesbian, gay, bisexual, transgender and transsexual plus (LGBT+); and those who have experienced adverse childhood experiences (ACEs). Health inequalities can be compounded amongst these groups of young people, making their health outcomes significantly worse than their peers (Government Equalities Office, 2019; Hagell & Shah, 2019). This means that any economic evaluation of programmes should be aware of the above likely variability of effectiveness and cost-effectiveness across different contexts (i.e. socioeconomic groups, ethnic communities, and neighbourhoods). There seems to be a real need to apply recent developments in distributional cost-effectiveness analysis to investigate interventions to address adolescent well-being and well-becoming (Cookson et al., 2020).

Connectedness, Positive Values, and Contribution to Society

Prior to the COVID-19 pandemic, in the UK, three quarters of young people aged thirteen to fifteen rated their life satisfaction as 'high' or 'very high' (Hagell & Shah, 2019). Approximately one in ten young people aged ten to twenty-four reported often feeling lonely—this incidence was found to decrease with age. The sexual health and behaviour of young people is a consistently high priority in adolescent public health, with important ramifications for well-being, education, and service provision (Hagell & Shah, 2019).

Exploration of sexual identity

Sexual identity in adolescents is a key factor determining healthy adolescent mental health development. Australian panel analysis has shown that having a non-heterosexual identity can cause a significant reduction in subjective well-being when compared to heterosexual individuals (Perales, 2016). In a small survey of fifty-three same-sex and opposite-sex attracted adolescents (average age fourteen years in both groups), it was found that same-sex attracted individuals were more likely to report drinking alcohol alone than their heterosexual peers; however, they were no more likely to engage in health-risk behaviours or use Class 1 or 2 drugs (Rivers & Noret, 2008). In terms of psychological well-being, same-sex attracted students scored significantly higher on a hostility-subscale than their opposite-sex attracted peers and were more likely to report feeling lonely (Rivers & Noret, 2008).

In a model of risk of resilience for LGBT adolescents in the US, Kosciw and colleagues (2015) found that being 'out' (acknowledging their sexuality to their peers and/or parents) was related to higher victimization, but also higher self-esteem and lower depression, suggesting an element of resilience in LGBT adolescence. The costs of victimization were projected onto negative academic outcomes, both directly and indirectly by diminished levels of well-being. These effects were exacerbated in adolescents living in rural areas. Kosciw and colleagues called for more policies that prohibit anti-LGBT bullying and encourage reporting of victimization.

In a national population-based study, Khanolkar and colleagues (2023) found that young people from sexual minority groups had significantly worse mental health compared with heterosexual peers. Over 9,700 young people aged seventeen years from the UK-wide Millennium Cohort Study, with data on self-identified sexual and ethnic identities, completed questionnaires on general health, mental health, and health-related behaviours. Findings showed that sexual minority adolescents from both White and ethnic minority groups experience significantly higher levels of psychological distress, emotional problems, self-harm, and attempted suicide, as well as poorer general health compared to heterosexual peers. Young people who are White and from a sexual minority group reported a higher prevalence of adverse health-related behaviours compared to young people from an ethnic minority and sexual minority group. This study highlights the need for accessible and affirming mental health support, particularly in educational settings such as schools and universities. Support should be tailored to address the unique experiences of young people with sexual minority identities (Khanolkar et al., 2023).

Gender identity in adolescence

'Gender non-conformity' describes an individual whose gender identity, role, or expression are not typical of individuals with the same assigned sex in a given society and historical era (Guss et al., 2015). 'Gender dysphoria' refers to the distress and discomfort that can occur when there is incongruence between an individual's biological sex and their gender identity (NHS, 2020). Non-conformity in gender identity can have a negative effect on adolescent mental health and well-being, with some evidence suggesting it has a larger effect than sexual identity on mental health. In Canada, Aspenlieder and colleagues (2009) examined whether peer victimization (physical, verbal, and relational) and gender non-conformity were connected for pre and early adolescent boys and girls ($n = 462$). They found that in both boys and girls, gender non-conformity was uniquely predictive of peer-reported victimization. The findings also showed that the relationship between physical and relational victimization was moderated by sex in reverse patterns. In the Netherlands, Baams and colleagues (2013) found that gender non-conformity predicted lower levels of psychological well-being in young adults aged nineteen to twenty-four years ($n = 192$), and that this was likely caused by the individual's experience of the perceived experience of stigmatization. Another study from Canada found that harassment due to gender non-conformity mediated the association between sexual minority status and depressive symptoms in college students ($n = 251$) (Martin-Storey & August, 2016).

Some evidence suggests that the mechanisms of interaction between gender non-conformity and well-being are more prevalent than those found for sexual orientation. For example, in a survey of high school seniors in the US (female, $n = 230$; male, $n = 245$), Rieger and Savin-Williams (2012) found that neither sexual orientation nor biological sex were a significant predictor of psychological well-being. This study concluded that gender atypical traits (both environmental and biological) may be more relevant for psychological health than a same-sex orientation (Rieger & Savin-Williams, 2012). More recently, NICE (2020) reviewed the evidence for the clinical effectiveness, safety, and cost-effectiveness of gender-affirming hormones for children and adolescents aged eighteen years or under with gender dysphoria. Results from five uncontrolled, observational studies suggested that gender-affirming hormones can improve symptoms of gender dysphoria, and may also improve depression, anxiety, quality of life, suicidality, and psychosocial functioning. The impact of treatment on body image was unclear. No cost-effectiveness evidence was found to determine whether gender-affirming hormones are a cost-effective treatment for children and adolescents with gender dysphoria

(NICE, 2020). This is probably one of the most challenging current areas for those designing and commissioning age-appropriate health services for children and young people.

Use of technology and social media

The use of information and communication technology and social media is one of the biggest changes of modern society, with over 4.59 billion active social media users worldwide in 2022 (Dixon, 2023). The way young people use information and communication technology has changed over recent decades. Young people watch less scheduled television than other age groups in favour of streamed and downloaded programmes (British Audience Research Board, 2018; Hagell & Shah, 2019). Ninety-five per cent of sixteen to twenty-four-year-olds in the UK own a smartphone (Statista, 2019). New technologies bring both challenges and opportunities. The risks are widely discussed; the opportunities less so. However, there is growing recognition that new media and communications devices offer platforms for health interventions that may be particularly suitable for young people (House of Commons Science and Technology Committee, 2019).

Though this may be the case, there is growing evidence demonstrating associations between social media use and a range of poor mental health outcomes, such as depressive symptoms and suicidal behaviour (Kelly et al., 2018; Twenge et al., 2018); most powerfully argued in *The anxious generation* (Haidt, 2024). In a review of empirical literature on social media use by adolescents, Allen and colleagues (2014) examined how social media affects social connectedness in terms of sense of belonging, psychological well-being, and identity development and processes. Mixed results were found: young people expressed both positive and negative psychological outcomes. The ease of creating new social groups and communities was found to increase well-being, but the potential of increased alienation and ostracism was a negative outcome of social media use (Allen et al., 2014). A more recent systematic review and thematic meta-analysis synthesis identified nineteen qualitative studies where adolescents shared their views and experiences of social media and well-being (Shankelman et al., 2021). Studies were generally considered of a high level of quality and represented adolescents from diverse geographical regions and a broad age range. Four themes emerged from the thematic meta-synthesis concerning well-being: connections, identity, learning, and emotions. These themes appeared to be connected with key developmental processes such as attachment, identity formation, attention, and emotional regulation, providing theoretical links between social media use and well-being (Shankelman et al., 2021).

During the COVID-19 pandemic, access to mental health support had increasingly been through an online basis. A systematic overview of digital mental health interventions for adolescents and young people found that interventions with a hybrid digital and in-person contact with professional, peer, or parent were associated with greater effectiveness and adherence as well as lower drop-out than fully automatized or self-administered interventions (Lehtimaki et al., 2021). Cost-effectiveness data were not reported in any of the eighteen systematic reviews and meta-analyses examined. Five systematic reviews reported on the low cost of interventions, for example, in terms of reduced time and personal expenses (Vigerland et al., 2016). Research on cost-effectiveness is needed when scaling up interventions in mental health services which have limited resources (Lehtimaki et al., 2021).

Safety and a Supportive Environment

Youth services work with children, young people, and families, and organize educational and recreational leisure activities. They provide 'a sense of belonging, a safe space, and the opportunity for young people to enjoy being young' (Young Men's Christian Association (YMCA), 2020, p. 2). These services support young people who want to attend a youth club; want to gain an award outside of school; are at risk of dropping out of school; are at risk of being involved in criminal activity; and are experiencing difficulty at home and require social work input. Spending on youth services has been cut over recent years in the UK. In 2010/2011, local authorities spent £1.36 billion on youth services in England. By 2018/2019, spending had reduced by £959 million (YMCA, 2020). Although the cuts in Wales have been less severe, Welsh services have seen a 38 per cent decrease in spending from £50 million in 2010/2011 to £19 million in 2018/2019 (YMCA, 2020). Over the past ten years, 760 youth centres have closed across the UK, with over 4,500 jobs being cut (Unison, 2019). Although additional funding has been allocated to buildings and refurbishments, the YMCA (2020) has called for funding to also be directed to the resources to deliver services for young people, and for the UK Government to take a strategic approach and create national strategies to repurpose existing buildings. Investment in age-appropriate health promotion, youth-friendly health services, and universal youth services, such as youth clubs, could help to improve young people's health and well-being (Hagell & Shah, 2019).

Box 4.1 presents a case study on Premier League Kicks, a community programme which began in 2006 to see football clubs work together with young people, local policy forces, and other stakeholders to help create safer and more inclusive communities.

Box 4.1 Premier League Kicks: A community programme using sport to inspire young people

Since 2006, Premier League Kicks has been working in local communities to inspire young people in the most high-need areas in England and Wales through 'the power of football and sport' (see www.premierleague.com). The programme includes sports, coaching, music, and educational and personal development sessions to increase participation in football and other sports, and has seen reductions in antisocial behaviour reported in participating areas. The programme vision is to encourage children and young people to achieve their potential and improve their well-being, while building stronger, safer, and more inclusive communities. Between 2019 and 2022, over 175,000 young people were engaged in the programme. The Tigers Trust, based in Hull, has delivered the Premier League Kicks programme since 2010, engaging with thousands of young local people, encouraging their participation in football and promoting positive activities. The programme aims to create safer and more respectful communities through a culture of volunteering, social activities, and role models (Tigers Trust, 2023). In 2019/2020, at a cost £200,000, Premier League Kicks generated over £3.7 million of social value, based on the social outcomes received by the beneficiaries and staff, as well as the fiscal and economic outcomes associated with staff employed through the programme (Tigers Trust, 2021).

Living conditions

Growing up in an impoverished environment can have a detrimental effect on the development of adolescents. Living in a deprived neighbourhood can lead to greater risk of teenage self-harm and suicide, increased symptoms of depression and anxiety, and increased externalization of problematic behaviours (Bozzini et al., 2020; Buckner et al., 2004; Fergusson et al., 2000). The effects of growing up in poverty can also be cumulative over the long term. Chronic exposure to poverty is linked to increased rates of mental health disorders (e.g. depression) and addictive behaviours (e.g. substance abuse; Fergusson et al., 2000); early sexual debut (McLeod & Knight, 2010; McLeod & Shanahan, 1996); criminal activity (Davis et al., 2004); and poor academic achievement (Wilkins et al., 2004). Mitigating the effects of poverty on mental health is an important consideration and a strong argument against austerity as a government policy. As discussed in Chapter 1, the landmark review by Marmot and colleagues (2010) introduced the 'Marmot curve', showing healthy life expectancy by neighbourhood deprivation. The Marmot curve shows that average life expectancy in the poorest areas in England was seven years lower than in the wealthiest areas. Individuals living in poorer communities not only die sooner, but they also live more of their lives with chronic disease and disability, with an average disability-free life expectancy difference of seventeen years (Marmot et al., 2010).

Qualitative research by Birch and colleagues (2020) explored how urban nature can support the mental health and well-being of young multi-ethnic urban residents living in Sheffield, a north-central city in England. These researchers undertook interviews and creative arts workshops with twenty-four people aged seventeen to twenty-seven years, nine of whom had lived experience of mental health difficulties. During the arts workshops, some participants undertook activities such as free writing, creating mood boards, word play, painting, handling nature objects, and walking in the outdoors. The study findings showed that engaging with urban nature, such as trees, water, open spaces, and views, fostered a stronger sense of self, feelings of escape, and connection and care with the human and non-human world. One participant expressed how she felt:

> [This nature place would] just like give me a hug basically, like 'here's a hug', this is a gift from me to you and like these are all of the resources that you'll ever need: you've got the ground to ground you, you've got the sky to inspire you, [laughs] you've got the trees and how well rooted they are and, that offer you security and like you can recognise the cycles of death and life and you can let them come and go as you please (Mina). (Birch et al., 2020, p. 1)

Birch and colleagues (2020) also found that deteriorating landscapes (e.g. greenspaces where antisocial behaviour takes place), young people's shifting identities, and perceived time pressures disrupted support for young people. They called for further qualitative research into how nature can care for young people as a heterogenous group with shifting identifies and relationships with the natural world.

Improving mental health literacy in schools

A systematic review of the effectiveness and cost-effectiveness of school-based mental health literacy programmes found that with a prevalence of one in eight children and young people aged five to nineteen years having at least one mental health disorder, the main barriers to mental health treatment include low perceived need and attitudinal barriers (Ma et al., 2022). Schools play a major part in improving mental health literacy and reducing stigma which may facilitate help-seeking behaviour and use of mental health services by young people. School-based interventions can improve mental health literacy and reduce stigma in the short-term; however, refresher interventions may be required to sustain the positive outcomes in the long term. Interventions comprising mental health education followed by contact with a person with lived experience of mental health disorders may be most effective. Live contact and filmed contact are equally effective (Ma et al., 2022). Ma and colleagues (2022) illustrate how challenging undertaking effectiveness and cost-effectiveness analyses in the area of primary and secondary prevention of mental health conditions in children and young people can be. Despite their review focusing on studies with randomized designs, intervention and methodological heterogeneity pose uncertainties around conclusions. They argue future research should focus on resolving methodological issues, particularly how outcomes are assessed and include process evaluations to better inform the design of an intervention in terms of its delivery and implementation (Ma et al., 2022).

Mindfulness in schools

During the COVID-19 pandemic, the UK Government imposed a series of national lockdowns. With the closure of school buildings, classes moved to an online format so that children could learn from home (Genie et al., 2020). In countries that are members of the Organisation for Economic Co-operation and Development (OECD), it was acknowledged that one of the most important challenges created by the pandemic was how to adapt a system of education built around physical schools (OECD Policy Brief, 2020). At the peak of the pandemic in 2020, more than 188 countries, encompassing 91 per cent of enrolled learners worldwide, closed their schools in an attempt to contain the spread of the COVID-19 virus (OECD Policy Brief, 2020). School closures had an impact on all students, but especially on the most vulnerable, who were more likely to face additional barriers to learning such as food insecurity, heating poverty, and access to technology and internet services (Sinha et al., 2020). Children and young people from low income and single-parent families, as well as children with special educational needs, were deprived of physical learning opportunities, social and emotional support available in schools, and extra services such as free school meals (Baraniuk, 2020).

Since the spring of 2021, although schools re-opened in the UK, there have been enduring mental health issues affecting children and young people (McCluskey et al., 2021). This has been referred to as 'the pandemic within the pandemic' (Qureshi, 2021). In order to deal with increased mental health issues experienced by children and young people, the UK Government has encouraged the implementation of mindfulness programmes in all schools to improve the learning, cognitive ability, and well-being of students. Mindfulness is an integrative, mind-body based approach that can help people to manage their thoughts, feelings and mental health (Kabat-Zinn, 2016). It is becoming widely used in a range of contexts. For example, mindfulness-based cognitive therapy is recommended by NICE (2009b, 2022b) as a preventative practice for people who have experienced three or more previous episodes of depression.

Mindfulness can be effective for children and young people, with school-based interventions having positive outcomes on well-being, reducing anxiety and distress, and improving behaviour (Crane & Kuyken, 2013). In school settings, mindfulness may be especially relevant to the anticipation of written and oral exams (Kozina, 2020). In North Wales, a study showed that the Paws b (pause be) mindfulness programme delivered by classroom teachers significantly reduced negative affect and enhanced meta-cognition in children aged seven to nine years at the three months follow-up, when compared to a control group receiving education as usual (Vickery & Dorjee, 2016). More recently, secondary analyses using data from the My Resilience in Adolescence (MYRIAD) trial, a two-arm parallel group cluster RCT that explored school-based mindfulness training in early adolescence, gave mixed evidence about its effectiveness (Montero-Marin et al., 2022). This universal intervention comprised psychoeducation, using mainstream educational methods and brief mindfulness practices delivered by schoolteachers who had undertaken bespoke training. Montero-Marin and colleagues (2022) questioned whether a more engaging format with a different focus (e.g. key mechanisms of risk/resilience), shorter but more frequent sessions, and delivered by more highly trained teachers would make the intervention more accessible, engaging, and effective. It is also important to understand if there are subgroups that do and do not benefit from mindfulness in schools. For example, Montero-Marin and colleagues noted that younger adolescents may have limited meta-cognitive ability so they experience some difficulty in reflecting on their experience and awareness, and have difficulty self-regulating their behaviour when being confronted by challenging emotions. Also, adolescents who experience mental health difficulties may have poorer executive function which might partly explain why this subgroup did not benefit from the intervention. These findings suggest that more targeted and intensive interventions might better suit some subgroups of adolescents in supporting their health and well-being (Montero-Marin et al., 2022).

Prior to the COVID-19 pandemic, Anna Freud (a mental health charity for children and families) was commissioned by the Department for Education to deliver the Education for Wellbeing programme, England's largest research trial of school-based mental health interventions (Anna Freud, 2018). For Year 7 students (aged eleven to twelve) and Year 8 students (aged twelve to thirteen), schools were randomly allocated to one of four groups: mindfulness; relaxation;

strategies for safety and well-being; or usual practice. For Year 9 students (aged thirteen to fourteen), schools were randomly allocated to one of three groups: youth aware of mental health; the mental health and high school curriculum guide; or usual practice. The delivery of Wave 1 of the programme took place in 2019, Wave 2 took place in 2020, Wave 3 took place in 2022, and results are expected in 2024. Although some schools in Wales already offer mindfulness sessions on an ad hoc basis, there is an opportunity for mindfulness to be part of the school curriculum in Wales from September 2022 (Mindfulness in Schools Project, 2023).

In Scotland, the National Improvement Hub provides information and support for teachers and early learning and childcare practitioners to improve their practice and enhance the quality of learners' experiences and outcomes. The Hub provides resources on health and well-being, including information about mindfulness for mental well-being and offers exercises for children to practise, such as keeping a sleep diary (National Improvement Hub, 2017). In Northern Ireland, mindfulness is taught to students at Key Stage 3 and 4 (aged eleven to sixteen) during modules about understanding well-being (Council for the Curriculum, Examinations and Assessment, 2020). Resources are available for students to practise a guided mindfulness meditation and they are encouraged to reflect on their experiences.

In Slovenia, a study investigating the role of emotional competencies (mindfulness and emotional self-efficacy) for psychological responding (mental well-being, general anxiety, and COVID–19 anxiety) was conducted during the COVID-19 pandemic (Kozina et al., 2021). This study also examined whether practising mindfulness with inner (meditation-based) and body (yoga-based) exercise supported emotional competencies. Kozina and colleagues (2021) found that such competencies were a viable source of support for psychological responses to the COVID-19 pandemic and that practising mindfulness fostered several aspects of emotional competencies. This work gave an overview of the education system's responsiveness and helped to identify efficient practices and initiatives to support students' learning and well-being (Kozina et al., 2021).

There are a number of trials and cost-effectiveness studies of mindfulness programmes in schools, such as the MYRIAD study (Kuyken et al., 2017; Montero-Marin et al., 2021). It is credible that mindfulness initiatives could be cost-effective in the long term. Reducing stress and anxiety may be cost-effective for society in terms of dealing with mental health issues before they intensify and start affecting education, physical health, and societal impact of unmanaged behaviour. The methodological design questions in Box 4.2 can shift our reference set in a life-course model and are considered in full by Edwards and colleagues (2015).

Box 4.2 Ten methodological design questions for mindfulness-based interventions that can shift our reference set in a life-course model

1. What is the specific research question being asked about the mindfulness-based intervention (MBI) under evaluation?

2. With what alternative intervention or situation is the MBI to be compared?

3. How is effectiveness to be measured, and what is an important change on such measures?

4. Which economic analysis method is most appropriate and from whose perspective is the MBI evaluation being conducted?

5. How are costs of an MBI to be measured, and what is the range of costs to be considered?

6. How should benefits of an MBI be measured for an economic evaluation?

7. Are the study results sensitive to changes to our assumptions?

8. Does the research consider equity as well as efficiency?

9. Is economic modelling going to be useful in MBI research?

10. How should results be compared with the findings of other studies and used to advise service commissioners and policymakers?

Source: data from Edwards, R. T., Bryning, L., & Crane, R. (2015). Design of economic evaluations of mindfulness-based interventions: Ten methodological questions of which to be mindful. *Mindfulness*, 6(3), 490–500. doi.org/10.1007/s12671-014-0282-6. Copyright (2015), Springer Nature. Reproduced under the Creative Commons License CC BY

Anti-bullying programmes

Bullying in childhood and adolescence is one of the most challenging but potentially addressable population-level mental health problems facing young people with a lifetime impact (Ford, 2014). Bullying has many definitions, but may be characterized by behaviour that is aggressive, intentional, repetitive, unprovoked, and involves a power imbalance in favour of the perpetrator (Ireland, 2002). The psychiatric morbidity arising from bullying is substantial. Population studies estimate that 25 per cent to 40 per cent of mental health problems including depression, anxiety, and self-harm in young adults may be attributable to childhood bullying (Bowes et al., 2015; Fisher et al., 2012). Bullied children access more school health services, primary care services, and specialist child mental health services, and experience poorer mental health into adulthood, than their counterparts who are not bullied (Brimblecombe et al., 2018; Takizawa et al., 2014). Bullying is associated with school absenteeism, impacting future educational attainment, and employment prospects (Brown et al., 2011; Kearney, 2008).

International evidence of the cost-effectiveness of anti-bulling programmes largely comes from Northern European countries. For example, between 2007 and 2009, 234 Finnish schools took part in an RCT of the KiVa programme, a whole-school programme with universal actions that places a strong emphasis on changing bystander behaviour. This programme was developed at the University of Turku, Finland, with funding from the Ministry of Education and Culture. The KiVa programme was found to significantly reduce all forms of bullying and victimization, including verbal, physical, racist, and cyberbullying, and reduce anxiety and depression in children aged seven to eleven years (Kärnä et al., 2011a; Salmivalli et al., 2011; Williford et al., 2012). Since 2009, KiVa has been scaled-up into over 90 per cent of Finnish public schools (approximately 2,700 schools) and demonstrated year-on-year positive effects (Kärnä et al., 2011b). A Swedish study assessing the cost-effectiveness of the KiVa programme reported an increased cost of €829 for a gain of 0.47 victim-free years per student, and a cost per quality-adjusted life year (QALY) gain of €13,823 (Persson et al., 2018). This was considered cost-effective when compared to the Swedish health policy threshold of around €50,000 per QALY. In the UK, trials are ongoing of the KiVa programme in secondary schools across England and Wales, though these were interrupted during the COVID-19 pandemic (Clarkson et al., 2022, 2016).

Exposure to childhood bullying heightens the risk of physical and mental health problems (e.g. obesity and depression), personal finance (e.g. debt), and social problems (e.g. divorce) in adulthood. These outcomes have been referred to as the 'long shadow of childhood bullying' (see Figure 4.2; Wolke, 2014). For children who are bullied at home and at school, there is limited opportunity to find a safe place away from bullying. Dantchev and colleagues (2019) suggested that interventions tailored towards reducing sibling bullying should be prioritized as this may help to prevent peer bullying. Health professionals could support young people who are being bullied by regularly enquiring about sibling and peer bullying experiences, as these may be early warning signs of poor mental health and well-being (Dantchev et al., 2019; Scott et al., 2016).

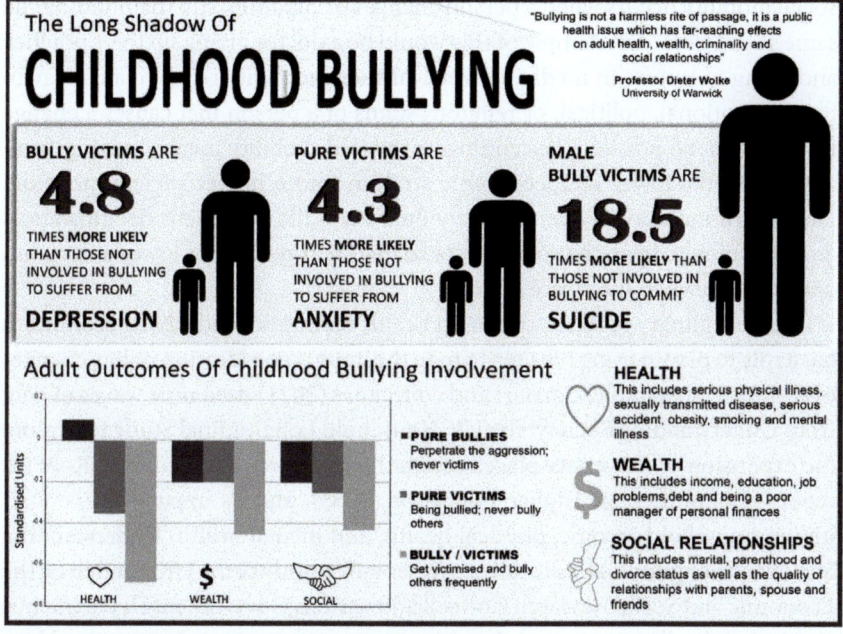

Figure 4.2 The long shadow of childhood bullying
Reproduced from Wolke, D. (2014, 20 May). *The long shadow of bullying*. https://warwick.
ac.uk/newsandevents/pressreleases/the_long_shadow_of_childhood_bullying1/. Copyright
© 2014 University of Warwick

Learning, Competence, Education, Skills, Employability, and Social Mobility

Education plays a key role in human development and reforms to educational systems and policy have been viewed as a social transformational lever of the second half of the twentieth century (Shavit et al., 2007). Education, especially access to university, is also considered as a powerful tool to promote 'social mobility' and reduce the gap in lifetime earning potential between individuals from different socioeconomic backgrounds. Social mobility, also called 'intergenerational mobility' by economists, measures the degree to which people's social status changes between and within generations. Social mobility reflects 'the extent to which parents influence the success of their children in later life or, on the flipside, the extent to which individuals can make it by virtue of their own talents, motivation and luck' (Blanden et al., 2005, p. 18). There are several types of social mobility, for example, 'horizontal mobility', 'vertical mobility', 'ascending or upward mobility', and 'downward mobility'. Horizontal social mobility occurs when a person changes occupation, still maintaining the same social class. An example of this would be a doctor giving up their practice and going to lecture in medicine. Vertical social mobility refers to a change in the occupational, political, or religious status of a person that causes a change in their societal position. Ascending or upward mobility means moving from a group in the lower socioeconomic stratum into a higher societal position. Downward mobility is when an individual starts life in affluent circumstances and later moves down the social strata so that their position is lower as an adult compared to when they were a child.

Interdisciplinary research spanning health economics and labour economics has a role to play in using big data to map the impact of education policy changes over time. For example, Carrieri and colleagues (2021) used nine waves of data from Understanding Society: the UK Household Longitudinal Study to explore the expansion of university places across the UK, since the landmark Robbins report (Committee on Higher Education, 1963), and its impact on inequalities in household income, physical health, and mental health. Understanding Society is a longitudinal, naturally representative study of the UK, funded by the Economic and Social Research Council and various Government Departments. Carrieri and colleagues found the university expansion was characterized by a large increase in the proportion of graduates, with higher rates of graduation among individuals from more advantaged socioeconomic backgrounds. This was evidenced by a persistent existing gradient of opportunity in society in the UK. Overall, they found the expansion of university places barely affected inequality of opportunity in household income. Paternal occupation was found to have the most influence on university participation, though over more recent years, maternal occupation has had an increasingly important effect (although paternal occupation remains dominant). These findings are in line with Heckman and Landersø (2021) who found that in Denmark, as in the US, higher income families were able to better access universal resources including education. They also found neighbourhood effects, which aligns with the work of Marmot and colleagues (2010) in the UK (discussed in Chapter 1 of this book).

Education

In the UK, the majority of young people stay in some type of education until the age of eighteen, with only 6.3 per cent of those aged sixteen to eighteen not in education, employment, or training (NEET) (Hagell & Shah, 2019). After age eighteen, young people tend to move into higher education, vocational training, or employment. Prior to the COVID-19 pandemic, youth unemployment rates were low, and young people were disproportionately dependent on casual employment such as seasonal work and zero-hours contracts (Hagell &

Shah, 2019). Youth unemployment rates reached a peak of 22.5 per cent in 2011 following the 2008 financial crisis and fell to 12.3 per cent at the start of the pandemic during January to March 2020. During July to September 2020, youth employment rates rose to 14.9 per cent, but since then have been falling steadily to 9.8 per cent during July to September 2022 (Francis-Devine et al., 2023).

Agency and Resilience

Resilience can be thought of as, 'the process of effectively negotiating, adapting to, or managing significant sources of stress or trauma. Assets and resources within the individual, their life, and environment facilitate this capacity for adaptation and 'bouncing back' in the face of adversity' (Windle, 2011, p. 163). Strengthening of resilience protective factors can reduce mental health difficulties (such as depression, anxiety, stress, and obsessive-compulsive symptoms) in adolescents (Hjemdal et al., 2011; Luthar & Cicchetti, 2000). Protective factors include strong family cohesion, high levels of prosocial behaviour at school and in the community, high social skills/competence, and strong moral beliefs (Bond et al., 2005; Hjemdal et al., 2011). A systematic review of universal resilience-focused interventions targeting child and adolescent mental health in school settings found that all interventions were effective relative to a control group in reducing four out of seven outcomes: depressive symptoms, internalizing problems, externalizing problems, and psychological distress (Dray et al., 2017). For short-term follow-up, these interventions were effective for managing depressive symptoms and anxiety symptoms, particularly when a cognitive behavioural therapy (CBT)-based approach was used. For long-term follow-up, interventions were effective for internalizing problems (Dray et al., 2017).

Well-being is influenced by the individual and the environment, and during adolescence, environmental factors can be critical to healthy development (Gómez-López et al., 2019). Building competence, confidence, connection, character, and caring can help adolescents to stay healthy and have the resilience to return to good health (WHO, 2020a, 2021a). WHO (2020b) considers adolescent mental health a public health concern worldwide, with suicide being the fourth leading cause of death in fifteen to nineteen-year-olds. The more risk factors adolescents are exposed to, the greater the potential impact on their mental health (WHO, 2020b). Hagell and Shah (2019) outlined nine reasons to invest in young people's health (see Box 4.3).

Preventative interventions for mental health can prove particularly effective when applied to vulnerable children (at risk of mental health problems or experiencing behavioural difficulties) and adolescents (Furlong et al., 2012). The

Box 4.3 Nine reasons to invest in young people's health

1. The health of young people is not improving enough compared to other age groups.

2. Young people are not getting the health services or information that are relevant to them.

3. Health inequalities are already prevalent by the time of transition to adulthood, and some health inequalities are widening.

4. Positive trends in health behaviour need to be supported so they can be maintained (e.g. decrease in teenage pregnancy).

5. Overlooking chronic adolescent disease costs money.

6. Effects of poor health care in adolescence can have an impact on health and well-being in later life-course stages.

7. Investing in young people's well-being has benefits beyond health.

8. Many mental health issues are diagnosed at this life-course stage.

9. Investment in young people maintains and reinforces successful health interventions delivered in early childhood.

Reproduced from Hagell, A., & Shah, R. (2019). *Highlights: Key data on young people 2019*. Association for Young People's Health. https://www.active-together.org/files/68190/ayph-kdyp2019-fullversion.pdf. Copyright © AYPH 2019 with permission.

positives of taking a preventative approach to depression are amplified when interventions are applied to mitigate the effect of poverty and inequality on mental health (Wahlbeck et al., 2017). In the US, targeted programmes have been shown to generate a positive return on investment (ROI) for health, education, and criminal justice, as well as on the labour market upon reaching adulthood (McDaid et al., 2019). These ranged between $1.80 and $3.30 for every $1 spent on programmes targeted at children with behavioural problems (Washington State Institute for Public Policy, 2017).

Digital mental health interventions

Digital mental health interventions use software programmes accessed via computers, tablets, smartphones, audio-visual and virtual reality equipment, gaming consoles, robots, and other devices to prevent or improve mental health difficulties. In an update to NICE guidance on depression in children and young people, evidence for the most effective psychological interventions was reviewed (NICE, 2019b). Digital and online interventions, such as CBT, were identified as effective treatments for mild depression in children and young people. NICE (2019b) highlighted that the choice of treatment should be based on clinical need as well as patient and carer preferences.

In a review of published economic studies on digital interventions for mental health and addiction problems, Gega and colleagues (2022) reviewed seventy-six economic evaluations, including eleven economic models and sixty-five within-trial evaluations. As the digital interventions were complex and heterogeneous, the results of the economic evaluations were not directly comparable. However, the authors concluded that, overall, digital interventions were likely to be cost-effective, compared with no intervention and non-therapeutic control, whereas the value of digital interventions compared with face-to-face therapy or printed manuals was unclear. The decision analytic model found that digital interventions for generalized anxiety disorder were associated with lower net monetary benefit than medication and face-to-face therapy, but greater monetary net benefit than non-therapeutic controls and no intervention. Stakeholders identified safety, sustainability, and reduction of waiting times as being important factors when assessing the value of digital interventions. Factors other than costs and outcomes that might influence stakeholders' decisions to use digital interventions included increasing patient choice, reaching underserved populations, enabling continuous care, and accepting the 'inevitability of going digital' (Gega et al., 2022).

Evidence from systematic reviews has demonstrated in more than ten studies with 720 participants that internet-based CBT (i-CBT) is a clinically acceptable alternative to face-to-face administered psychotherapy, although can be associated with a higher drop-out rate (Simon, et al., 2019). i-CBT offers a range of programmes for people experiencing post-traumatic stress disorder (PTSD), including standard CBT and trauma-focused CBT (TF-CBT) methods, offering a cost-effective alternative method of administration for potential interventions already discussed (Gratzer & Khalid-Khan, 2016). For anxiety, school-administered universal preventative programmes have been found to be as effective as a targeted programme—both producing a small positive effect. Out-of-school delivered anxiety interventions appear to have a similar effect as school programmes, unlike for depression where the out-of-school programmes produced a more beneficial effect (Werner-Seidler et al., 2017).

Reactive therapies for generalized anxiety disorder can be an effective form of treatment when preventative approaches are not effective. Similarly, when attempting to prevent anxiety symptoms, CBT appears to be a popular and effective method for mitigating anxiety. In a UK-based meta-analysis of anxiety treatments (studies, $n = 41$; participants, $n = 2{,}132$), Cuijpers and colleagues (2014) found that the pooled effect of psychotherapies (mostly CBT studies) versus a control group (waiting list) was larger with low to moderate heterogeneity. The effects of psychotherapies on depression were also large, supporting CBT as a potential intervention for both generalized anxiety and depression (Cuijpers et al., 2014). Cost-effectiveness evidence for psychologist-issued CBT as a treatment for anxiety is sparse. An Australian cost-effectiveness study found that using disability-adjusted life years (DALYs), CBT conducted by a psychologist was the most cost-effective intervention for both generalized anxiety disorder ($6,900 per DALY saved) and panic disorder ($6,800 per DALY saved). CBT was found to create a higher total health benefit than drug interventions (Heuzenroeder, et al., 2004). The DALY is a single measure used to quantify the burden of diseases, injuries, and risk factors (Murray, 1996). One DALY represents the loss of the equivalent of one year of full health. DALYs for a disease or health condition are the sum of the years of life lost (YLLs) due to premature mortality and the years lived with a disability (YLDs) due to prevalent cases of the disease or health condition in a population (WHO, 2020b). In the UK, an RCT investigating computer-delivered CBT was found to be effective in treating anxiety and depression and was shown to have an 81 per cent chance of being cost-effective under the NICE threshold of £20,000 to £30,000 per QALY (Claxton et al., 2015; McCrone et al., 2004).

The Costs of Late Intervention in Children and Young People

The costs of late intervention have been defined as the range of acute or statutory services that are required when children and young people experience significant difficulties in life, as well other support they may draw upon such as welfare benefits, which might have been prevented. The cost of late intervention has been estimated to be nearly £17 billion per year for England and Wales (Chowdry & Fitzsimons, 2016). This figure covers crime and anti-social behaviour, school absence and exclusion, children's social care, child injuries and mental health problems, youth substance misuse, and youth economic inactivity. It does not reflect the longer-term cumulative impact

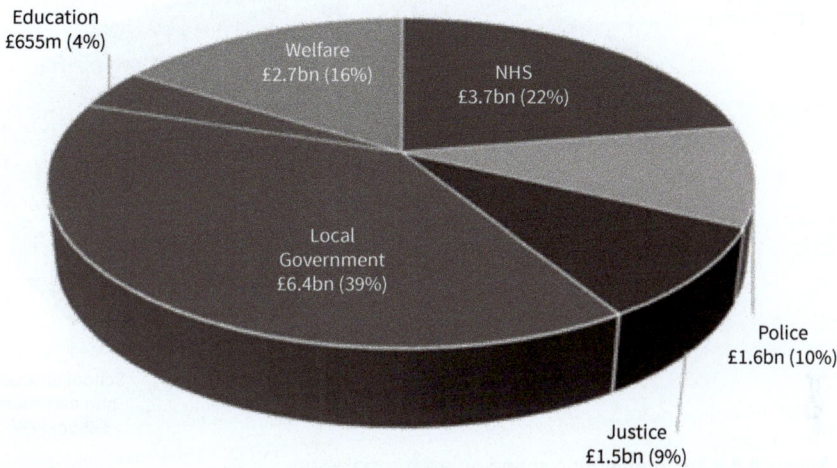

Total annual spend: £16.6bn (2016–2017 prices)

Figure 4.3 Late intervention spend by budget area
Reproduced from Chowdry, H., & Fitzsimons, P. (2016). *The cost of late intervention: EIF analysis 2016.* Early Intervention Foundation. https://www.eif.org.uk/files/pdf/cost-of-late-intervention-2016.pdf

of late intervention for children and adolescents, for example, lasting effects into adult life and subsequent generations, as well as the wider social and economic costs. The £17 billion spent on late prevention is spread across different public agencies at national and local level, including local govern-ment (£6.4 billion); the NHS (£3.7 billion); the Department for Work and Pensions (£2.7 billion); police (£1.6 billion); the criminal justice system (£1.5 billion); and education (£655 million) (see Figure 4.3). The amount spent on late intervention varies significantly across England and Wales. On average, £298 is spent per person in each local authority, but can range from £164 to £531, depending on the level of deprivation in the area. Rural areas are more likely to show lower levels of both late intervention spend and deprivation, while urban areas are more likely to show higher levels of both (Chowdry & Fitzsimons, 2016).

Figure 4.4 shows the cost of late intervention spend on different social issues. Late intervention associated with crime and antisocial behaviour accounts for just over a third of the total spend (£5.9 billion), as does spending on children's social care (£6.2 billion). In other areas, spending is as follows: youth economic inactivity (£2.7 billion); child injuries and mental health problems (£774 mil-lion), and youth substance misuse (£443 million) (Chowdry & Fitzsimons, 2016).

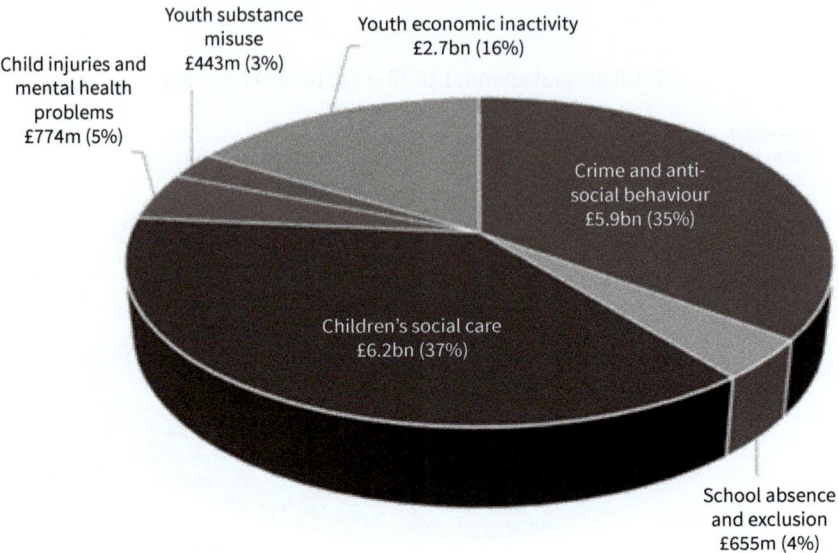

Total annual spend: £16.6bn (2016–17 prices)

Youth substance misuse £443m (3%)

Youth economic inactivity £2.7bn (16%)

Child injuries and mental health problems £774m (5%)

Crime and anti-social behaviour £5.9bn (35%)

Children's social care £6.2bn (37%)

School absence and exclusion £655m (4%)

Figure 4.4 Late intervention spend on each social issue
Reproduced from Chowdry, H., & Fitzsimons, P. (2016). *The cost of late intervention: EIF analysis 2016.* Early Intervention Foundation. https://www.eif.org.uk/files/pdf/cost-of-late-intervention-2016.pdf

Summary

For adolescents and young adults, well-being is multidimensional, and this includes health. Programmes to improve adolescent well-being require a multisectoral approach. The measurement of adolescent well-being (including cost-effectiveness) requires multidimensional indicators that encompass, for example, all five domains of adolescent well-being shown in the Introduction to Chapter 4, and should include both subjective and objective measures (Ross et al., 2020). In Chapter 3, we explored the benefits of investment in the early years. Those substantial investments and subsequent health gains are at risk of being lost if we do not continue to invest in the health and well-being of adolescents and young people. In Chapter 5, we focus on the next life-course stage—adulthood—and the well-being and well-becoming of the workforce.

Curiosity Questions

- What are the most cost-effective interventions, programmes, and policies to promote or mitigate barriers to positive well-being for adolescents and young people?
- The evidence shows that most interventions developed to tackle adolescent obesity are multi-component, spanning physical activity and

dietary intake. How can such multi-component interventions be adequately accounted for in future cost-effectiveness studies?

- What evidence is there that interventions that are cost-effective in the short run—in terms of promoting well-being in adolescents and young people—have a lasting impact into adulthood?

- In the example of evaluation of the effectiveness and cost-effectiveness of school-based anti-bullying programmes, how would it be possible to identify, measure, and value wider cultural impact to schools, families, and communities of such programmes in the longer term?

- How can we apply recent developments in distributional cost-effectiveness analysis to investigate interventions to address adolescent well-being with a focus on place, ethnicity, and poverty?

- How can health economists contribute to the evidence base of mitigating transference of intergenerational barriers to joining the workforce, good parenting, and lifestyles that promote better life-time health?

References

Abu-Omar, K., Rütten, A., Burlacu, I., Schätzlein, V., Messing, S., & Suhrcke, M. (2017). The cost-effectiveness of physical activity interventions: A systematic review of reviews. *Preventive Medicine Reports*, 8, 72–78. https://doi.org/10.1016/j.pmedr.2017.08.006

Allen, K. A., Ryan, T., Gray, D. L., McInerney, D. M., & Waters, L. (2014). Social media use and social connectedness in adolescents: The positives and the potential pitfalls. *The Australian Educational and Developmental Psychologist*, 31(1), 18–31. https://doi.org/10.1017/edp.2014.2

Anna Freud. (2018, February). *Schools wanted for new research programme*. https://www.annafreud.org/news/schools-wanted-for-new-research-programme/

Appleby, L., Richards, N., Ibrahim, S., Turnbull, P., Rodway, C., & Kapur, N. (2021). Suicide in England in the COVID-19 pandemic: Early observational data from real time surveillance. *The Lancet Regional Health-Europe*, 4, 1–7. https://doi.org/10.1016/j.lanepe.2021.100110

Aslam, R. W., Hendry, M., Booth, A., Carter, B., Charles, J. M., Craine, N., Edwards, R. T., Noyes, J., Ntambwe, L. I., Pasterfield, D., Rycroft-Malone, J., Williams, N., & Whitaker, R. (2017). Intervention now to eliminate repeat unintended pregnancy in teenagers (INTERUPT): A systematic review of intervention effectiveness and cost-effectiveness, and qualitative and realist synthesis of implementation factors and user engagement. *BMC Medicine*, 15(1), 1–13. https://bmcmedicine.biomedcentral.com/articles/10.1186/s12916-017-0904-7

Aspenlieder, L., Buchanan, C. M., McDougall, P., & Sippola, L. K. (2009). Gender nonconformity and peer victimization in pre-and early adolescence. *International Journal of Developmental Science*, 3(1), 3–16. https://doi.org/10.3233/DEV-2009-3103

Baams, L., Beek, T., Hille, H., Zevenbergen, F. C., & Bos, H. M. (2013). Gender nonconformity, perceived stigmatization, and psychological well-being in Dutch sexual minority youth and young adults: A mediation analysis. *Archives of Sexual Behavior*, 42, 765–773. https://doi.org/10.1007/s10508-012-0055-z

Baraniuk, C. (2020). Fears grow of nutritional crisis in lockdown UK. *BMJ*, 370, m3193. https://doi.org/10.1136/bmj.m3193

Birch, J., Rishbeth, C., & Payne, S. R. (2020). Nature doesn't judge you—how urban nature supports young people's mental health and wellbeing in a diverse UK city. *Health & Place*, 62, 102296, 1–13. https://doi.org/10.1016/j.healthplace.2020.102296

Blanden, J., Gregg, P., & Machin, S. (2005, February). *Social mobility in Britain: Low and falling* [Paper No. CEPCP172]. CentrePiece. Centre for Economic Performance, London School of Economics and Political Science. https://cep.lse. ac.uk/pubs/download/cp172.pdf

Bond, L., Toumbourou, J. W., Thomas, L., Catalano, R. F., & Patton, G. (2005). Individual, family, school, and community risk and protective factors for depressive symptoms in adolescents: A comparison of risk profiles for substance use and depressive symptoms. *Prevention Science*, 6(2), 73–88. https://doi.org/10.1007/s11121-005-3407-2

Borde, R., Smith, J. J., Sutherland, R., Nathan, N., & Lubans, D. R. (2017). Methodological considerations and impact of school-based interventions on objectively measured physical activity in adolescents: A systematic review and meta-analysis. *Obesity Reviews*, 18(4), 476–490. https://doi.org/10.1111/obr.12517

Bowes, L., Joinson, C., Wolke, D., & Lewis, G. (2015). Peer victimisation during adolescence and its impact on depression in early adulthood: Prospective cohort study in the United Kingdom. *BMJ*, 350, h2469. https://doi.org/10.1136/bmj.h2469

Bozzini, A. B., Bauer, A., Maruyama, J., Simões, R., & Matijasevich, A. (2020). Factors associated with risk behaviors in adolescence: A systematic review. *Brazilian Journal of Psychiatry*, 43, 210–221. https://doi.org/10.1590/1516-4446-2019-0835

Brimblecombe, N., Evans-Lacko, S., Knapp, M., King, D., Takizawa, R., Maughan, B., & Arseneault, L. (2018). Long term economic impact associated with childhood bullying victimisation. *Social Science & Medicine*, 208, 134–141. https://doi.org/10.1016/j.socsci med.2018.05.014

British Audience Research Board. (2018). *The viewing report: Our annual exploration of the UK's viewing habits*. https://www.barb.co.uk/download/?file=/wp-content/uploads/ 2018/04/Barb-Viewing-Report-2017_FINAL_LR-May-2018.pdf

British Pregnancy Advisory Service. (2018). *Social media, SRE, and sensible drinking: Understanding the dramatic decline in teenage pregnancy*. https://www.bpas. org/media/3037/bpas-teenage-pregnancy-report.pdf

Broad, K. L., Sandhu, V. K., Sunderji, N., & Charach, A. (2017). Youth experiences of transition from child mental health services to adult mental health services: A qualitative thematic synthesis. *BMC Psychiatry*, 17, 1–11. https://doi.org/10.1186/s12 888-017-1538-1

Brown, V., Clery, E., & Ferguson, C. (2011). *Estimating the prevalence of young people absent from school due to bullying*. National Centre for Social Research. http://archive. anti-bullyingalliance.org.uk/sites/default/files/field/attachment/estimating-prevalence-young-people.pdf

Buckner, J. C., Beardslee, W. R., & Bassuk, E. L. (2004). Exposure to violence and low-income children's mental health: Direct, moderated, and mediated relations. *American Journal of Orthopsychiatry*, **74**(4), 413–423. https://doi.org/10.1037/0002-9432.74.4.413

Carrieri, V., Davillas, A., & Jones, A. M. (2021). *Equality of opportunity and the expansion of higher education in the UK*. Understanding Society. https://www.understandingsociety.ac.uk/research/publications/546997

Charles, J. M., Harrington, D. M., Davies, M. J., Edwardson, C. L., Gorely, T., Bodicoat, D. H., Khunti, K., Sherar, L. B., Yates, T., & Edwards, R. T. (2019). Micro-costing and a cost-consequence analysis of the 'Girls Active' programme: A cluster randomised controlled trial. *PLoS One*, **14**(8), e0221276. https://doi.org/10.1371/journal.pone.0221276

Chowdry, H., & Fitzsimons, P. (2016). *The cost of late intervention: EIF analysis 2016*. Early Intervention Foundation. https://www.eif.org.uk/files/pdf/cost-of-late-intervention-2016.pdf

Clark, D. (2023a, 9 March). *Population of England 2021, by age group*. Statista. https://www.statista.com/statistics/281208/population-of-the-england-by-age-group/

Clark, D. (2023b, 9 March). *Population of Northern Ireland 2021, by age group*. Statista. https://www.statista.com/statistics/533486/northern-ireland-population-by-age/

Clark, D. (2023c, 9 March). *Population of Scotland 2021, by age group*. Statista. https://www.statista.com/statistics/533482/scotland2-population-by-age/

Clark, D. (2023d, 9 March). *Population of Wales 2021, by age group*. Statista. https://www.statista.com/statistics/533485/population-of-wales-by-age/

Clarkson, S., Axford, N., Berry, V., Edwards, R. T., Bjornstad, G., Wrigley, Z., Charles, J., Hoare, Z., Ukoumunne, O. C., Matthews, J., & Hutchings, J. (2016). Effectiveness and micro-costing of the KiVa school-based bullying prevention programme in Wales: study protocol for a pragmatic definitive parallel group cluster randomised controlled trial. *BMC Public Health*, **16**(1), 1–11. https://doi.org/10.1186/s12889-016-2746-1

Clarkson, S., Bowes, L., Coulman, E., Broome, M. R., Cannings-John, R., Charles, J. M., Edwards, R. T., Ford, T., Hastings, R. P., Hayes, R., Patterson, P., Sergott, J., Townson, J., Watkins, R., Badger, J., Hutchings, J., & the Stand Together Team. (2022). The UK Stand Together trial: Protocol for a multicentre cluster randomised controlled trial to evaluate the effectiveness and cost-effectiveness of KiVa to reduce bullying in primary schools. *BMC Public Health*, **22**(1), 608. https://doi.org/10.1186/s12889-022-12642-x

Claxton, K., Martin, S., Soares, M., Rice, N., Spackman, E., Hinde, S., Devlin, N., Smith, P. C., & Sculpher, M. (2015). Methods for the estimation of the National Institute for Health and Care Excellence cost-effectiveness threshold. *Health Technology Assessment*, **19**(14), 1–503. https://doi.org/10.3310/hta19140

Committee on Higher Education. (1963, 23 September). *Higher education: Report of the Committee appointed by the Prime Minister under the Chairmanship of Lord Robbins 1961–63*. Cmnd. 2154. Her Majesty's Stationery Office.

Conroy, K. (2016). Promoting uptake of long-acting reversible contraception among teen mothers. *Journal of Adolescent Health*, **58**(6), 598–599. https://doi.org/10.1016/j.jadohealth.2016.03.031

Cookson, R., Griffin, S., Norheim, O. F., & Culyer, A. J. (Eds.). (2020). *Distributional cost-effectiveness analysis: Quantifying health equity impacts and trade-offs*. Oxford University Press.

Corder, K., Sharp, S. J., Jong, S. T., Foubister, C., Brown, H. E., Wells, E. K., & van Sluijs, E. M. (2020). Effectiveness and cost-effectiveness of the GoActive intervention to increase physical activity among UK adolescents: A cluster randomised controlled trial. *PLoS Medicine*, 17(7), e1003210. https://doi.org/10.1371/journal.pmed.1003210

Council for the Curriculum, Examinations and Assessment. (2020). *Understanding Homelessness. Understanding wellbeing*. https://ccea.org.uk/learning-resources/unders tanding-homelessness/key-stages-3-4/understanding-wellbeing#section-5894

Crane, R. S., & Kuyken, W. (2013). The implementation of mindfulness-based cognitive therapy: Learning from the UK health service experience. *Mindfulness*, 4, 246–254. https://doi.org/10.1007/s12671-012-0121-6

Cuijpers, P., Sijbrandij, M., Koole, S., Huibers, M., Berking, M., & Andersson, G. (2014). Psychological treatment of generalized anxiety disorder: a meta-analysis. *Clinical Psychology Review*, 34(2), 130–140. https://doi.org/10.1016/j.cpr.2014.01.002

Dantchev, S., Hickman, M., Heron, J., Zammit, S., & Wolke, D. (2019). The independent and cumulative effects of sibling and peer bullying in childhood on depression, anxiety, suicidal ideation, and self-harm in adulthood. *Frontiers in Psychiatry*, 10(651), 1–12. https://doi.org/10.3389/fpsyt.2019.00651

Davis, M., Banks, S., Fisher, W., & Grudzinskas, A. (2004). Longitudinal patterns of offending during the transition to adulthood in youth from the mental health system. *The Journal of Behavioral Health Services & Research*, 31, 351–366. https://doi.org/10.1007/BF02287689

Department for Work & Pensions. (2022, 31 March). *Children in low income families: Local area statistics, financial year ending 2021*. https://www.gov.uk/government/statistics/children-in-low-income-families-local-area-statistics-2014-to-2021/children-in-low-income-families-local-area-statistics-financial-year-ending-2021

Department of Health. (2010). *Teenage pregnancy strategy: Beyond 2010*. Department for Children, Schools and Families. https://dera.ioe.ac.uk/id/eprint/11277/1/4287_Teen age%20pregnancy%20strategy_aw8.pdf

Dixon, S. J. (2023, 29 August). *Number of global social media users from 2017 to 2027*. Statista. https://www.statista.com/statistics/278414/number-of-worldwide-social-netw ork-users/

Dray, J., Bowman, J., Campbell, E., Freund, M., Wolfenden, L., Hodder, R. K., McElwaine, K., Tremain, D., Bartlem, K., Bailey, J., Small, T., Palazzi, K., Oldmeadow, C., & Wiggers, J. (2017). Systematic review of universal resilience-focused interventions targeting child and adolescent mental health in the school setting. *Journal of the American Academy of Child & Adolescent Psychiatry*, 56(10), 813–824. https://doi.org/10.1016/j.jaac.2017.07.780

Edwards, R. T., Bryning, L., & Crane, R. (2015). Design of economic evaluations of mindfulness-based interventions: Ten methodological questions of which to be mindful. *Mindfulness*, 6(3), 490–500. https://doi.org/10.1007/s12671-014-0282-6

Fergusson, D. M., Woodward, L. J., & Horwood, L. J. (2000). Risk factors and life processes associated with the onset of suicidal behaviour during adolescence and early adulthood. *Psychological Medicine*, 30(1), 23–39. https://doi.org/10.1017/S003329179900135X

Fisher, H. L., Moffitt, T. E., Houts, R. M., Belsky, D. W., Arseneault, L., & Caspi, A. (2012). Bullying victimisation and risk of self harm in early adolescence: Longitudinal cohort study. *BMJ*, **344**, e2683. https://doi.org/10.1136/bmj.e2683

Ford, T., Mitrofan, O., & Wolpert, M. (2014). Life course: Children and young people's mental health. In **N. Mehta, O. Murphy, & C. Lillford-Wildman** (Eds.), *Annual report of the Chief Medical Officer 2013* (pp. 99–131). Department of Health. https://assets.pub lishing.service.gov.uk/government/uploads/system/uploads/attachment_data/file/413 196/CMO_web_doc.pdf

Francis-Devine, B., Powell, A., & Buchanan, I. (2023). *Youth unemployment statistics.* House of Commons Library. https://commonslibrary.parliament.uk/research-briefings/sn05871/

Frech, A. (2012). Healthy behavior trajectories between adolescence and young adulthood. *Advances in Life Course Research*, **17**(2), 59–68. https://doi.org/10.1016/j.alcr.2012.01.003

Furlong, M., McGilloway, S., Bywater, T., Hutchings, J., Smith, S. M., & Donnelly, M. (2012). Behavioural and cognitive-behavioural group-based parenting programmes for early-onset conduct problems in children aged 3 to 12 years. *Campbell Systematic Reviews*, **8**(1), 39. https://doi.org/10.4073/csr.2012.12

Gega, L., Jankovic, D., Saramago Goncalves, P. R., Marshall, D., Dawson, S., Brabyn, S., Nikolaidis, G. F., Melton, H., Churchill, R., & Bojke, L. (2022). Costs and outcomes of digital interventions (CODI) in mental health: Evidence synthesis, economic modelling and knowledge exchange. *Health Technology Assessment*, **26**(1), 1–182. https://doi.org/10.3310/RCTI6942

Genie, M. G., Loría-Rebolledo, L. E., Paranjothy, S., Powell, D., Ryan, M., Sakowsky, R. A., & Watson, V. (2020). Understanding public preferences and trade-offs for government responses during a pandemic: A protocol for a discrete choice experiment in the UK. *BMJ Open*, **10**(11), e043477. https://doi.org/10.1136/bmjopen-2020-043477

Gómez-López, M., Viejo, C., & Ortega-Ruiz, R. (2019). Psychological well-being during adolescence: Stability and association with romantic relationships. *Frontiers in Psychology*, **10**, 1772, 1–13. https://doi.org/10.3389/fpsyg.2019.01772

Government Equalities Office. (2019). *LGBT action plan: Annual progress report 2018 to 2019.* Government Equalities Office. https://dera.ioe.ac.uk/id/eprint/33740/1/20190702__LGBT_Action_Plan__Annual_Report__WESC.pdf

Gratzer, D., & Khalid-Khan, F. (2016). Internet-delivered cognitive behavioural therapy in the treatment of psychiatric illness. *Canadian Medical Association Journal*, **188**(4), 263–272. https://doi.org/10.1503/cmaj.150007

Guss, C., Shumer, D., & Katz-Wise, S. L. (2015). Transgender and gender nonconforming adolescent care: Psychosocial and medical considerations. *Current Opinion in Pediatrics*, **26**(4), 421–426. https://doi.org/10.1097/MOP.0000000000000240

Hagell, A., & Rigby, E. (2015). Looking at the effectiveness of prevention and early intervention. *British Journal of School Nursing*, **10**(1), 26–30. https://doi.org/10.12968/bjsn.2015.10.1.26

Hagell, A., & Shah, R. (2019). *Highlights: Key data on young people 2019.* Association for Young People's Health. https://www.active-together.org/files/68190/ayph-kdyp2019-full version.pdf

Haidt, J. (2024). *The anxious generation: How the great rewiring of childhood is causing an epidemic of mental illness.* Random House.

Harrington, D. M., Davies, M. J., Bodicoat, D. H., Charles, J. M., Chudasama, Y. V., Gorely, T., Khunti, K., Plekhanova, T., Rowlands, A. V., Sherar, L. B., Edwards, R. T., Yates, T., & Edwardson, C. L. (2018). Effectiveness of the 'Girls Active' school-based physical activity programme: A cluster randomised controlled trial. *International Journal of Behavioral Nutrition and Physical Activity*, 15(1), 1–18. https://doi.org/10.1186/s12966-018-0664-6

Hartmann-Boyce, J., McRobbie, H., Butler, A. R., Lindson, N., Bullen, C., Begh, R., Theodoulou, A., Notley, C., Rigotti, N. A., Turner, T., Fanshawe, T. R., & Hajek, P. (2022). Electronic cigarettes for smoking cessation. *Cochrane Database of Systematic Reviews*, 11, CD010216. https://doi.org/10.1002/14651858.CD010216.pub7

Heckman, J. J., & Landersø, R. (2021). *Lessons from Denmark about inequality and social mobility*. [Working paper 28543]. National Bureau of Economic Research. https://doi.org/10.3386/w28543

Heuzenroeder, L., Donnelly, M., Haby, M. M., Mihalopoulos, C., Rossell, R., Carter, R., Andrews, G., & Vos, T. (2004). Cost-effectiveness of psychological and pharmacological interventions for generalized anxiety disorder and panic disorder. *Australian & New Zealand Journal of Psychiatry*, 38(8), 602–612. https://doi.org/10.1080/j.1440-1614.2004.01423.x

Hjemdal, O., Vogel, P. A., Solem, S., Hagen, K., & Stiles, T. C. (2011). The relationship between resilience and levels of anxiety, depression, and obsessive-compulsive symptoms in adolescents. *Clinical Psychology & Psychotherapy*, 18(4), 314–321. https://doi.org/10.1002/cpp.719

House of Commons Science and Technology Committee. (2019). *Impact of social media and screen-use on young people's health*. HC 822. House of Commons. https://publications.parliament.uk/pa/cm201719/cmselect/cmsctech/822/822.pdf

Ireland, J. L. (Ed.). (2002). *Bullying among prisoners: Evidence, research and intervention strategies* (2013, digital ed.). Routledge. https://doi.org/10.4324/9781315783239

Kabat-Zinn, J. (2016). *Wherever you go, there you are: Mindfulness meditation for everyday life*. Piatkus.

Kärnä, A., Voeten, M., Little, T. D., Poskiparta, E., Alanen, E., & Salmivalli, C. (2011a). Going to scale: A nonrandomized nationwide trial of the KiVa antibullying program for grades 1–9. *Journal of Consulting and Clinical Psychology*, 79(6), 796. https://doi.org/10.1037/a0025740

Kärnä, A., Voeten, M., Little, T. D., Poskiparta, E., Kaljonen, A., & Salmivalli, C. (2011b). A large-scale evaluation of the KiVa antibullying program: Grades 4–6. *Child Development*, 82(1), 311–330. https://doi.org/10.1111/j.1467-8624.2010.01557.x

Kearney, C. A. (2008). School absenteeism and school refusal behavior in youth: A contemporary review. *Clinical Psychology Review*, 28(3), 451–471. https://doi.org/10.1016/j.cpr.2007.07.012

Kelly, Y., Zilanawala, A., Booker, C., & Sacker, A. (2018). Social media use and adolescent mental health: Findings from the UK Millennium Cohort Study. *EClinicalMedicine*, 6, 59–68. https://doi.org/10.1016/j.eclinm.2018.12.005

Khanolkar, A. R., Frost, D. M., Tabor, E., Redclift, V., Amos, R., & Patalay, P. (2023). Ethnic and sexual identity-related inequalities in adolescent health and well-being in a national population-based study. *LGBT Health*, **10**(1), 26–40. https://doi.org/10.1089/lgbt.2021.0473

Kosciw, J. G., Palmer, N. A., & Kull, R. M. (2015). Reflecting resiliency: Openness about sexual orientation and/or gender identity and its relationship to well-being and educational outcomes for LGBT students. *American Journal of Community Psychology*, **55**(1), 167–178. https://doi.org/10.1007/s10464-014-9642-6

Kozina, A. (2020). School-based prevention of anxiety using the 'My FRIENDS' emotional resilience program: Six-month follow-up. *International Journal of Psychology*, **55**, 70–77. https://doi.org/10.1002/ijop.12553

Kozina, A., Vidmar, M., Veldin, M., Pivec, T., & Peras, I. (2021). The role of emotional competencies in psychological responding to COVID–19 pandemic. *Psihologija*, **54**(4), 423–440. https://doi.org/10.2298/PSI200723006K

Kuyken, W., Nuthall, E., Byford, S., Crane, C., Dalgleish, T., Ford, T., Greenberg, M. T., Ukoumunne, O. C., Viner, R. M., Williams, J. M. G., & the MYRIAD team. (2017). The effectiveness and cost-effectiveness of a mindfulness training programme in schools compared with normal school provision (MYRIAD): Study protocol for a randomised controlled trial. *Trials*, **18**(1), 1–17. https://doi.org/10.1186/s13063-017-1917-4

Laine, J., Kuvaja-Köllner, V., Pietilä, E., Koivuneva, M., Valtonen, H., & Kankaanpää, E. (2014). Cost-effectiveness of population-level physical activity interventions: A systematic review. *American Journal of Health Promotion*, **29**(2), 71–80. https://doi.org/10.4278/ajhp.131210-LIT-622

Lanigan, J., Tee, L., & Brandreth, R. (2019). Childhood obesity. *Medicine*, **47**(3), 190–194. https://doi.org/10.1016/j.mpmed.2018.12.007

Lehnert, T., Sonntag, D., Konnopka, A., Riedel-Heller, S., & König, H. H. (2012). The long-term cost-effectiveness of obesity prevention interventions: Systematic literature review. *Obesity Reviews*, **13**(6), 537–553. https://doi.org/10.1111/j.1467-789X.2011.00980.x

Lehtimaki, S., Martic, J., Wahl, B., Foster, K. T., & Schwalbe, N. (2021). Evidence on digital mental health interventions for adolescents and young people: Systematic overview. *JMIR Mental Health*, **8**(4), e25847. https://doi.org/10.2196/25847

Lewis, C. E., Ubido, J., Holford, R., & Scott-Samuel, A. (2010). *Prevention programmes cost-effectiveness review: Physical activity*. Liverpool Public Health Observatory. https://researchonline.ljmu.ac.uk/id/eprint/2004/1/83_28th_Feb_Physical_activity_and_cost_FINAL.pdf

Love, R., Adams, J., & van Sluijs, E. M. (2019). Are school-based physical activity interventions effective and equitable? A meta-analysis of cluster randomized controlled trials with accelerometer-assessed activity. *Obesity Reviews*, **20**(6), 859–870. https://doi.org/10.1111/obr.12823

Luthar, S. S., & Cicchetti, D. (2000). The construct of resilience: Implications for interventions and social policies. *Development and Psychopathology*, **12**(4), 857–885. https://doi.org/10.1017/S0954579400004156

Ma, K. K. Y., Anderson, J. K., & Burn, A. M. (2022). Review: School-based interventions to improve mental health literacy and reduce mental health stigma—a systematic review. *Child and Adolescent Mental Health*, **28**(2), 230–240. https://doi.org/10.1111/camh.12543

Magnus, A., Haby, M. M., Carter, R., & Swinburn, B. (2009). The cost-effectiveness of removing television advertising of high-fat and/or high-sugar food and beverages to Australian children. *International Journal of Obesity*, 33(10), 1094–1102. https://doi.org/10.1038/ijo.2009.156

Marmot, M., Allen, J., Goldblatt, P., Boyce, T., McNeish, D., Grady, M., & Geddes, I. (2010). *Fair society, healthy lives: The Marmot review. Strategic review of health inequalities in England post-2010*. https://www.instituteofhealthequity.org/resources-reports/fair-society-healthy-lives-the-marmot-review

Martin-Storey, A., & August, E. G. (2016). Harassment due to gender nonconformity mediates the association between sexual minority identity and depressive symptoms. *The Journal of Sex Research*, 53(1), 85–97. https://doi.org/10.1080/00224499.2014.980497

McCluskey, G., Fry, D., Hamilton, S., King, A., Laurie, M., Mcara, L., & Stewart, T.M. (2021). School closures, exam cancellations and isolation: The impact of Covid-19 on young people's mental health. *Emotional and Behavioural Difficulties*, 26(1), 46–59. https://doi.org/10.1080/13632752.2021.1903182

McCrone, P., Knapp, M., Proudfoot, J., Ryden, C., Cavanagh, K., Shapiro, D. A., Ilson, S., Gray, J. A., Goldberg, D., Mann, A., & Marks, I. (2004). Cost-effectiveness of computerised cognitive-behavioural therapy for anxiety and depression in primary care: Randomised controlled trial. *The British Journal of Psychiatry*, 185(1), 55–62. https://doi.org/10.1192/bjp.185.1.55

McDaid, D., Park, A. L., & Wahlbeck, K. (2019). The economic case for the prevention of mental illness. *Annual Review of Public Health*, 40, 373–389. https://doi.org/10.1146/annurev-publhealth-040617-013629

McLeod, J. D., & Knight, S. (2010). The association of socioemotional problems with early sexual initiation. *Perspectives on Sexual and Reproductive Health*, 42(2), 93–101. https://doi.org/10.1363/4209310

McLeod, J. D., & Shanahan, M. J. (1996). Trajectories of poverty and children's mental health. *Journal of Health and Social Behavior*, 37(3), 207–220. https://doi.org/10.2307/2137292

Mindfulness in Schools Project. (2023). *Mindfulness as part of the curriculum for Wales 2022*. https://mindfulnessinschools.org/mindfulness-as-part-of-the-curriculum-for-wales-2022/

Montero-Marin, J., Allwood, M., Ball, S., Crane, C., De Wilde, K., Hinze, V., Jones, B., Lord, L., Nuthall, E., Raja, A., Taylor, L., Tudor, K., MYRIAD Team, Blakemore, S-J., Byford, S., Dalgleish, T., Ford, T., Greenberg, M., Ukoumunne, O., . . . Kuyken, W. (2022). School-based mindfulness training in early adolescence: What works, for whom and how in the MYRIAD trial? *Evidence-based Mental Health*, 25(3), 117–124. http://dx.doi.org/10.1136/ebmental-2022-300439

Montero-Marin, J., Nuthall, E., Byford, S., Crane, C., Dalgleish, T., Ford, T., Ganguli, P., Greenberg, M. T., Ukoumunne, O.C., Viner, R. M., Williams, J. M. G., MYRIAD team, & Kuyken, W. (2021). Update to the effectiveness and cost-effectiveness of a mindfulness training programme in schools compared with normal school provision (MYRIAD): Study protocol for a randomised controlled trial. *Trials*, 22(254), 1–5. https://doi.org/10.1186/s13063-021-05213-9

Moodie, M., Haby, M., Galvin, L., Swinburn, B., & Carter, R. (2009). Cost-effectiveness of active transport for primary school children—Walking School Bus program. *International Journal of Behavioral Nutrition and Physical Activity*, 6(1), 1–11. https://doi.org/10.1186/1479-5868-6-63

Mulvale, G. M., Nguyen, T. D., Miatello, A. M., Embrett, M. G., Wakefield, P. A., & Randall, G. E. (2016). Lost in transition or translation? Care philosophies and transitions between child and youth and adult mental health services: A systematic review. *Journal of Mental Health*, 28(4), 1–10. https://doi.org/10.3109/09638 237.2015.1124389

Murray, C. J. L. (1996). Rethinking DALYs. In C. L. J. Murray & A. D. López (Eds.), *The global burden of disease: A comprehensive assessment of mortality and disability from diseases, injuries and risk factors in 1990 and projected to 2020* (pp. 1–18). Harvard University Press.

National Health Service. (2020, 28 May). *Overview: Gender dysphoria.* https://www.nhs.uk/conditions/gender-dysphoria/

National Health Service. (2022, 10 October). *Using e-cigarettes to stop smoking.* https://www.nhs.uk/live-well/quit-smoking/using-e-cigarettes-to-stop-smoking/

National Improvement Hub. (2017, 1 January). *Mental, emotional, social and physical wellbeing.* https://education.gov.scot/parentzone/learning-at-home/supporting-health-and-wellbeing/mental-emotional-social-and-physical-wellbeing/

National Institute for Health and Care Excellence. (2009a). *Physical activity for children and young people* (PH17). https://www.nice.org.uk/guidance/ph17/resources/physical-activity-for-children-and-young-people-pdf-1996181580229

National Institute for Health and Care Excellence. (2009b). *NICE guideline. Depression in adults: Recognition and management* (CG90). https://www.nice.org.uk/guidance/cg90

National Institute for Health and Care Excellence. (2013). *Weight management: Lifestyle services for overweight or obese children and young people* (PH47). https://www.nice.org.uk/guidance/ph47

National Institute for Health and Care Excellence. (2014). *Smoking: Preventing uptake in children and young people* (PH14). https://www.nice.org.uk/guidance/ph14

National Institute for Health and Care Excellence. (2015). *Obesity in children and young people: Prevention and lifestyle weight management programmes* (QS94). https://www.nice.org.uk/guidance/qs94

National Institute for Health and Care Excellence. (2019a). *Sexual health* (QS178). https://www.nice.org.uk/guidance/qs178/resources/sexual-health-pdf-75545667625669

National Institute for Health and Care Excellence. (2019b). *Depression in children and young people: Identification and management* (NG134). https://www.nice.org.uk/guidance/NG134

National Institute for Health and Care Excellence. (2020). *Evidence review: Gender-affirming hormones for children and adolescents with gender dysphoria.* https://cass.independent-review.uk/wp-content/uploads/2022/09/20220726_Evidence-review_Gender-affirming-hormones_For-upload_Final.pdf

National Institute for Health and Care Excellence. (2022a). *Lifestyle weight management services for overweight or obese children and young people overview.* https://pathways.nice.org.uk/pathways/lifestyle-weight-management-services-for-overweight-or-obese-children-and-young-people

National Institute for Health and Care Excellence. (2022b). *Depression in adults: Treatment and management* (NG222). https://www.nice.org.uk/guidance/ng222

Nuffield Trust. (2021). *Teenage pregnancy*. https://www.nuffieldtrust.org.uk/resource/teen age-pregnancy

Office for Health Improvement and Disparities. (2022a). *Nicotine vaping in England: 2022 evidence* update. https://www.gov.uk/government/publications/nicotine-vaping-in-engl and-2022-evidence-update

Office for Health Improvement and Disparities. (2022b). *Making smoking obsolete: Summary*. https://www.gov.uk/government/publications/the-khan-review-making-smoking-obsolete/making-smoking-obsolete-summary

Office for Health Improvement and Disparities. (2023). *Youth vaping: Call for evidence*. https://www.gov.uk/government/consultations/youth-vaping-call-for-evidence/youth-vaping-call-for-evidence

Office for National Statistics. (2021, 27 May). *Young people not in education, employment or training (NEET), UK: May 2021*. https://www.ons.gov.uk/employmentandlabourmar ket/peoplenotinwork/unemployment/bulletins/youngpeoplenotineducationemplo ymentortrainingneet/may2021

Office for National Statistics. (2022a, 7 March). *Avoidable mortality in Great Britain: 2020*. https://www.ons.gov.uk/peoplepopulationandcommunity/healthandsocialcare/causes ofdeath/bulletins/avoidablemortalityinenglandandwales/latest#avoidable-mortal ity-by-cause

Office for National Statistics. (2022b, 6 September). *Suicide in England and Wales: 2021 registrations*. https://www.ons.gov.uk/peoplepopulationandcommunity/birthsdeathsa ndmarriages/deaths/bulletins/suicideintheunitedkingdom/2021registrations#suicide-patterns-by-age

Organisation for Economic Co-operation and Development Policy Brief. (2020). *The impact of COVID-19 on student equity and inclusion: Supporting vulnerable students during school closures and school re-openings*. https://www.oecd.org/coronavirus/policy-responses/the-impact-of-covid-19-on-student-equity-and-inclusion-supporting-vul nerable-students-during-school-closures-and-school-re-openings-d593b5c8/

Paul, M., Street, C., Wheeler, N., & Singh, S. P. (2015). Transition to adult services for young people with mental health needs: a systematic review. *Clinical Child Psychology and Psychiatry*, 20(3), 436–457. https://doi.org/10.1177/1359104514526603

Perales, F. (2016). The costs of being 'different': Sexual identity and subjective wellbeing over the life course. *Social Indicators Research*, 127, 827–849. https://doi.org/10.1007/s11 205-015-0974-x

Persson, M., Wennberg, L., Beckman, L., Salmivalli, C., & Svensson, M. (2018). The cost-effectiveness of the Kiva antibullying program: Results from a decision-analytic model. *Prevention Science*, 19(6), 728–737. https://doi.org/10.1007/s11121-018-0893-6

Polos, J., Koning, S., & McDade, T. (2021). Do intersecting identities structure social contexts to influence life course health? The case of school peer economic disadvantage and obesity. *Social Science & Medicine*, 289, 114424. https://doi.org/10.1016/j.socsci med.2021.114424

Ponsford, R., Bragg, S., Meiksin, R., Tilouche, N., Van Dyck, L., Sturgess, J., Allen, E., Elbourne, C., Hadley, A., Lohan, M., Mercer, C.H., Melendez Torres, G., Morris, S., Young, H., & Bonell, C. (2022a). Feasibility and acceptability of a whole-school social-marketing intervention to prevent unintended teenage pregnancies and promote sexual health: Evidence for progression from a pilot to a phase III randomised trial in English secondary schools. *Pilot and Feasibility Studies*, **8**(1), 1–15. https://doi.org/10.1186/s40814-022-00971-y

Ponsford, R., Meiksin, R., Allen, E., Melendez-Torres, G. J., Morris, S., Mercer, C., Campbell, R., Young, H., Lohan, M., Coyle, K., & Bonell, C. (2022b). The Positive Choices trial: Update to study protocol for a phase-III RCT trial of a whole-school social-marketing intervention to promote sexual health and reduce health inequalities. *Trials*, **23**(1), 287. https://doi.org/10.1186/s13063-022-06191-2

Public Health England. (2018). *Teenage pregnancy prevention framework supporting young people to prevent unplanned pregnancy and develop healthy relationships*. https://www.gov.uk/government/publications/teenage-pregnancy-prevention-framework

Qureshi, S. (2021). Pandemics within the pandemic: Confronting socio-economic inequities in a datafied world. *Information Technology for Development*, **27**(2), 151–170. https://doi.org/10.1080/02681102.2021.1911020

Rieger, G., & Savin-Williams, R. C. (2012). Gender nonconformity, sexual orientation, and psychological well-being. *Archives of Sexual Behavior*, **41**, 611–621. https://doi.org/10.1007/s10508-011-9738-0

Rivers, I., & Noret, N. (2008). Well-being among same-sex-and opposite-sex-attracted youth at school. *School Psychology Review*, **37**(2), 174–187. https://doi.org/10.1080/02796015.2008.12087892

Ross, D. A., Hinton, R., Melles-Brewer, M., Engel, D., Zeck, W., Fagan, L., Herat, J., Phaladi, G., Imbago-Jácome, D., Anyona, P., Sanchez, A., Damji, N., Terki, F., Baltag, V., Patton, G., Silverman, A., Fogstad, H., Banerjee, A., & Mohan, A. (2020). Adolescent well-being: A definition and conceptual framework. *Journal of Adolescent Health*, **67**(4), 472–476. https://doi.org/10.1016/j.jadohealth.2020.06.042

Salmivalli, C., Kärnä, A., & Poskiparta, E. (2011). Counteracting bullying in Finland: The KiVa program and its effects on different forms of being bullied. *International Journal of Behavioral Development*, **35**(5), 405–411. https://doi.org/10.1177/0165025411407457

Scott, E., Dale, J., Russell, R., & Wolke, D. (2016). Young people who are being bullied—do they want general practice support? *BMC Family Practice*, **17**(1), 1–9. https://doi.org/10.1186/s12875-016-0517-9

Shavit, Y., Arum, R., & Gamoran, A. (Eds.). (2007). *Stratification in higher education: A comparative study*. Stanford University Press.

Simon, N., McGillivray, L., Roberts, N. P., Barawi, K., Lewis, C. E., & Bisson, J. I. (2019). Acceptability of internet-based cognitive behavioural therapy (i-CBT) for post-traumatic stress disorder (PTSD): A systematic review. *European Journal of Psychotraumatology*, **10**(1), 1646092. https://doi.org/10.1080/20008198.2019.1646092

Sinha, I. P., Lee, A. R., Bennett, D., Mcgeehan, L., Abrams, E. M., Mayell, S. J., Harwood, R., Hawcutt, D. B., Gilchrist, F. J., Auth, M. K., Simba, J. M., & Taylor-Robinson, D. C. (2020). Child poverty, food insecurity, and respiratory health during the COVID-19 pandemic. *The Lancet Respiratory*, **8**(8), 762–763. https://doi.org/10.1016/S2213-2600(20)30280-0

Shankleman, M., Hammond, L., & Jones, F. W. (2021). Adolescent social media use and well-being: A systematic review and thematic meta-synthesis. *Adolescent Research Review*, **6**, 471–492. https://doi.org/10.1007/s40894-021-00154-5

Statista. (2019). *UK: Smartphone ownership by age from 2012–2018*. https://www.statista. com/statistics/271851/smartphone-owners-in-the-united-kingdom-uk-by-age

Takizawa, R., Maughan, B., & Arseneault, L. (2014). Adult health outcomes of childhood bullying victimization: Evidence from a five-decade longitudinal British birth cohort. *American Journal of Psychiatry, 171*(7), 777–784. https://doi.org/10.1176/appi. ajp.2014.13101401

Tammelin, T., Näyhä, S., Hills, A. P., & Järvelin, M. R. (2003). Adolescent participation in sports and adult physical activity. *American Journal of Preventive Medicine, 24*(1), 22–28. https://doi.org/10.1016/s0749-3797(02)00575-5

Telama, R., Yang, X., Viikari, J., Välimäki, I., Wanne, O., & Raitakari, O. (2005). Physical activity from childhood to adulthood: A 21-year tracking study. *American Journal of Preventive Medicine, 28*(3), 267–273. https://doi.org/10.1016/j.amepre.2004.12.003

Tigers Trust. (2021). *Tigers Trust—PL Kicks/Kicks Targeted Programme. Social value report 2019–2021*. https://www.tigerstrust.co.uk/_webedit/uploaded-files/All%20Files/ FINAL_SPC_TigersTrust_KicksImpactReport2021%5B5132%5D.pdf

Tigers Trust. (2023). *Premier League Kicks*. https://www.tigerstrust.co.uk/activities-courses/ young-people-13-17/premier-league-kicks/

Twenge, J. M., Joiner, T. E., Rogers, M. L., & Martin, G. N. (2018). Increases in depressive symptoms, suicide-related outcomes, and suicide rates among US adolescents after 2010 and links to increased new media screen time. *Clinical Psychological Science, 6*(1), 3–17. https://doi.org/10.1177/2167702617723376

Unison. (2019). *Youth services at breaking point*. https://www.unison.org.uk/content/uplo ads/2019/04/Youth-services-report-04-2019.pdf

United Kingdom Parliament. (2021, 13 July). *Mental health services: Children and young people*. UIN 32561. https://questions-statements.parliament.uk/written-questions/det ail/2021-07-13/32561

Vickery, C. E., & Dorjee, D. (2016). Mindfulness training in primary schools decreases negative affect and increases meta-cognition in children. *Frontiers in Psychology, 6*, 1–13. https://doi.org/10.3389/fpsyg.2015.02025

Vigerland, S., Lenhard, F., Bonnert, M., Lalouni, M., Hedman, E., Ahlen, J., Olén, O., Serlachius, E., & Ljótsson, B. (2016). Internet-delivered cognitive behavior therapy for children and adolescents: A systematic review and meta-analysis. *Clinical Psychology Review, 50*, 1–10. https://doi.org/10.1016/j.cpr.2016.09.005

Wahlbeck, K., Cresswell-Smith, J., Haaramo, P., & Parkkonen, J. (2017). Interventions to mitigate the effects of poverty and inequality on mental health. *Social Psychiatry and Psychiatric Epidemiology, 52*, 505–514. https://doi.org/10.1007/s00127-017-1370-4

Warburton, D. E., & Bredin, S. S. (2016). Reflections on physical activity and health: What should we recommend? *Canadian Journal of Cardiology, 32*(4), 495–504. https://doi. org/10.1016/j.cjca.2016.01.024

Washington State Institute for Public Policy. (2017). *Benefit-cost results*. https://www.wsipp. wa.gov/BenefitCost/WsippBenefitCost_AllPrograms

Werner-Seidler, A., Perry, Y., Calear, A. L., Newby, J. M., & Christensen, H. (2017). School-based depression and anxiety prevention programs for young people: A systematic review and meta-analysis. *Clinical Psychology Review, 51*, 30–47. https://doi.org/ 10.1016/j.cpr.2016.10.005

Whitaker, R., Hendry, M., Aslam, R., Booth, A., Carter, B., Charles, J. M., Craine, N., Edwards, R. T., Noyes, J., Ntambwe, L. I., Pasterfield, D., Rycroft-Malone, J., & Williams, N. (2016). Intervention now to eliminate repeat unintended pregnancy in teenagers (INTERUPT): A systematic review of intervention effectiveness and cost-effectiveness, and qualitative and realist synthesis of implementation factors and user engagement. *Health Technology Assessment*, 20(16), 1–214. https://doi.org/10.3310/hta20160

Wilkins, A. J., O'Callaghan, M. J., Najman, J. M., Bor, W., Williams, G. M., & Shuttlewood, G. (2004). Early childhood factors influencing health-related quality of life in adolescents at 13 years. *Journal of Paediatrics and Child Health*, 40(3), 102–109. https://doi.org/10.1111/j.1440-1754.2004.00309.x

Williford, A., Boulton, A., Noland, B., Little, T. D., Kärnä, A., & Salmivalli, C. (2012). Effects of the KiVa anti-bullying program on adolescents' depression, anxiety, and perception of peers. *Journal of Abnormal Child Psychology*, 40(2), 289–300. https://doi.org/10.1007/s10802-011-9551-1

Windle, G. (2011). What is resilience? A review and concept analysis. *Reviews in Clinical Gerontology*, 21(2), 152–169. https://doi.org/10.1017/S0959259810000420

Wolke, D. (2014, 20 May). *The long shadow of bullying*. https://warwick.ac.uk/newsandevents/pressreleases/the_long_shadow_of_childhood_bullying1

World Health Organization. (2020a). *Adolescent mental health*. https://www.who.int/news-room/fact-sheets/detail/adolescent-mental-health

World Health Organization. (2020b). *WHO methods and data sources for global burden of disease estimates 2000–2019*. https://cdn.who.int/media/docs/default-source/gho-documents/global-health-estimates/ghe2019_daly-methods.pdf

World Health Organization. (2021a). *Adolescent health*. https://www.who.int/health-topics/adolescent-health

World Health Organization. (2021b). *Obesity*. https://www.who.int/health-topics/obesity

World Health Organization. (2021c). *Obesity and overweight*. https://www.who.int/news-room/fact-sheets/detail/obesity-and-overweight

World Health Organization. (2023). *Adolescent health*. https://www.who.int/health-topics/adolescent-health

Wu, S., Cohen, D., Shi, Y., Pearson, M., & Sturm, R. (2011). Economic analysis of physical activity interventions. *American Journal of Preventive Medicine*, 40(2), 149–158. https://doi.org/10.1016/j.amepre.2010.10.029

Young Men's Christian Association. (2020). *Out of service. A report examining local authority expenditure on youth services in England and Wales*. https://www.ymca.org.uk/wp-content/uploads/2020/01/YMCA-Out-of-Service-report.pdf

Zanganeh, M., Adab, P., Li, B., & Frew, E. (2019). A systematic review of methods, study quality, and results of economic evaluation for childhood and adolescent obesity intervention. *International Journal of Environmental Research and Public Health*, 16(3), 485. https://doi.org/10.3390/ijerph16030485

Chapter 5

Well-being of the Workforce

Bethany F. Anthony, Llinos H. Spencer,
Lucy Bryning, Huw Lloyd-Williams,
Catherine L. Lawrence, and
Rhiannon T. Edwards

Introduction

The working years are also often parenting years and years spent caring for older relatives or family members with a disability. Themes of caring appear in all chapters of this book. We felt it important to devote a whole chapter to the well-being and well-becoming of the workforce so affected by the coronavirus disease 2019 (COVID-19) pandemic and crucial to future recovery from the current period of low economic growth in the United Kingdom (UK). In Chapter 4, we focused on the well-being and well-becoming of adolescents and young adults. Promoting healthy behaviour during this life-course stage can establish a pattern of healthy lifestyles that individuals carry into adulthood. Mitigating risk factors such as mental health problems and health-harming lifestyle choices can, amongst other things, improve employee health and well-being, creating substantial savings to the UK National Health Service (NHS) and wider economy.

We first presented Maslow's (2017, 1943) hierarchy of needs model in Chapter 2 (see Figure 2.1). Maslow argued that humans are motivated by five essential needs: biological and psychological; safety; love/belonging; esteem; and self-actualization/self-fulfilment. This model has been applied to the workplace relating to employee motivation and development (Sodexo, n.d.). Applying this model to the workplace can help us think about the design, implementation, and evaluation of interventions that focus on employee health and well-being, reduce presenteeism, absenteeism, and improve rates of retention and productivity (see Figure 5.1). For example:

- The biological and psychological needs of an employee include having a place of work and receiving a regular salary.

Bethany F. Anthony, Llinos H. Spencer, Lucy Bryning, Huw Lloyd-Williams, Catherine L. Lawrence, and Rhiannon T. Edwards, *Well-being of the Workforce* In: *Health Economics of Well-being and Well-becoming across the Life-course*. Edited by: Rhiannon T. Edwards and Catherine L. Lawrence, Oxford University Press. © Oxford University Press 2024. DOI: 10.1093/9780191919336.003.0005

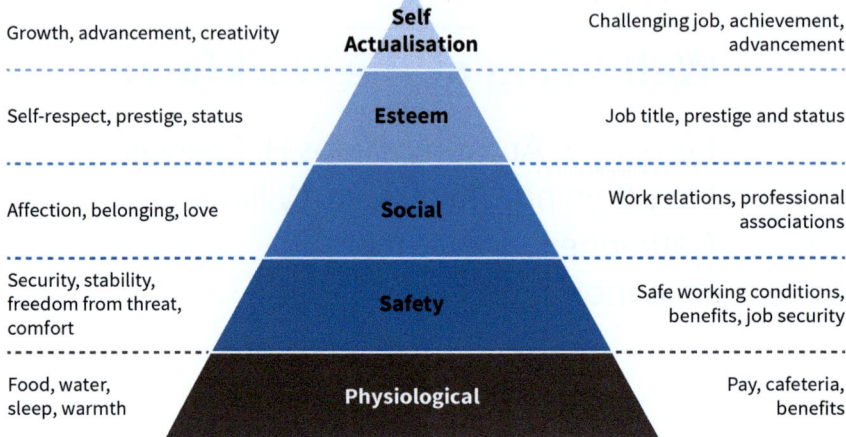

Figure 5.1 Maslow's hierarchy of needs model applied to the workplace
Reproduced from Sodexo. (n.d.). *Applying Maslow's hierarchy of needs theory to HR responsibilities.* Sodexo Quality of Life Services. https://www.sodexoengage.com/blog/rewards-recognition/apply ing-maslows-hierarchy-of-needs-theory-to-hr-responsibilities

- The safety needs of an employee include having access to a formal employment contract, sick pay, and a pension scheme, as well as health and safety regulations in the work environment.
- The love/belonging needs of an employee include having colleagues to work with for team building and networking opportunities, social activities, and peer support.
- The esteem needs of an employee include having a culture of respect, praise, and recognition of employee value and achievement in the workplace, which could be achieved through supportive annual performance reviews and be undertaken through 360-degree feedback and appraisal during line management meetings and coaching schemes.
- The self-actualization/self-fulfilment needs of an employee include development plans, training, secondment, mentoring, and promotion (Sodexo, n.d.).

The Chartered Institute of Personnel and Development (Findlay et al., 2021) created the Good Work Index, which captures data on the following seven dimensions of good work: pay and benefits; contracts; work-life balance; job design and the nature of work; relationships at work; employee voice; and health and well-being (see Table 5.1). We have structured this chapter around these dimensions. Health economists are increasingly involved in the evaluation of workplace interventions. This has mainly been limited to the evaluation of

Table 5.1 Dimensions of good work: The Good Work Index

Dimension	Areas included
1 Pay and benefits	Subjective feelings regarding pay, employer pension contributions, and other employee benefits.
2 Contracts	Contract type, underemployment, and job security.
3 Work-life balance	Overwork, commuting time, how much work encroaches on personal life and vice versa, and human resources provision for flexible working.
4 Job design and the nature of work	Workload or work intensity, autonomy or how empowered people are in their jobs, how well resourced they are to carry out their work, job complexity and how well this matches the person's skills and qualifications, how meaningful people find their work, and what development opportunities are provided.
5 Relationships at work	Social support and cohesion. The quality of relationships at work, psychological safety, and the quality of people management.
6 Employee voice	Channels and opportunities for feeding views to one's employer and managers' openness to employee views.
7 Health and well-being	Positive and negative impacts of work on physical and mental health. Often considered as an outcome of job quality.

Adapted from Findlay, P., Lindsay, C., McIntyre, S., Roy, G., Stewart, R. and Dutton, E. (2021). *CIPD Good Work Index 2021: Survey report.* Chartered Institute of Personnel and Development. https://www.cipd. org/globalassets/media/zzz-misc---to-check/good-work-index-survey-report-2021-1_tcm18-96105.pdf. With the permission of the publisher, the Chartered Institute of Personnel and Development in London (www.cipd.co.uk).

interventions, programmes, and policies directed towards employee health and well-being, largely but not exclusively delivered in the workplace, which we can see from the list above is one of the seven dimensions of job quality.

A systematic review found thirty-two cost-effectiveness workplace health and well-being interventions (Anthony et al., forthcoming). The interventions targeted a number of different areas, including but not limited to, mental health, substance abuse, smoking, health promotion, weight management, and physical activity (Anthony et al., forthcoming). This systematic review has informed an economic evidence report (Edwards et al., 2024) and the following sections of this chapter.

Social Mobility and Access to Good Work

Economists and social commentators have produced overarching evidence of social mobility and opportunities for both good and bad work which can have a 'long shadow' through life. In areas of low social mobility, up to 33 per cent of the pay gap is driven by family background and local market factors, over and beyond educational achievement (Carniero et al., 2020). In the 'Health equity in England: The Marmot review 10 years on' report, the importance of 'place' as a basis for the socioeconomic gradient was emphasized (Marmot et al., 2020; see Chapter 1, Figure 1.2). Areas of low social mobility typically have fewer professional and managerial occupations, fewer outstanding schools, more areas of deprivation, and moderate population density (Carniero et al., 2020).

Skills Development Programmes

Improving the skills base of the population is fundamental to increasing prosperity in the UK and is associated with economic growth and an inclusive society (Evans & Egglestone, 2019). Entry-level, low-skill opportunities are a necessity, not just for existing employees, but also for unemployed individuals who have been economically inactive for a great length of time. These individuals may lack basic employability skills such as timekeeping, safety awareness, following instructions, engaging with others in authority, and co-operation with others in the workplace. A large proportion of young people, particularly those from disadvantaged backgrounds, can have difficulty entering employment due to a shortfall in basic skills and capabilities (Impetus—Private Equity Foundation, 2014). The Ready for Work programme in England and Scotland helps to support disadvantaged groups, including people who have experienced homelessness, to equip themselves with the skills they need to enter and sustain employment (Impetus—Private Equity Foundation, 2014). Over a five-year period, for every £1 invested in the Ready for Work programme, £3.12 was generated to society (Inge et al., 2012).

More recently, a social return on investment (SROI) analysis was undertaken on the impact of the WeMindTheGap programme on the lives of young people taking part in the programme (Hatch Regeneris, 2020). WeMindTheGap is a charity which supports under-served people aged eighteen to thirty in North Wales and North West England to live independent lives. The charity offers a holistic programme of work experience, skills training, and mental health and well-being support. The SROI analysis found that between 2014 and 2020, the programme delivered £5.5 million in social value to the young people on the programme. This equates to a social value return of over £60,000 per person. This value reflects the impact of completing the programme, gaining employment, improved confidence, improved general health, and improved life choices. This is an SROI of £3.20 for every £1 invested. The programme also generated £2.4 million in public cost savings in terms of avoided costs related to employment and support allowance for people who were not in education, employment, or training (NEET). The charity plans to extend its programmes to include new communities across North Wales and North West England (Hatch Regeneris, 2020).

Young People and Employment

The lives of young people can be improved by working or volunteering to gain employment skills. Being in employment can give young people a sense of belonging to a community, and businesses are keen to support young people as they are viewed as future employees as well as future customers (UK Government, 2010, 2021).

At the start of the COVID-19 pandemic, from March to May 2020, the number of young people aged eighteen to twenty-four claiming unemployment-related benefits more than doubled. In June 2023, the number of young people claiming unemployment-related benefits increased to 273,000 (Office for National Statistics (ONS), 2023a; Ward et al., 2023). The Chartered Institute of Personnel and Development (CIPD, 2021) undertook an online survey of over 2,000 young people aged between eighteen and thirty years in the UK, exploring their attitudes and experiences of education and accessing employment. They found that:

- Over a quarter of young people thought that they were over qualified for their current role, and that the qualifications they hold were more necessary to *get* their current job rather than to carry out their job effectively.
- Paid work during education was beneficial for developing employability skills as opposed to gaining subsequent employment.
- Only half of young people received face-to-face careers guidance at school, and of those who did, 41 per cent reported that they found the guidance effective in helping them to understand and plan their future education, training, or work options.
- Less than one in ten young people were currently unemployed, of which, half had been unemployed for over twelve months and 42 per cent had applied for more than ten jobs, and where they had not been successful at interview, young people frequently did not receive feedback from the interviewers.
- Just over half of respondents were satisfied with their job, with those working in wholesale and retail reporting the lowest job and life satisfaction levels.
- Twenty-nine per cent of young people reported that career progression had failed to meet their expectations, with poor-quality line management,

lack of effective training programmes, and access to graduate programmes as the most commonly reported barriers.

- Forty-three per cent of young people reported that the pandemic has harmed their long-term career prospects, with younger workers more likely to report the negative impact of homeworking (e.g. easily distracted and missing out on social interaction) (CIPD, 2021).

In response to these findings, the CIPD launched the One Million Chances campaign with the aim of getting employers to create one million employment-related opportunities for young people (aged sixteen to thirty) through jobs, internships, work experience, apprenticeships, technical-based qualifications (T-Levels), or the Kickstart Scheme (CIPD, 2021). The CIPD called for:

- The UK Government to increase funding for careers advice so that every young person is guaranteed at least one face-to-face interview with a qualified career guidance professional by the age of sixteen.
- Employers to collaborate with local schools and colleges to ensure young people are equipped with the skills that businesses need, so they are ready to join the workforce when they leave education.
- More senior professionals from all sectors to volunteer for the Enterprise Advisers programme in England, run by The Careers and Enterprise Company. The programme matches individuals with a school to help them develop a careers advice strategy and connect them with local employers.

Below we draw on a wider example across Europe recognizing the longer-term impact of the support young people may need and can benefit from to move into work (see Box 5.1).

A report assessing the costs and benefits of apprenticeship schemes used data from Switzerland and Germany, due to a lack of data from the UK, to forecast the increasing opportunities for apprenticeships in the UK since Brexit (Wolter & Joho, 2018). The report forecast a higher return in the following areas:

- for programmes that run for three years;
- for younger employees (under nineteen years) because minimum wages increase substantially afterwards;
- for larger firms, whereas micro-companies (less than ten employees) may sometimes even face net costs in scenarios where the average firm can expect net benefits;
- for apprenticeship schemes in the retail sector and the catering and hospitality sector (cooks, retail cashiers, and waiters) it would prove difficult for firms to break even; and

Box 5.1 Case study: The Youth Employment Initiative

The European Union (EU) launched the Youth Employment Initiative (YEI) in 2013 to provide support to young people living in regions where youth unemployment was higher than 25 per cent (European Commission, 2022). The YEI supports young people who are considered to be not in education, employment, or training (NEET), including those who are long-term unemployed and who are not registered as job seekers. The YEI funds the provision of apprenticeships, traineeships, job placements, and further education leading to a qualification. Research undertaken by Ecorys UK, on behalf of the Department for Work and Pensions, evaluated the effectiveness, efficiency, and impact of the YEI (Department for Work and Pensions, 2022). Findings indicated that the YEI had a positive impact on the employment prospects of young people. On average, YEI participants were in employment for an additional fifty-six days in the twelve months following support. There was no statistically significant effect on the likelihood of claiming Jobseekers' Allowance or Employment and Support Allowance following YEI. While the programme had a social return in the range of £1.50 to £1.55 per £1 spent, the fiscal return is in the range of £0.13 to £0.17 per £1 spent. It is acknowledged in the report that these are likely to be underestimates with the true value for money being higher. The advantages of moving a young person into employment include: increases in earnings to the young person; increases in tax receipts to the government; reductions in costs to the government from paying out unemployment-related benefits; and health benefits to the young person (Department for Work and Pensions, 2022).

- for companies if they improved the quality of their training programmes that would improve the labour market outcomes of apprentices.

In a rural town in Australia, a benefit-cost analysis was conducted of BackTrack, a multi-component, community intervention aimed at young people deemed at 'high risk' in terms of criminal activity, lack of employment, mental health issues, alcohol and substance abuse, and lack of engagement with the health care system (Deeming et al., 2022). Work-related benefits of the intervention included educational attendance or completion, increased employment, and economic productivity. The BackTrack intervention yielded a net social benefit of over $3 million, with a return on investment (ROI) of $2.03 for every $1 invested (Deeming et al., 2022).

Older People and Employment

In the UK, prior to April 2011, employers could force workers to retire at age sixty-five, known as the Default Retirement Age. This practice was abolished through the Employment Equality (Repeal of Retirement Age Provisions) Regulations 2011 Act, which gave workers more choice about when to stop working. The percentage of the UK population aged over sixty-five who are economically active has grown substantially as the population has aged (ONS, 2019a). In 2000, 5 per cent of people aged sixty-five and over were economically active, a rate that more than doubled in 2022 (ONS, 2019a, 2022a). In April to June 2022, there was a record level of 1.468 million people aged sixty-five and over in employment. This increase was driven by rises in part-time work. Industries where informal employment is more common, such as hospitality and arts, entertainment and recreation, witnessed some of the largest increases in employment in this age group (ONS, 2022a).

Paid employment can help maintain well-being into later life for older people (Modini et al., 2016; van der Noordt et al., 2014). Worklessness may have detrimental effects on the well-being of an older person because of missing social connections, mental stimulation, maintaining confidence, feeling valued, and making a positive contribution to society (Hildon et al., 2008). Recognizing the skills and experience of older workers and valuing the contribution that older people make to the workplace and society is important in preventing worklessness for older people who are able and want to keep working. Older workers should have the same access to training, progression, mentoring, and leadership as younger workers. This includes well-being support and appropriate physical adjustments, equipment, flexible working arrangements, and all forms of adaptation that are usual in the workplace (Marvell & Cox, 2017). Flexible working arrangements, reduced hours, or ability to adjust the time and place of work are fundamental to making paid work more age-friendly for those over fifty who may also have caring responsibilities for family or friends. Self-employment can have benefits for older people as they may be able to work more flexibly.

Despite a global pandemic, entrepreneurialism appears to be rising among the older population (Lewis, 2020). Self-employed individuals have been particularly affected by the COVID-19 pandemic, with the risk of losing their employment being twice as high as individuals in paid employment (Henley & Reuschke, 2020). Unlike paid employees who were able to immediately claim the Coronavirus Job Retention Scheme (the furlough scheme) at the beginning of the pandemic in March 2020, it took longer for the UK Government to bring in practical support for the self-employed workforce (Henley & Reuschke,

2020). A large proportion of the self-employed workforce may not have been eligible for government support due to factors such as the absence of recent self-assessment tax returns or second job self-employment (Henley & Reuschke, 2020). Despite this, an increase in entrepreneurialism among the older population has emerged since the pandemic in response to reported age discrimination. The full impact of the pandemic on older people in employment is not yet known, however, transition to working from home using potentially unfamiliar technologies, the need to shield on the basis of age and health conditions, and furlough schemes will all have likely had an impact on older people continuing in employment.

Work and Caring Responsibilities

Women have historically assumed unequal responsibility for unpaid care work. Before the COVID-19 pandemic, women dedicated one to three hours or more per day to complete housework than men, and two to ten times the amount of time per day for caring responsibilities compared to men (The World Bank, 2012, 2018). These gender role differences have been found to reduce women's leisure, welfare, and well-being, and their capacity to take up economic opportunities (United Nations (UN) Women, 2016). The 'gender pension gap' is the percentage difference in pension income for female pensioners compared to male pensioners. In 2019/2020, the pension gap was 37.9 per cent, with men receiving a higher pension income than women (Prospect, 2023). This difference in pension wealth and income in retirement is driven by:

- different labour market experiences due to the gender pay gap or differences in the length of working life between men and women;
- different saving rates as men and women may be offered different pension schemes by their employer, work for employers offering different contributions, or make different contributions themselves; and
- different investment strategies as men and women may choose to invest in schemes with a different expected rate of return.

(Crawford & O'Brien, 2021)

In 2019, 75.1 per cent of mothers with dependent children were in work in the UK, compared to 92.6 per cent of fathers (ONS, 2019b). The UK Government has committed up to thirty hours of free childcare for working parents of three and four-year-olds during the school year (UK Government, 2022). The schemes available to parents vary across the devolved nations of England, Wales, Scotland, and Northern Ireland, although all areas have some provision for funded early years childcare (see Chapter 3). In Wales, there are early signs that the Childcare Offer launched in 2018 has been supporting working parents to continue working and also to work more hours (Glover et al., 2018). Findings from a parental survey indicated that some women, and to a lesser extent men, are working more hours and this is especially true for those who earn up to £41,599 (Glover et al., 2018). In England, the Free Early Education Entitlement offers 570 free hours of childcare per year for three and four-year-olds. An independent evaluation of the free childcare scheme found increased working hours, greater flexibility, and improved finances among the benefits for parents (Paull et al., 2017). The extended hours also have a positive impact on the child's continuity of care, the child's mood, more development opportunities, opportunities to socialize, and support with specific needs (Paull et al., 2017).

Caring responsibilities can have a substantial impact on women's employment and earnings. Working carers often have to attend hospital appointments with the person they are caring for, and this has an 'opportunity cost' to them (e.g. of working time) which can impact on how much they can contribute economically (NHS England, 2017). Opportunity cost is the value of benefits foregone by not using resources in their next best alternative use. Women do not just lose out on potential earnings from employment when taking up caring roles for children and dependent adults. There are also long-term consequences such as a reduction in experience and promotion prospects, and a reduction in pension contributions playing a role in the vertical segregation and gender pay gap experienced by women. This has implications for later life with more than a third of both male and female carers who had left work to undertake caring roles reporting that they were unable to save for a pension (Yeandle et al., 2014). There is a strong financial case, both for businesses and the wider economy, for supporting parents and carers in employment (Cottell & Harding, 2018; NHS England, 2017).

In 2021, there were five million unpaid carers over the age of five years across England and Wales (ONS, 2023b). Unpaid care in England has an estimated economic contribution of £54 billion to £86 billion per year (New Economics Foundation (NEF) Consulting, 2022). The wider social and economic costs associated with unpaid carers' labour is between £24 billion and £37 billion per year. These costs take into account lost earnings (to the carer and to the state); monetized estimates of the pain/discomfort, anxiety/depression, and social isolation that carers can experience, and the costs they represent to society and the NHS (NEF Consulting, 2022). The rise in unpaid care has been linked to a reduction in health and social care budgets, with some services reducing in areas of the UK. For example, in England, local authority budget cuts have had a knock-on effect on the provision of care (Buckner & Yeandle, 2015). The System of National Accounts, which provides information on important macroeconomic indicators such as gross domestic product (GDP), household disposable income, and final consumption, typically excludes the value of unpaid household activities (see van de Ven et al., 2018).

Fifteen per cent of workers are unpaid carers (Carers UK, 2019). Balancing these dual roles often results in carers reducing working hours, with carers more likely to work in part-time roles than those without care responsibilities (Carers UK, 2015a, 2015b). Difficulty switching to part-time working is also highlighted as a reason for carers leaving employment altogether (Carers UK, 2015a, 2015b). The number of informal carers reducing their participation in the labour market (both completely or partially) is expected to rise alongside the rising demand for carers in an aging population (Carers in Employment Task and Finish Group, 2013). Figure 5.2 summarizes the experience of unpaid carers in the workplace. The top three interventions that workers identified as being most helpful if they were caring for others alongside paid employment were: a supportive employer/line manager; flexible working; and additional paid care leave of between five and ten days per year (Carers UK, 2019).

In England, 345,000 working age carers (both men and women) were unable to work due to their caring responsibilities before the COVID-19 pandemic, costing the UK Government up to £2.9 billion per year in benefits including Carer's Allowance payments and lost tax revenues (NHS England, 2017; Pickard et al., 2018). Typically, employees leave employment due to caring responsibilities (for children, parents, or friends) between the ages of forty-five and sixty-four years, representing a substantial loss of highly skilled workers (in whom employers have likely invested time and money; Carers in Employment Task and Finish Group, 2013). Replacing staff or reorganizing work responsibilities amongst existing employees can incur further costs to employers through recruitment and staff training (Carers in Employment Task and Finish Group, 2013). In general terms, there are many examples of organizational and government policy and practice recommendations for supporting parents and carers in employment including:

- increasing flexible and part-time working opportunities, including at the higher earning end of careers, considering options such as job sharing;
- protecting the rights of mothers to return to work after maternity leave and exploring opportunities to extend this to carers;
- providing access to paid or unpaid temporary leave for parents and carers; and
- increasing provision of paternity leave to support more equity in caring responsibilities.

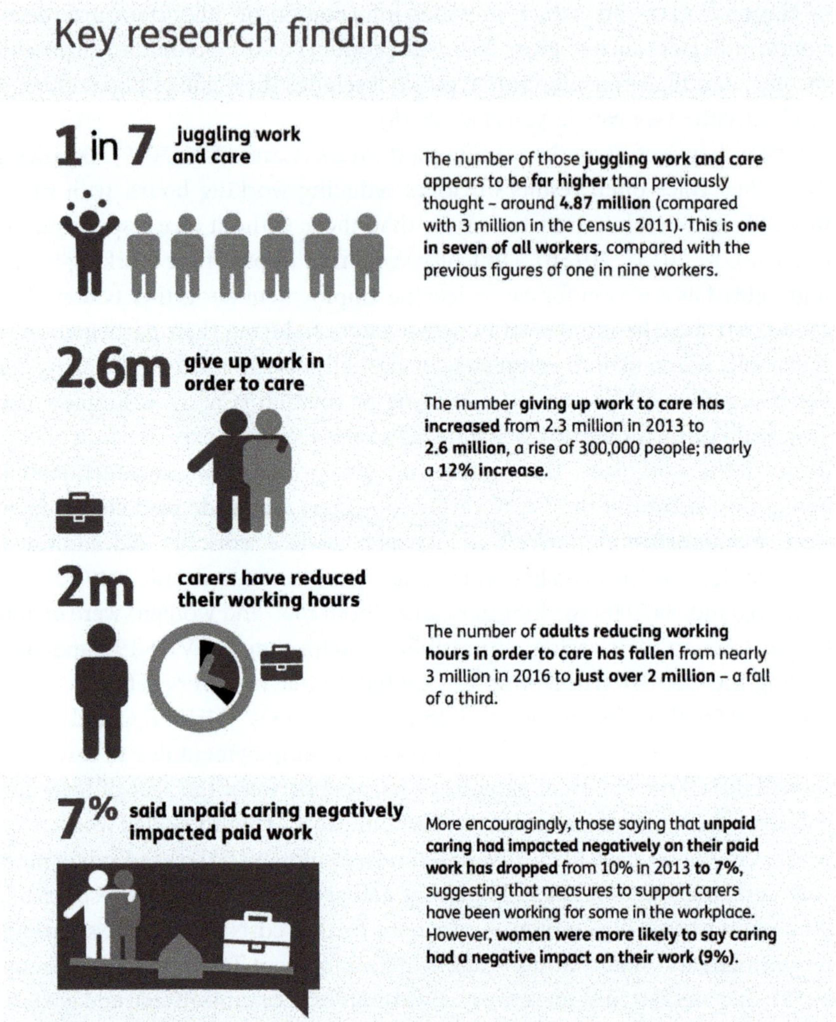

Key research findings

1 in 7 juggling work and care

The number of those **juggling work and care** appears to be **far higher** than previously thought – around **4.87 million** (compared with 3 million in the Census 2011). This is **one in seven of all workers**, compared with the previous figures of one in nine workers.

2.6m give up work in order to care

The number **giving up work to care has increased** from 2.3 million in 2013 to **2.6 million**, a rise of 300,000 people; nearly a **12% increase**.

2m carers have reduced their working hours

The number of **adults reducing working hours in order to care has fallen** from nearly 3 million in 2016 to **just over 2 million** – a fall of a third.

7% said unpaid caring negatively impacted paid work

More encouragingly, those saying that **unpaid caring had impacted negatively on their paid work has dropped** from 10% in 2013 **to 7%**, suggesting that measures to support carers have been working for some in the workplace. However, **women were more likely to say caring had a negative impact on their work (9%)**.

Figure 5.2 The experience of unpaid carers in the workplace

Reproduced with permission from Carers UK. (2019). *Juggling work and unpaid care: A growing issue*. Centrica. https://www.carersuk.org/media/no2lwyxl/juggling-work-and-unpaid-care-report-final-web.pdf. Copyright © 2019 Carers UK

Key research findings

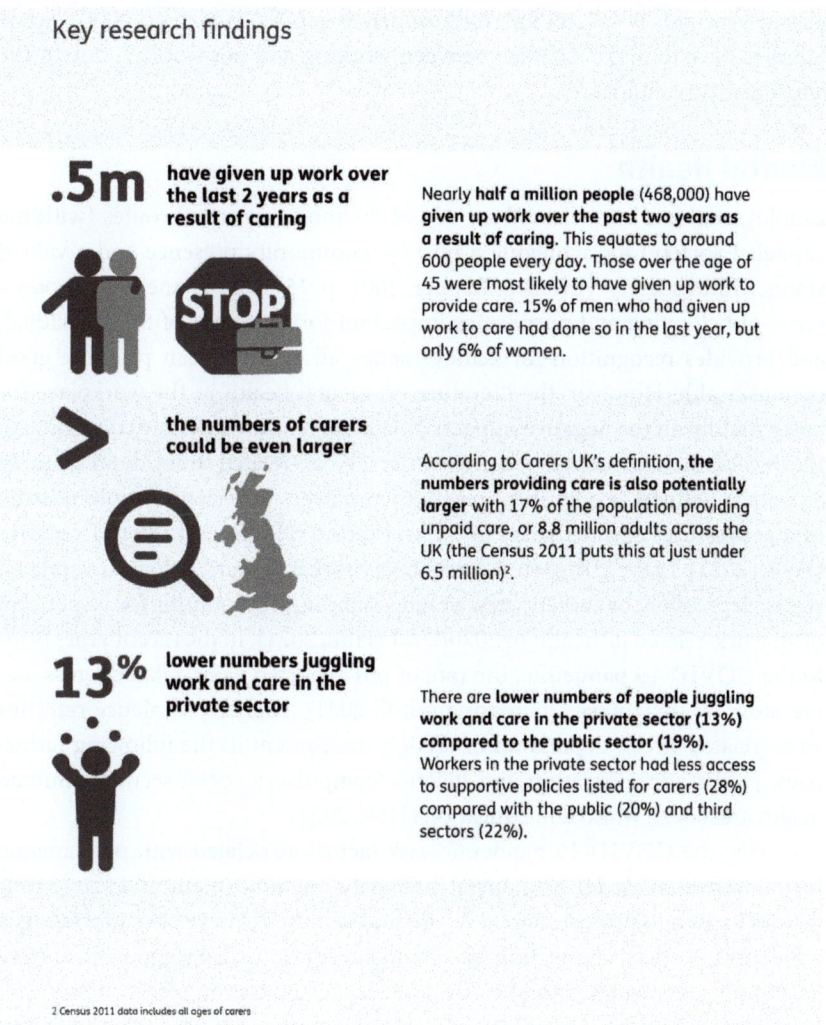

.5m have given up work over the last 2 years as a result of caring

Nearly **half a million people** (468,000) have **given up work over the past two years as a result of caring**. This equates to around 600 people every day. Those over the age of 45 were most likely to have given up work to provide care. 15% of men who had given up work to care had done so in the last year, but only 6% of women.

> the numbers of carers could be even larger

According to Carers UK's definition, **the numbers providing care is also potentially larger** with 17% of the population providing unpaid care, or 8.8 million adults across the UK (the Census 2011 puts this at just under 6.5 million)[2].

13% lower numbers juggling work and care in the private sector

There are **lower numbers of people juggling work and care in the private sector (13%) compared to the public sector (19%).** Workers in the private sector had less access to supportive policies listed for carers (28%) compared with the public (20%) and third sectors (22%).

2 Census 2011 data includes all ages of carers

Figure 5.2 Continued

The COVID-19 pandemic has caused the wealth gap to widen due to lack of childcare provision in some areas. For example, even before the pandemic, two in five local authorities in Wales reported that there was not enough childcare for those working atypical hours (Matejic, 2020). In England, only 16 per cent of local authorities reported sufficient childcare for parents working atypical hours in 2021 (Coleman et al., 2022). The average cost of childcare decreases after a child enters full-time education, but the bill can be very costly for some working families. The weekly price of an after-school club for five to eleven-year-olds is £61.16; for childminders it is £70.02 (Matejic, 2020). Some families have to make a choice between working and not working due to the affordability of childcare.

Mental Health

Employment has been classed as, 'one of the most important routes (within a capitalist society) for achieving a positive community presence and a valued status within society' (Evans & Repper, 2001, p. 15). Employment promotes a sense of belonging and purpose, is important for the status of the individual, and provides recognition for achievements; all of which can promote good mental health. However, the literature on mental health in the workplace focuses mainly on the negative impacts of work and how work may contribute to the development of mental health disorders. Work-related stress, depression, or anxiety is defined as a harmful reaction employees experience resulting from undue pressures and demands in the workplace (Health and Safety Executive (HSE), 2021). In the UK, there were 822,000 workers experiencing work-related stress, depression, or anxiety (new or long-standing), accounting for 50 per cent of all work-related ill-health in 2020/2021 (HSE, 2021). In the recent years prior to the COVID-19 pandemic, the rate of self-reported work-related stress, depression, or anxiety was increasing (HSE, 2021). Higher prevalence rates for work-related stress, depression or anxiety are present in the following industries: public administration and defence/compulsory social security; human health and social work, and education (HSE, 2021).

During the COVID-19 pandemic, risk factors associated with poor mental health were increased (e.g. financial insecurity, unemployment, and fear), while factors known to protect mental health and well-being were also affected (e.g. daily routine, social connection, employment, educational engagement, and access to physical exercise and health services) (Organisation for Economic Co-operation and Development (OECD), 2021). Employed individuals and people with childcare responsibilities were among the most affected groups in terms of mental health during the first months of the COVID-19 pandemic. Pierce and colleagues (2020) analysed personal well-being data from Understanding Society—The UK Household Longitudinal Study 2020. Well-being was measured using the General Health Questionnaire (GHQ)—an increase in GHQ score suggests a decrease in mental health. Pierce and colleagues performed repeated cross-sectional analysis and fixed-effects estimation to investigate the impact of the pandemic on subgroups of individuals by comparing the mental health of workers in 2017 and April 2020. Figure 5.3 illustrates the effect of the pandemic on people's mental health. While average mental health improved

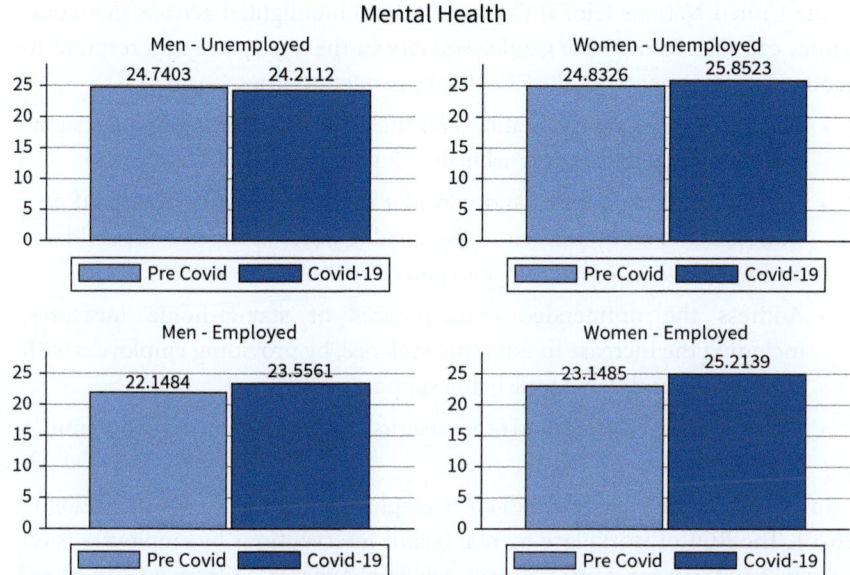

Figure 5.3 General Health Questionnaire score before and during the COVID-19 pandemic by gender and employment status

Note: A high General Health Questionnaire (GHQ) score indicates a low level of mental health

Source: Pierce, M., Hope, H., Ford, T., Hatch, S., Hotopf, M., John, A., Kontopantelis, E., Webb, R., Wessely, S., McManus, S., & Abel, K. M. (2020). Mental health before and during the COVID-19 pandemic: A longitudinal probability sample survey of the UK population. *The Lancet Psychiatry*, 7(10), 883–892. https://doi.org/10.1016/S2215-0366(20)30308-4 Copyright © 2023 Elsevier Inc

for men who were unemployed at baseline (February 2020), it decreased for men who were employed at baseline and for women regardless of their employment status. This is likely due to the increased pressure experienced by women during the pandemic (Hupkau & Petrongolo, 2020). While mental health for employed individuals is still better on average than for unemployed individuals, the former have seen a greater impact on their mental health during the pandemic. Possible explanations are the increased difficulty in managing childcare responsibilities, home-schooling, and working from home during national lockdowns imposed by the government, as well as the negative impact of redundancies and furlough schemes on well-being. For working parents, mothers were more likely than fathers to spend their time working while caring for children (Andrew et al., 2020). Women also accounted for the majority of health professionals and essential workers working at the frontlines of the COVID-19 response. In doing so, they risked their own health and safety as well as those of their families.

The United Nations Global Compact (2020) highlighted actions that companies can take to improve gender equality in the workplace and respond to gender-specific impacts of the COVID-19 pandemic. These include:

- Ensure women's representation and inclusion in planning and decision-making so that more sustainable decisions are made.
- Support working parents and consider that the majority of unpaid care work is taken on by women—offer flexible work arrangements, childcare options, and equal maternity and paternity leave.
- Address the unintended consequences of stay-at-home measures, including the increase in domestic violence, by providing employees with appropriate health and well-being support.
- Liaise with government and other sectors to support recovery programmes for women.

In the UK, poor mental health costs employers £45 billion a year (Deloitte, 2020). The ROI of workplace mental health interventions by employers is on average £5 return for every £1 spent, which has increased from a £4 to £1 return identified in 2017 (Deloitte, 2017). Employers are talking more openly about mental health and providing greater support to staff, helping to reduce stigma associated with taking time off work for mental health reasons (Deloitte, 2020; Stevenson & Farmer, 2017). The National Institute for Health and Care Excellence (NICE; 2022) recommends that organizations adopt a strategic, tiered approach to mental well-being in their policies and practices using organizational-level approaches as the foundation for good mental well-being, followed by individual approaches, and then targeted approaches. One of the key foundations of mental well-being in the workplace is an organizational commitment to it, recognizing that mental well-being is a spectrum (from good mental well-being to poor mental well-being), and that poor mental well-being is not a weakness (NICE, 2022). Organizations can take a preventative and proactive approach to mental well-being by actively promoting mental well-being rather than solely addressing poor mental well-being when it happens. NICE (2022) also recommends the need to view mental well-being in the workplace as equally important to physical well-being in the workplace. A supportive, inclusive work environment and culture can help promote good mental well-being, and can be achieved in part by positive social interactions between managers and employees. During the COVID-19 pandemic, many employees were required to work from home. While technology enabled many employers to do so effectively, an 'always on' culture can have a negative impact on employee well-being. This not only contributes to 'presenteeism', but also 'leaveism', where employees feel they must engage in work activities outside of their normal working hours (Deloitte, 2020).

Below are three examples of studies exploring the cost-effectiveness of workplace interventions to support mental health, getting people into work, and staying in work. The first is a European study which looked at an employment intervention (Individual Placement and Support (IPS)) to help people with poor mental health into paid employment (Knapp et al., 2013). The researchers found by comparing the two groups (IPS and standard vocational rehabilitation), a difference in net benefit of £19,407 was found in favour of IPS, showing that the intervention demonstrated a better use of resources than its comparator (Knapp et al., 2013). Another example is a cost-effectiveness analysis (CEA) alongside a randomized controlled trial (RCT) to investigate the cost-effectiveness of a web-based stress management intervention (Ebert et al., 2014). Work-related stress was associated with a myriad of mental health problems and led to substantial costs in terms of lost productivity and absenteeism. A cost-benefit analysis (CBA) yielded a net benefit of €181 per participant. With a willingness-to-pay (WTP) ceiling of €2,000, there was a 98 per cent probability of the intervention being cost-effective over and above its comparator. Note, this is not a recognized threshold as used by NICE. The third example is a CBA of a problem solving-based intervention (PSI) delivered by a workplace occupational health service to target common mental health issues or occupational stress compared with care as usual (Keus Van De Poll et al., 2020). Care as usual consisted of a one-hour general introduction to psychosocial factors and mental health at work. Intervention delivery costs and costs for long-term sickness absence were higher for care as usual compared with PSI. CBA conducted from a societal perspective demonstrated favourable results for the intervention and found that a one-day reduction of long-term sickness absence cost on average €101 for the intervention group and was associated with a reduction in socioeconomic burden compared with care as usual (Keus Van De Poll et al., 2020).

A systematic review published in 2020 of workplace nature-based interventions on the mental health and well-being of employees found consistently positive effects on mental health indices and cognitive ability (Gritzka et al., 2020). The effects of workplace nature-based interventions on recovery and restoration, work and life satisfaction, and psychophysiological indicators were less consistent. These authors argued that larger studies are needed when interpreting the current evidence in this emerging research field due to the diversity of nature-based interventions and the overall high risk of bias in the individual studies. The ten studies included in the systematic review had a large degree of heterogeneity in terms of design, nature exposure, assessed outcomes, and measurement tools (Gritzka et al., 2020).

Burnout

'Burnout' can be defined as a state of vital exhaustion (International Classification of Diseases-10 (ICD-10), 2016). It results from chronic workplace stress that has not been successfully managed and is characterized by three dimensions:

- feelings of energy depletion or exhaustion;
- increased mental distance from one's job, or feelings of negativity or cynicism related to one's job; and
- reduced personal efficacy (World Health Organization (WHO), 2018).

Burnout affects many employees in the UK and especially in the health care sector (Imo, 2017). In primary care settings, stress is reported in over half of working-age adults, especially among women, and symptoms of burnout and exhaustion are common (Coventry & White, 2018). A review of the evidence on burnout in the UK reported moderate evidence that individually oriented interventions produce positive results in relation to burnout and stress prevention in workplaces (Public Health England, 2016a). The return-to-work interventions that included a full economic evaluation aimed at depressed employees did not appear to be cost-effective (Public Health England, 2016a). In other cases, such as frontline health care workers, the costs associated with sickness absenteeism can be more than monetary.

Workforce burnout across the NHS and social care reached an emergency level and posed a risk to the future functioning of both services (Health and Social Care Committee (HSSC), 2021). Staff shortages across the NHS and social care have been identified as a main cause of workforce burnout. Even before the COVID-19 pandemic, one-third of doctors were experiencing burnout, particularly those working in emergency medicine and general practice (McKinley et al., 2020). Burnout has additional costs to the NHS and social care because locums and agency staff are employed to cover absenteeism, and locums are more expensive than filled posts. Jeremy Hunt, Chair of the HSCC, said:

> Achieving a long-term solution demands a complete overhaul of workforce planning. Those plans should be guided by the need to ensure that the long-term supply of doctors, nurses and other clinicians is not constrained by short-term deficiencies in the number trained. Failure to address this will lead to not just more burnout but more expenditure on locum doctors and agency nurses. (UK Parliament, 2021)

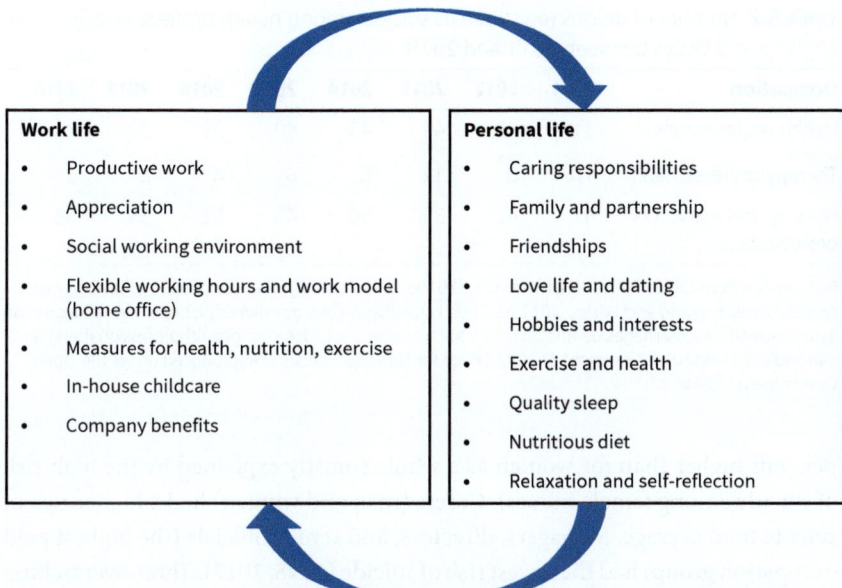

Work life	Personal life
• Productive work	• Caring responsibilities
• Appreciation	• Family and partnership
• Social working environment	• Friendships
• Flexible working hours and work model (home office)	• Love life and dating
	• Hobbies and interests
• Measures for health, nutrition, exercise	• Exercise and health
• In-house childcare	• Quality sleep
• Company benefits	• Nutritious diet
	• Relaxation and self-reflection

Figure 5.4 Work-life balance: The balance between work and personal life
Source: IONOS. (2019). *Work-life balance.* https://www.ionos.co.uk/startupguide/productivity/work-life-balance/. Copyright © 2023 IONOS Cloud Ltd

Figure 5.4 outlines some of the dimensions of a good work-life balance (IONOS, 2019).

Suicide

In 2021, there were 6,319 deaths registered in Great Britain where the cause was registered as suicide (Baker, 2022). Although being employed has a protective effect on suicide behaviour, the risk of suicide in England and Wales is highest among people aged between forty-five and fifty-four. Suicide in England and Wales is three times more common among men than women. This gap between sexes has increased over time. People living in the most deprived areas of England have a higher risk of suicide than those living in the least deprived areas (Baker, 2022). Men and women working in certain occupations are at a higher risk of suicide. In a study of suicide rates by occupation based on deaths registered in England between 2011 and 2015, the ONS (2017) found that men working in the lowest-skilled occupations had a 44 per cent higher risk of suicide than men as a whole. The risk of suicide among men who were labourers was three times higher than men as a whole. For women, the risk of suicide among professionals was 24

Table 5.2 Number of deaths registered as suicide among health professionals in England and Wales between 2011 and 2018

Occupation	2011	2012	2013	2014	2015	2016	2017	2018
Health professionals	31	30	44	43	40	39	32	36
Therapy professionals	10	8	12	8	6	4	8	9
Nursing and midwifery professionals	47	43	39	56	45	52	33	58

Reproduced from Office for National Statistics. (2019c, 3 September). *Number of suicides among health professionals, England and Wales, 2011 to 2018.* https://www.ons.gov.uk/peoplepopulationandcommun ity/birthsdeathsandmarriages/deaths/adhocs/10471numberofsuicidesamonghealthprofessionalsenglan dandwales2011to2018. Copyright © 2022 Office for National Statistics. Reproduced under the Open Government License 3.0.

per cent higher than for women as a whole (mostly explained by the high risk of suicide among female nurses). Carers (men and women) had a higher risk of suicide than average. Managers, directors, and senior officials (the highest paid occupation group) had the lowest risk of suicide (ONS, 2017). Three overarching characteristics have been identified to explain why some occupations may carry a high risk of suicide: 1) job-related features such as low pay and low job security; 2) people at high risk of suicide may selectively go into particular occupations; and 3) having access to, or knowledge of, a method of suicide may increase risk (ONS, 2017). Table 5.2 shows the number of deaths by suicide among health professionals in England and Wales between 2011 and 2018 (ONS, 2019c). The NHS Long Term Plan's Mental Health Implementation Plan set out plans to invest £57 million in suicide prevention.

Non-fatal suicide behaviour where a person has harmed themselves can impact the workplace as workers may be fully incapacitated or require a short absence from work. Kinchin and Doran (2017) quantified the economic cost of suicide and non-fatal suicide behaviour in the Australian workforce and examined the potential impact of introducing a workplace suicide prevention intervention to reduce this burden. Mates in Construction is a multifaceted workplace suicide prevention and early intervention programme. It has three main components: 1) general awareness training to improve knowledge of warning signs and encourage workers to seek support; 2) connector training where staff learn how to keep co-workers safe while connecting them to help; and 3) applied suicide intervention skills training. The findings demonstrated a positive ROI in excess of $1.50 ($1.11–$3.07) for every $1 invested in the intervention. Kinchin and Doran (2017) called for workplace strategies to be used within a multifaceted approach to reflect the complex nature of self-harming behaviour.

Reducing Presenteeism

When employees develop a health condition it does not always lead to absence from work, but can lead to reduced performance in work. Working whilst sick is called 'presenteeism'. Presenteeism can cause exhaustion, loss in productivity, and lead to workplace outbreaks where the health condition is transmissible (e.g. flu). The cost of presenteeism to businesses associated with mental health problems is estimated at £21.2 billion, with 1.5 days of work time lost due to presenteeism for every one day lost due to absenteeism (Parsonage & Saini, 2017). An integral part of fostering co-production for health at work relies on individuals taking responsibility for their own health and well-being. This is alongside employers carrying out workplace health promotion activities, including improving working environments and encouraging personal development, promoting the active participation of all stakeholders in the process (European Agency for Safety and Health at Work, 2012). Factors that are likely to hinder co-production of good health relevant to the workplace include heavy alcohol consumption on work nights, not getting enough sleep, and poor diet (Ford et al., 2011; Public Health England, 2019; Varney, 2018). Figures 5.5 and 5.6 show the synergistic benefits of a healthy and happy workforce, and the health and financial benefits of moving individuals into employment, respectively (Public Health England, 2019; WHO & Burton, 2010).

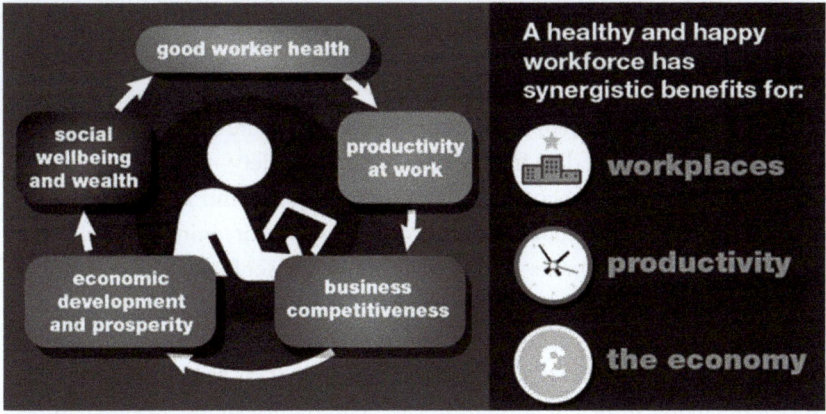

Figure 5.5 Health and work cycle
Reproduced from Public Health England. (2019, 31 January). *Health matters: Health and work.* https://www.gov.uk/government/publications/health-matters-health-and-work/health-matters-health-and-work. Copyright © 2019. Reproduced under the Open Government License 3.0
Source: World Health Organization & Burton, J. (2010) . *WHO healthy workplace framework and model: Background and supporting literature and practices.* World Health Organization. https://apps.who.int/iris/handle/10665/113144. Copyright © 2021 World Health Organization

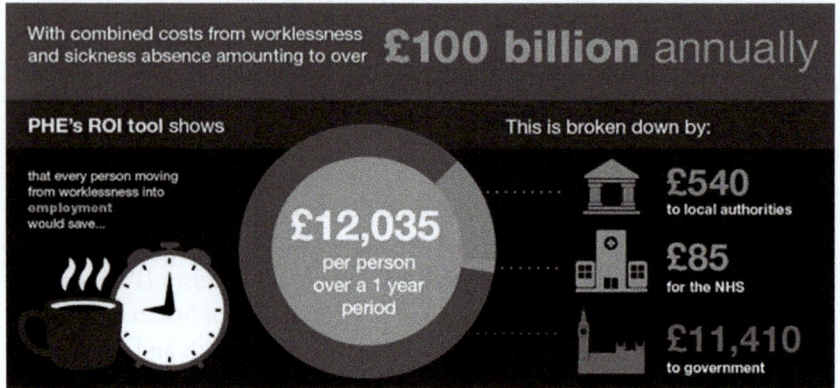

Figure 5.6 Health and financial benefits of moving individuals into employment
Reproduced from Public Health England. (2019). *Health matters: Health and work.* https://www.gov.uk/government/publications/health-matters-health-and-work/health-matters-health-and-work. Copyright © 2019. Reproduced under the Open Government License 3.0.

Kigozi and colleagues (2017) reviewed cost of illness studies to explore the methods used to take account of presenteeism. On the basis of twenty-eight studies that met the review criteria, they concluded that presenteeism was rarely accounted for in full economic studies and that methods varied. They argued that the potential impact of presenteeism costs needs to be highlighted and greater consideration given to including these in economic evaluations and cost of illness studies. National economic guidelines should emphasize the importance of identifying, measuring, and valuing presenteeism costs (Kigozi et al., 2017).

Bryan and colleagues (2020) produced the first estimate of the cost of presenteeism in the UK. Using data from Understanding Society—The UK Household Longitudinal Study, they concluded that both physical and mental health significantly predict the probability of presenteeism. Worsening of health over time significantly increases the probability of presenteeism. The effects of mental health problems seem to be worse than physical health. In comparison, changes to other work circumstances had little effect on presenteeism other than job security. Conducive working conditions, such as being in part-time work and having sufficient autonomy, can help to mitigate the negative impact of health on productivity (Bryan et al., 2020).

Sleep Deprivation and Employment

In general, adults need between six and nine hours of sleep to function well in day-to-day life (Basner, 2011). Sleep is linked to memory consolidation and immune system supporting effects (Besedovsky et al., 2019). Conversely, sleep debt impairs immune responses by disrupting circadian rhythms, which has a negative effect on the endocrine system (important for producing and releasing hormones) and on some cytokines (important for immune and inflammation responses in the body; Mônico-Neto et al., 2020). People in the UK get on average six and a half hours of sleep per night, and on an annual basis, the UK workforce loses 200,000 working days due to insufficient sleep, which corresponds to 1.65 million working hours (National Sleep Foundation, 2013). Insufficient sleep can be caused by a variety of different individual-level and workplace factors such as smoking, physical inactivity, stress and anxiety, unrealistic time pressures at work, working irregular hours, and long commuting times.

There is a relationship between income and sleep, with 71 per cent of those who earn a household income of £80,001 to £100,000 sleeping for more than six hours on an average night, compared with 50 per cent of those who earn under £10,000 (The Sleep Council, 2017). People who experience unrealistic time pressures and stress in the workplace sleep on average eight minutes less per day compared to colleagues reporting low levels of time pressure (Hafner et al., 2017). This amounts to nearly one hour less sleep per week. According to a 2016 cross-country comparative analysis exploring the economic costs of insufficient sleep, the UK sustained an economic productivity loss of £40.2 billion per year (1.86 per cent of its GDP) due to insufficient sleep (Hafner et al., 2017). This is expected to rise to £47 billion by 2030. During the COVID-19 pandemic, many people reported trouble sleeping and having more nightmares. This sleep deprivation may be the result of increased stress due to experiencing a traumatic situation (Lin et al., 2021).

Alcohol Misuse and Employment

People working whilst hungover or under the influence of alcohol costs the UK economy between £1.2 billion and £1.4 billion a year (Bhattacharya, 2019). The impact of alcohol misuse has a high cost to society each year due to productivity losses resulting from alcohol-related absenteeism, presenteeism, unemployment, and premature death (Institute of Alcohol Studies, 2020; Knapp et al., 2011). In a survey of 3,400 British workers about how their work has been affected by alcohol, 42 per cent reported they had gone to work hungover or under the influence of alcohol, and rated their work performance to be 39 per cent less effective than usual (Bhattacharya, 2019). Specific cognitive functions may still be impaired the morning following binge drinking, even when there is little or no alcohol content present in the bloodstream (Gunn et al., 2018). The economic burden of alcohol use is estimated to be between 1.3 per cent and 2.7 per cent of annual GDP (Burton et al., 2016).

Government policies such as taxation and price regulation on alcohol are likely to be the most effective and cost-effective methods of prevention and health improvement (Public Health England, 2016b). Between 2013 and 2018, cuts in alcohol duty are estimated to have reduced income to the Exchequer by £5 billion (Burton et al., 2016). Minimum unit pricing of alcohol has been found to have little effect on the consumption of alcohol by moderate drinkers (regardless of income) (Holmes et al., 2014). Importantly, minimum unit pricing has been found to have a significant impact on heavy drinkers, especially for those living on low incomes (Holmes et al., 2014).

Smoking and Employment

Smoking breaks and smoking-related sick days cost businesses in England £6.8 billion a year (Public Health England, 2018). Shift workers are more likely than other workers to engage in riskier behaviour including smoking and misuse of drugs and alcohol, and do not engage as much in physical activity (Nabe-Nielsen et al., 2011). Reducing levels of smoking among workers could help reduce illnesses and conditions such as cardiovascular and respiratory disease, which are linked to sickness absence. This can, in turn, lead to improved productivity and a reduced burden on employers and employees (Public Health England, 2018).

Workplaces can be important settings for promoting smoking cessation interventions because large numbers of people can be reached (including groups which may not routinely consult health professionals, e.g. young men), peer support groups can be established, and a non-smoking environment can encourage people who smoke to quit (Public Health England, 2018). NICE (2021, updated in 2023) recommends that behavioural interventions (e.g. behaviour support and advice) and medicinally licensed products (e.g. nicotine replacement therapy) are accessible to adults who smoke. In particular in the workplace, NICE recommends that employers make information about local stop-smoking support easily available and allow employees to attend stop-smoking support during working hours without loss of pay. Employers should be responsive to the individual needs and preferences of employees, and provide on-site stop-smoking support if feasible. Recommendations also called for employees to negotiate a smoke-free workplace policy with employers, for example, covering whether smoking breaks can be taken during working hours (NICE, 2021).

In the Netherlands, a trial-based CEA and cost-utility analysis (CUA) was conducted comparing a work-based smoking cessation training programme with incentives with a work training programme without incentives (van den Brand et al., 2020). From a societal perspective, the intervention was found to be cost-effective at a WTP of €11,546 per additional employee who stopped smoking. The cost-effectiveness acceptability curve demonstrated an 80 per cent probability of the intervention being cost-effective at €20,000 per employee who stopped smoking. Secondary CUA revealed similar quality-adjusted life years (QALYs) between the intervention and control groups (van der Brand et al., 2020).

E-cigarettes, known as vapes, produce an aerosol by heating a liquid that usually contains nicotine, flavourings, and other chemicals (e.g. propylene glycol and vegetable glycerine; NHS, 2022). As e-cigarettes do not burn tobacco or produce tar or carbon monoxide, they are thought to be safer than smoking cigarettes, although the long-term risks of vaping are currently unclear (NHS, 2022). In 2021, vaping prevalence in England was between 6.9 per cent and 7.1 per cent (i.e. between 3.1 million and 3.2 million adults; Office for Health Improvement & Disparities, 2022). Early evidence suggests that e-cigarettes are a cost-effective smoking cessation tool (Thomas et al., 2021). A Cochrane systematic review found that vapes were more effective than nicotine therapy in helping people to stop smoking (Hartmann-Boyce et al., 2022). Maintaining access to vaping devices for current smokers is crucial in reducing smoking rates and contributes to 50,000 to 70,000 fewer smokers every year (Office for Health Improvement & Disparities, 2023).

Illicit Drug Use, Prescription Drug Abuse, and Employment

Illicit drug use and prescription drug abuse can have an impact on workplace productivity. In the year ending June 2022, one in eleven adults aged sixteen to fifty-nine years (three million people) reported taking drugs, with 2.7 per cent of adults reporting Class A drug use (ONS, 2022b). During this period there were decreases in the use of Class A drugs, ecstasy, and nitrous oxide, thought to be a result of the COVID-19 pandemic and government restrictions on social contact (ONS, 2022b). Use of illicit drugs can impair a person's performance at work through poor time-keeping, poor decision-making, and impaired reaction times causing lost productivity, inferior goods/services, errors, and accidents (Nicholson & Mayho, 2016). Drugs testing is not commonplace in UK workforces, although it is used in the construction, transport, and energy generation industries, and in sport (Trades Union Congress (TUC), 2019). The TUC, a trade union in the UK, noted that the most effective way of ensuring that drug-taking is not a problem in the workplace is to have a comprehensive drugs and alcohol policy that seeks to support those who need help in a non-judgemental way (TUC, 2019). However, when illicit drug use does interfere with safety at work, the use and possession of illicit drugs falls under several criminal laws (Nicholson & Mayho, 2016). Employers have a general duty under the Health and Safety at Work Act 1974 to ensure, as far as is reasonably practicable, the health, safety, and welfare at work of their employees and others affected by their work activities (Nicholson & Mayho, 2016). Employers are breaking the law (Misuse of Drugs Act 1971, cl. 38) if they knowingly allow drug-related activities in the workplace and fail to act (HSE, 2019). Before the first COVID-19 lockdown, many people stockpiled alcohol and drank more alcohol in the period from March to April of 2020 than before the pandemic (Wright et al., 2021). It has been suggested that increased alcohol consumption could have been due to stress, and that this stress level lowered as employees became more familiar with the new normal way of working in their workplace or working from home. Working from home may have enabled alcohol consumption that otherwise would not have happened (Monteiro et al., 2020).

Workers who report misuse of prescription drugs (e.g. painkillers) are more likely to report absenteeism in the previous month compared to workers who do not report prescription drug misuse (Van Hasselt et al., 2015). There are many serious health risks to misuse of prescription drugs and continued usage can result in dependency with possible long-term damage to the body (Welsh Government, 2019). Prescription drug misuse can be caused by stress at work due to long working hours, frantic work pace, and poor management. A London-based study found that NHS consultants who drank alcohol and took non-prescription drugs in response to job stress were at a greatly increased risk of psychiatric morbidity (Graham et al., 2001). Employers have a duty of care for their employees and could raise awareness of the positive and negative impacts of different strategies to manage work-related stress (Clarke & Cooper, 2004; Graham et al., 2001). In the United States (US), Orme and colleagues (2023) assessed the costs and cost-effectiveness of substance abstinence contingent wage supplements to tackle substance abuse and unemployment. Abstinence contingent wage supplements were associated with increased employment rates and negative drug tests among participants. Following the twelve-month intervention period, the incremental cost-effectiveness ratio (ICER) was $1,437 per additional participant with a negative drug test result and $915 per additional participant in employment (Orme et al., 2023). These researchers called for further research to determine whether abstinence contingent wage supplements offer benefits beyond health care costs and to better understand what decision-makers may be willing to spend (Orme et al., 2023).

Social Networks at Work

Research has been conducted on the relationship between employment and social network membership in older people. For example, Haynes and colleagues

(2014) found that those employed were more likely to participate in a community organization and have a greater number of friends. This challenges previous research which claimed that employment tended to reduce social network activity (e.g. Ferring et al., 2004). Being in employment can provide a wider 'transformative potential', providing people with an identity, improving social contact and self-respect, and reducing loneliness (Bailey, 2017; Patrick, 2012).

Employee Voice

Mentoring in the workplace involves a senior-level employee (mentor) working with a junior-level employee (mentee), usually on a one-to-one basis. The mentor shares their knowledge, skills, and connections, motivating and empowering the mentee to identify and achieve work-related goals (Clutterbuck, 2014). For example, successful mentoring schemes can help junior nurses to develop their skills, increase career satisfaction, and decrease turnover rates (Gazaway et al., 2016; Gruber-Page, 2016). The mentoring relationship is more than a dyad experience between the mentor and mentee as the organization also invests and benefits from the mentoring process. A healthy workplace and good mentoring process are necessary for cultivating a successful mentoring relationship. Table 5.3 lists the structural factors, process, and outcomes vital in creating an effective mentoring scheme in a hospital setting (Goodyear & Goodyear, 2018).

We could not find many examples of CEA of mentoring or coaching programmes in the workplace. We found a few examples relating to reducing teacher turnover. For example, in California, US, using actual programme cost information and data on student achievement, teacher retention, and mentor evaluations, Villar and Strong (2007) performed a benefit-cost analysis to find out whether comprehensive mentoring for new teachers made financial sense. The findings showed that increases in teacher effectiveness yielded greater savings than the reduction in costs associated with teacher attrition. Overall, the benefit-cost analysis showed that, after five years, an investment of $1 produced a positive return to society, the school district, the teachers, and the students. Assuming the costs of hiring a replacement represent 50 per cent of a new teacher's salary, investment in the mentoring programme paid $1.50 for every $1 spent (Villar & Strong, 2007).

In light of the increased demand for mental health services following the COVID-19 pandemic, Makanjuola and colleagues (2023) examined whether lifestyle coaching could be a potential cost-effective intervention to address the backlog for mental health counselling. While mental health counselling often requires a long-term approach to mental health conditions such as anxiety and depression, lifestyle coaching offers a short to medium-term, goal-focused approach that can empower clients to develop skills and increase personal

Table 5.3 Structural factors, process aspects, and outcomes for mentoring success in a hospital setting

Structural factors	Process aspects	Outcomes
Mentor characteristics	Quality of mentoring relationship	Mentee benefits
Mentee characteristics	Details of mentoring takes place	Mentor benefits
Hospital environmental factors, including: • Support for mentoring programmes • Culture of growth and development • Time for mentoring • Mentoring programme and resources available • Healthy work environments	Quantity of mentoring (how often, how long)	Hospital benefits, including: • Improved culture of growth and development • Identification of potential leaders • Development of new leaders • Succession planning • Employee engagement and satisfaction • Increased retention • Improved culture of feedback • Possible positive patient outcomes, including patient satisfaction

fulfilment. Following a rapid review of relevant literature, ten papers were evaluated. These papers focused on the cost-effectiveness of counselling and other talking therapies, such as cognitive behavioural therapy (CBT); no papers considered the cost-effectiveness or efficacy of lifestyle coaching (Makanjuola et al., 2023). These researchers called for a feasibility RCT to evaluate the effectiveness and cost-effectiveness of lifestyle coaching compared with treatment as usual (i.e. counselling).

Supporting Women in the Workplace through Menopause Transition

In 2021, the UK Government undertook a consultation exercise to develop their Women's Health Strategy (Department of Health and Social Care, 2021). The call was launched to ensure that the strategy was evidence-based and reflected what women identify as priorities, focusing on the inequalities in women's health. The call sought views on six core themes that connected different areas of women's health across the life-course, including maximizing women's health in the workplace. Female-specific health conditions, such as heavy menstrual bleeding, endometriosis, pregnancy-related issues, and the menopause, can affect women's workforce participation, productivity, and outcomes (Department of Health and Social Care, 2021). Research commissioned by Health & Her® and conducted by Censuswide found that menopause symptoms, such as hot flushes, memory loss, joint aches, and anxiety, costs the UK economy fourteen million working days per year (Health & Her®, 2021). This equates to £1.8 billion in GDP loss to the UK economy. To compensate for the (possibly perceived) productivity loss, over half of women aged between fifty and sixty-four choose to work extra hours to make up for the time lost. Over 370,000 working women aged between fifty and sixty-four reported they have left or considered leaving their job because they found managing symptoms in the workplace too difficult. The number of days lost to the UK as a result of symptoms can be difficult to assess as remaining social taboos mean that many women may give other reasons for time-off work that are actually menopause-related (Baker, 2020).

In a review of the most clinical and cost-effective treatment for the relief of menopause symptoms, transdermal oestradiol and progestogen was the most cost-effective treatment in women with a uterus, and non-oral oestradiol was cost-effective in women without a uterus (NICE, 2015). St John's Wort is a cost-effective treatment for women with breast cancer, though it might interact with other medicines (e.g. tamoxifen) (NICE, 2015). More recently, a review of economic evaluations of menopausal hormone therapy found that for women aged fifty to sixty years, menopausal hormone therapy was cost-effective and below the NICE WTP threshold (Velentzis et al., 2017). However, three analyses based the quality of life benefit for symptom relief on one small primary study, suggesting further research is needed in this area.

Disability and the Workplace

In 2019, 4.2 million people with a disability were in employment in the UK (ONS, 2019d). The current definition of 'disability' includes people who have a long-term physical or mental health condition that affects their day-to-day activities (Government Statistical Service, 2019). People with disabilities are over a third less likely to be employed than people who are not disabled, with an employment rate of 53.2 per cent (aged sixteen to sixty-four years) for people with disabilities compared to 81.8 per cent for people who are not disabled (ONS, 2019d). Two of the main reasons for absenteeism are musculoskeletal problems (e.g. back ache) and mental health problems (e.g. stress). One in five of the working-age population is classed as disabled (Department for Work & Pensions, 2021). Since 2013 (the earliest comparable year using the current definition) up to the start of the COVID-19 pandemic, there has been a general positive trend in the number of people with a disability finding employment. The number and rate of people with disabilities in employment was increasing, resulting in a narrowing of the gap between the rate of people with and without disabilities in employment (Department for Work & Pensions, 2021). This is in line with the UK Government's goal of reducing the disability employment gap. The increasing number of people with disabilities in employment is driven by disability prevalence, the disability employment gap, and the non-disabled

---

Box 5.2 Case study: The Access to Work programme supporting people with disabilities in the workplace

Access to Work is a UK Government publicly funded employment support programme that aims to support people who have a disability or physical or mental health condition to start working, stay in work, move into self-employment, or start a business. Access to Work provides practical advice and support to people with disabilities and their employers to help them overcome work-related barriers resulting from disability. For example, Access to Work can help pay for assistive technology, a support worker, or travel costs.

The Royal National Institute of Blind People (RNIB) is one of the UK's leading sight loss charities. They commissioned the Centre for Economic and Social Inclusion to conduct a cost-benefit analysis (CBA) of the Access to Work scheme. They found that the potential benefits for participants from Access to Work included reduced sickness, improved attendance, retained employment, development of working skills, increased income, and improved health and well-being (Melville et al., 2015). Employers benefitted from Access to Work through improved productivity, lower employee turnover, a better understanding of the needs of their employee, and the increased well-being of employees. Melville and colleagues (2015) estimated that the overall benefits of Access to Work to society outweighed its costs by a considerable margin with ratios of these benefits to the costs of 3.86 for Access to Work as a whole and 2.48 for the part of the programme that assists blind and partially sighted individuals. From 2011/2012 to 2013/2014, the Access to Work programme generated on average £1.14 in fiscal flow backs per £1 spent on the programme (Melville et al., 2015). The equivalent figure for the part of the programme assisting blind and partially sighted individuals is £0.72.

employment rate. Today, more people are reporting a long-term health condition or disability compared to eight years ago, which is largely driven by an increase in prevalence of mental health conditions. People with disabilities are more likely than people without disabilities to be working in lower-skilled occupations, working part-time, working in the public sector, temporarily away from work, and self-employed (Department for Work & Pensions, 2021). An important aspect of the government strategy is for a more healthy and inclusive society (OECD, 2015). Some people enter employment with pre-existing conditions or challenging social conditions. Box 5.2 describes the UK Government's Access to Work scheme that supports people with disabilities in the workplace.

Health and Well-being in the Workplace

Interventions to help employees thrive (i.e. to be successful and achieve) at work may need to be targeted and tailored (Stevenson & Farmer, 2017). For example, the thriving at work framework proposed by Stevenson and Farmer (2017) argues that all employees may need some support to thrive, but those who are struggling need targeted support, and those who are ill and possibly off work need tailored support to return to work and thrive in the work environment (see Figure 5.7).

Keeping people healthy and in work prevents loss of productivity and profit (Black, 2008). Workplace health programmes are concerned with efforts to maintain, protect, and improve the health of people at their place of work (European Network for Workplace Health Promotion, 2007). The needs of employees can be complex and different levels of support may be required. Good quality work contributes to the well-being of employees by meeting the basic psychological needs of self-efficacy, self-esteem, sense of belonging, and meaningfulness (Hunter, 2010). This is illustrated earlier in this chapter in Figure 5.1 (Sodexo, n.d.). There has been an emphasis on promoting good quality jobs for good health, with some of the key characteristics of good work being autonomy, fair pay, a good work-life balance, and the absence of bullying or harassment (Public Health England, 2015; Stevenson & Farmer, 2017).

More highly paid work is associated with better health outcomes (Marmot et al., 2010). The nature of work can adversely affect health through adverse physical conditions, such as exposure to chemicals or other hazards, long hours, and shift work. Adverse psychosocial conditions include conflict and lack of autonomy or control, poor pay, or insufficient hours (e.g. zero hours contracts) (Public Health England, 2015). Temporary work and risk of redundancy can affect stress levels, job satisfaction levels, and the well-being of employees (Public Health England, 2015).

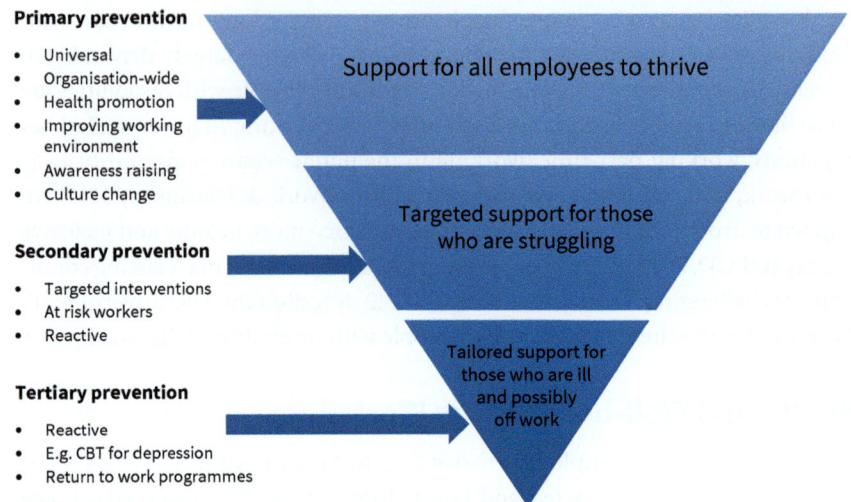

Primary prevention

- Universal
- Organisation-wide
- Health promotion
- Improving working environment
- Awareness raising
- Culture change

Secondary prevention

- Targeted interventions
- At risk workers
- Reactive

Tertiary prevention

- Reactive
- E.g. CBT for depression
- Return to work programmes

Support for all employees to thrive

Targeted support for those who are struggling

Tailored support for those who are ill and possibly off work

Figure 5.7 Thriving at work framework

Reproduced from Stevenson, D., & Farmer, P. (2017) *Thriving at work: The Stevenson/Farmer review of mental health and employers*. Department for Work and Pensions and Department of Health and Social Care. https://assets.publishing.service.gov.uk/government/uploads/system/uploads/attachment_data/file/658145/thriving-at-work-stevenson-farmer-review.pdf. Copyright © 2017 Department for Work and Pensions and Department of Health and Social Care. Reproduced under the Open Government License 3.0.

A review of published economic evaluations found positive findings on the cost-effectiveness of interventions to promote health and well-being in the workplace (Anthony et al., forthcoming). An example of an economic evaluation of a primary prevention intervention is a CBA of a voluntary influenza vaccination programme in Italy (Ferro et al., 2020). Monthly mean costs of absenteeism per employee were significantly greater for employees who did not receive the influenza vaccination (€129.00) in comparison to vaccinated employees (€54.00). Findings from the CBA revealed that the intervention produced an overall net saving of €314.00 per vaccinated employee (Ferro et al., 2020). A CEA and CUA of a secondary prevention weight management programme implemented in the workplace in the US assessed the cost-effectiveness of three interventions: telephone coach, small group coach, or self-study (Corso et al., 2019). All three groups received a manual on healthy eating, physical activity, and problem-solving advice, and an initial orientation session with a coach. Participants in the telephone coach and small group coach conditions also received eight sessions with a coach. The telephone coach condition had the highest delivery cost at $589 to $601 per employee, and the self-study intervention was the least costly condition at a cost of $143 to $145 per employee (Corso et al., 2019). The small group coach condition was more costly and no more effective in terms of weight loss when compared to the self-study condition. The telephone condition was significantly more costly and produced significantly lower QALYs compared to the small group coach condition. When compared to self-study, the small group coach intervention was cost-effective at a cost of $22,400 per QALY. The group intervention was more cost-effective than telephone consultation or self-study (Corso et al., 2019). Another study from the US found that a tertiary prevention intervention which involved a supported employment programme for veterans with spinal injury to help individuals return to work and improve their quality of life produced positive economic benefits (Sutton et al., 2020). Total costs were similar between the intervention and control groups, but QALYs were significantly higher in the intervention group at both the one-year and two-year follow-up (Sutton et al., 2020).

Reducing Work-related Musculoskeletal Disorders

Musculoskeletal disorders are injuries or disorders of the muscles, nerves, tendons, joints, cartilage, and spinal discs that work environments can make worse. They are a frequent cause of work-related disability with considerable economic impact (ONS, 2019e). Musculoskeletal conditions are the second main cause of short-term and long-term sickness absence in the UK, and the leading contributor to disability worldwide (CIPD, 2020). Studies investigating the economic costs of musculoskeletal disorders in workplaces worldwide have shown that some interventions were clinically effective and cost-effective, some were only clinically effective, and others were neither clinically effective nor cost-effective. For example, there is early economic evidence that interventions such as yoga can be cost-effective when delivered to NHS staff (Hartfiel et al., 2012, 2017). Programmes such as these not only have beneficial clinical outcomes from promoting healthy lifestyle choices, but also result in beneficial workplace outcomes, such as reduced absenteeism and increased productivity. For example, over a six-month period, a yoga intervention delivered to NHS Wales staff resulted in a 95 per cent reduction in absenteeism due to work-related musculoskeletal disorders (Hartfiel et al., 2017). These programmes may also reduce future disease burden and associated costs.

In Sweden, a cluster-RCT, WorkUp, was conducted to facilitate participants at risk of sick leave or on short-term sick leave due to acute/subacute neck and/or back pain to stay at work or return to work (Saha et al., 2019). Participants in the intervention group and control group both received structured evidence-based physiotherapy, while participants in the intervention group also received a workplace dialogue with the employer. This workplace dialogue involved three steps: 1) the participant was interviewed by the physiotherapist to identify factors that could affect their work ability; 2) the participant's supervisor/manager was interviewed by the physiotherapist to identify workplace adjustments that could facilitate remaining at work or return to work; and 3) a meeting was held with the participant, supervisor/manager, and physiotherapist to identify workplace adjustments to support work ability and agree a plan for this. Structured evidence-based physiotherapeutic care along with workplace dialogue was found to be cost-effective from both a societal and a health care perspective. From a health care perspective, the ICER was €23,666 per QALY gain. From the societal perspective, the intervention was less costly and more effective than the control group at a €50,000 WTP threshold per QALY (Saha et al., 2019). With more people working from home since the COVID-19 pandemic there is concern that musculoskeletal problems could increase if staff do not have adequate equipment or home-working set-ups (Hupkau & Petrongolo, 2020).

Autism Spectrum Disorder and Employment

Autism spectrum disorder is a lifelong developmental disability which affects how people communicate and interact with the world (National Autistic Society, 2021). In the UK, there are 700,000 people living with autism (one in one hundred people; National Autistic Society, 2021). Seventy-seven per cent of unemployed people with autism want to work (Knapp et al., 2019). However, people with this condition are often excluded from the labour market, with only 21.7 per cent of people with autism in employment (Jacob et al., 2015; ONS, 2021). People with autism may have difficulties in understanding nuances in job advertisements and interviews, experience lack of support in the workplace, and face employer discrimination (Knapp et al., 2019). As previously discussed in this chapter, being employed brings the advantage of social integration, increased satisfaction, higher self-esteem, more independent living, and reduced family burden, which leads to lower service costs (Heffernan & Pilkington, 2011). People living with autism can make excellent employees as they often have a good work ethic (e.g. tend to be punctual and reliable), can think more logically and understand connections, and can have good attention to detail (National Autistic Society, 2021; Scott et al., 2017).

Employment support interventions provide tailored training and guidance for adults with autism through the application process to maintaining employment. Research shows a strong economic case for supported employment from both a health and social care perspective, as well as a broader societal perspective, which includes productivity gains (based on employment support for the general population; Knapp et al., 2019). For example, Mavranezouli and colleagues (2014) compared the cost-effectiveness of supported employment with standard care (day services) for adults with autism in the UK. Supported employment was provided by support workers who assessed the person with autism (e.g. level of functioning, past education, and job history), identified employment opportunities, and checked the person with autism could cope with the social and occupational requirements of the employment. The support workers also educated potential and existing employers about autism. The researchers found that supported employment resulted in better outcomes at an extra cost of £18 per additional week in employment or £5,600 per QALY. Supported employment dominated standard care (i.e. supported employment produced better outcomes at a lower total cost). This study demonstrated that supported employment schemes for adults with autism can be cost-effective (Mavranezouli et al., 2014).

Organizational and Individual Outcomes of Health Promotion Strategies

A systematic review found that workplace health promotion interventions led to a positive change in the health behaviour of employees and effected an organizational change. Financial benefits resulting from the implementation of workplace health promotion interventions were noted in eleven studies. However, they rarely led to savings or a reduction in costs resulting from sickness absenteeism, presentism, and turnover (Basińska-Zych & Springer, 2021).

A separate study, a CUA of the Food Choice at Work study in Ireland, assessed the cost-effectiveness of a system-level dietary modification intervention (consisting of menu modification, fruit discounts, portion size control, and positioning of healthy food options in the cafeteria) in comparison with a nutritional advice intervention and a control group (no intervention; Fitzgerald et al., 2018). Cost-utility results found that the system-level intervention was the dominant intervention when compared to the nutritional advice intervention and control. In comparison with the control group, the system-level intervention produced a cost per QALY of €101.37 and was therefore deemed as a cost-effective strategy when compared to the national cost-effective threshold in Ireland of €45,000 per QALY (Fitzgerald et al., 2018).

In another example, a CBA was conducted to compare the costs and benefits of an organizational-level workplace intervention to decrease absenteeism amongst public sector employees in Sweden (Severin et al., 2022). The programme involved a monetary support approach as well as a combined monetary and facilitator support approach, and included a number of different interventions targeting workplace structures, policies, procedures, routines, and management practices at a large public sector organization with 55,000 employees. The cost per employee for monetary support approach and facilitator support approach were 1,560 kr and 3,410 kr, respectively (Severin et al., 2022). Based on productivity loss, the facilitator support approach yielded a net benefit of 5,850 kr per employee per year, whereas the monetary support approach produced a net loss (-60 kr per employee). The researchers concluded that the organizational-level programme was deemed as cost-effective with respect to a reduction in productivity loss, but was not economically viable in terms of reducing direct sick pay associated with short-term sickness absence (Severin et al., 2022).

Summary

This chapter set out a model of factors determining well-being in work. The chapter focused on factors within the CIPD Good Work Index such as pay and benefits, contracts, work-life balance, job design and the nature of work, relationships at work, employee voice, and health and well-being in the workplace (Findlay et al., 2021). This chapter covered a range of topics such as women and menopause relating to the workplace, addiction behaviours and the workplace, burnout and presenteeism, and working and caring responsibilities.

The UK population is ageing. This is due to a combination of factors, such as improvements in life expectancy, people having fewer children, and people having children later in life (ONS, 2018). The number of pensioners per person of working age is increasing (ONS, 2019f). Since people of working age pay the bulk of taxes which support public spending, including state pensions, this potentially impacts on the provision of future health and care services.

In the next chapter, Chapter 6, we explore ageing well and the economic case for investing in older people as assets. Though the relationship between the number of older people to the number of people of working age is important to the economy, it is a misnomer that older people are a net cost to society. The 'grey pound', the value of informal care of grandchildren enabling working age adults to go out to work, plus the volunteering work that older people do, is an enormous value to society, as explored in the next chapter.

Curiosity Questions

- How can large employers, including public sector organizations (e.g. higher education institutions), measure the cost-effectiveness of interventions they put in place to improve staff well-being? What are the challenges of capturing changes in work culture that promote better staff well-being?

- What is the best way to estimate and include overheads in the evaluation of workplace interventions, programmes, or policies? These can be physical overheads relating to office accommodation, heating, lighting etc., but also managerial or supervisory overheads, and now overheads of people working from home.

- What is the most appropriate perspective of analysis to take? Largely this comes down to who is paying for an intervention, programme, or policy aimed to improve workplace health and well-being, enable people into work, or support people of working age in other activities. This means that the relevant perspective might be the employer themselves, the public sector, or as the National Institute for Health and Care Excellence refers to this, the perspective of health and personal social services. Or, it might be the perspective of the third sector if a study is an intervention or programme being run by a charity. Sometimes shared budgets are being explored in prevention, and these require a shared perspective (Barry, 2021).

- What evidence is there that interventions that are cost-effective in the short run, in terms of promoting workplace health, have a lasting impact into early old age?

References

Andrew, A., Cattan, S., Dias, M. C., Farquharson, C., Kraftman, L., Krutikova, S., Phimister, S., & Sevilla, A. (2020, 27 May). *Parents, especially mothers, paying heavy price for lockdown*. Institute for Fiscal Studies. https://ifs.org.uk/news/parents-especia lly-mothers-paying-heavy-price-lockdown

Anthony, B. F., Spencer, L. H., Davies, J., Makanjuola, K., Lloyd-Williams, H., Pisavadia, K., & Edwards, R. T. (forthcoming). Systematic review of cost-effectiveness of interventions to promote wellness in work.

Bailey, N. (2017). Employment, poverty and social exclusion. In G. Bramley & N. Bailey (Eds.), *Poverty and social exclusion in the UK: Volume 2—the dimensions of disadvantage* (Vol. 2. 159–178). Policy Press.

Baker, C. (2022, 2 December). *Suicide statistics*. UK Parliament. House of Commons Library. https://commonslibrary.parliament.uk/research-briefings/cbp-7749/

Baker, S. (Ed.) (2020). *The shift: How I (lost and) found myself after 40—and you can too.* Coronet.

Barry, M. M. (2021). Transformative health promotion: What is needed to advance progress? *Global Health Promotion, 28*(4), 8–16. https://doi.org/10.1177/17579759211013766

Basińska-Zych, A., & Springer, A. (2021). Organizational and individual outcomes of health promotion strategies—a review of empirical research. *International Journal of Environmental Research and Public Health, 18*(2), 383. https://doi.org/10.3390/ijerph18020383

Basner, M. (2011). Sleep duration and chronic sleep debt: Are 6 hours enough? *Biological Psychology, 87*(1) 15–16. https://doi.org/10.1016/j.biopsycho.2011.02.015

Besedovsky, L., Lange, T., & Haack, M. (2019). The sleep-immune crosstalk in health and disease. *Physiological Reviews, 99*(3), 1325–1380. https://doi.org/10.1152/physrev.00010.2018

Bhattacharya, A. (2019). *Financial headache: The cost of workplace hangovers and intoxication to the UK economy.* Institute of Alcohol Studies. https://www.drugsandalcohol.ie/30712/1/Financial_headache.pdf

Black, C. M. (2008). *Working for a healthier tomorrow: Dame Carol Black's review of the health of Britain's working age population.* Department for Work and Pensions. https://www.gov.uk/government/publications/working-for-a-healthier-tomorrow-work-and-health-in-britain

Bryan, M. L., Bryce, A. M., & Roberts, J. (2020, May). *Presenteeism in the UK: Effects of physical and mental health on worker productivity.* The Sheffield Economic Research Paper Series (SERPS). Department of Economics, The University of Sheffield. https://eprints.whiterose.ac.uk/160936/8/paper_2020005.pdf

Buckner, L. & Yeandle, S. (2015). *Valuing carers 2015: The rising value of carers' support.* Carers UK. https://socialcare.wales/cms-assets/documents/hub-downloads/Valuing_Carers_2015.pdf

Burton, R., Henn, C., Lavoie, D., O'Connor, R., Perkins, C., Sweeney, K., Greaves, F., Ferguson, B., Beynon, C., Belloni, A., Musto, V., Marsden, J., Sheron., N., & Wolff, A. (2016). *The public health burden of alcohol and the effectiveness and cost-effectiveness of alcohol control policies: An evidence review.* Public Health England. https://assets.publishing.service.gov.uk/government/uploads/system/uploads/attachment_data/file/733108/alcohol_public_health_burden_evidence_review_update_2018.pdf

Carers in Employment Task and Finish Group. (2013). *Supporting working carers: The benefits to families, business and the economy.* Carers UK. HM Government. https://assets.publishing.service.gov.uk/government/uploads/system/uploads/attachment_data/file/232303/Supporting_Working_Carers_Final_Report__accessible_.pdf

Carers UK. (2015a). *Unpaid carers save the UK £132 billion a year—the cost of a second NHS.* https://www.leeds.ac.uk/news-health/news/article/3790/unpaid-carers-save-the-uk-132-billion-a-year-the-cost-of-a-second-nhs

Carers UK. (2015b). *Policy briefing October 2015: Facts about carers.* https://www.carersuk.org/for-professionals/policy/policy-library/facts-about-carers-2015.

Carers UK. (2019). *Juggling work and unpaid care: A growing issue.* Centrica. https://www.carersuk.org/media/no2lwyxl/juggling-work-and-unpaid-care-report-final-web.pdf

Carniero, P., Cattan, S., Dearden, L., van der Erve, L., Krutikova, S., & Macmillan, L. (2020). *The long shadow of deprivation: Differences in opportunities across England.* Social Mobility Commission Research Report. https://assets.publishing.service.gov. uk/government/uploads/system/uploads/attachment_data/file/923623/SMC_Long_ shadow_of_deprivation_MAIN_REPORT_Accessible.pdf

Chartered Institute of Personnel and Development. (2020). *Health and well-being at work. Survey report.* https://www.cipd.org/globalassets/media/comms/news/eehealth-and-well-being-2020-report_tcm18-73967.pdf

Chartered Institute of Personnel and Development. (2021). *Youth employment in the UK 2021.* https://www.cipd.co.uk/Images/youth-employment-UK_tcm18-103279.pdf

Clarke, S., & Cooper, C. (2004). *Managing the risk of workplace stress: Health and safety hazards* (1st ed.). Routledge.

Clutterbuck, D. (2014). *Everyone needs a mentor* (5th ed.). CIPD—Kogan Page. https:// www.perlego.com/book/1589542/everyone-needs-a-mentor-pdf

Coleman, L., Shorto, S., & Ben-Galim, D. (2022). *Childcare survey 2022.* Coram Family Childcare. https://www.familyandchildcaretrust.org/sites/default/files/Resource%20 Library/Final%20Version%20Coram%20Childcare%20Survey%202022_0.pdf

Corso, P. S., Ingels, J. B., Padilla, H. M., Zuercher, H., DeJoy, D. M., Vandenberg, R. J., & Wilson, M. G. (2019). Cost effectiveness of a weight management program implemented in the worksite: Translation of fuel your life. *Journal of Occupational and Environmental Medicine,* 60(8), 683–687. https://doi.org/10.1097/JOM.0000000000001 343

Cottell, J., & Harding, C. (2018). *Holding on or moving up? Supporting carers and parents in employment.* Coram Family and Childcare. UNISON. https://www.familyandchildca retrust.org/holding-or-moving-supporting-carers-and-parents-employment

Coventry, P. A., & White, P. C. (2018). Are we ready to use nature gardens to treat stress-related illnesses? *The British Journal of Psychiatry,* 213(1), 396–397. https://doi.org/ 10.1192/bjp.2018.82

Crawford, R., & O'Brien, L. (2021, 11 May). *Understanding the gender pension gap.* Institute of Fiscal Studies. https://ifs.org.uk/articles/understanding-gender-pension-gap

Deeming, S., Edmunds, K., Knight, A., Searles, A., Shakeshaft, A. P., & Doran, C. M. (2022). A benefit-cost analysis of BackTrack, a multi-component, community-based intervention for high-risk young people in a rural Australian setting. *International Journal of Environmental Research and Public Health,* 19(16), 10273. https://doi.org/ 10.3390/ijerph191610273

Deloitte. (2017). *Mental health and employers: The case for investment.* Monitor Deloitte. https://www2.deloitte.com/content/dam/Deloitte/uk/Documents/public-sector/deloi tte-uk-mental-health-employers-monitor-deloitte-oct-2017.pdf

Deloitte. (2020). *Mental health and employers. Refreshing the case for investment.* https:// www2.deloitte.com/uk/en/pages/consulting/articles/mental-health-and-employers-ref reshing-the-case-for-investment.html

Department for Work & Pensions. (2021, 11 February). *The employment of disabled people 2021.* https://www.gov.uk/government/statistics/the-employment-of-disabled-people-2021/the-employment-of-disabled-people-2021

Department for Work and Pensions. (2022, 2 March). *Youth Employment Initiative—Impact Evaluation* (DWP research report no. 1011). Government Social Research Profession.

https://www.gov.uk/government/publications/youth-employment-initiative-impact-evaluation/youth-employment-initiative-impact-evaluation

Department of Health and Social Care. (2021). *Women's health strategy: Call for evidence.* https://www.gov.uk/government/consultations/womens-health-strategy-call-for-evidence

Ebert, D. D., Lehr, D., Smit, F., Zarski, A. C., Riper, H., Heber, E., Cuijpers, P., & Berking, M. (2014). Efficacy and cost-effectiveness of minimal guided and unguided internet-based mobile supported stress-management in employees with occupational stress: A three-armed randomised controlled trial. *BMC Public Health,* 14(1), 1–11. https://doi.org/10.1186/1471-2458-14-807

Edwards, R. T., Spencer, L., Anthony, B., Davies, J., Pisavadia, K., Makanjuola, A., Lloyd-Williams, H., Fitzsimmons, D., Collins, B., Charles, J. M., Lewis, R., Cooper, A., Barutcu, S., & McKibben, M.-A., & Edwards, A. (2024). Wellness in work—supporting people in work and assisting people to return to the workforce: An economic evidence review. *medRxiv.* https://doi.org/10.1101/2024.01.17.23300197

European Agency for Safety and Health at Work. (2012). *Motivation for employers to carry out workplace health promotion literature review.* https://osha.europa.eu/en/publications/motivation-employers-carry-out-workplace-health-promotion

European Commission. (2022). *Youth Employment Initiative (YEI).* https://ec.europa.eu/social/main.jsp?catId=1176

European Network for Workplace Health Promotion. (2007). *Luxembourg Declaration on Workplace Health Promotion in the European Union.* Luxembourg Declaration. https://www.enwhp.org/resources/toolip/doc/2018/05/04/luxembourg_declaration.pdf

Evans, J., & Repper, J. (2001). Employment, social inclusion and mental health. *Journal of Psychiatric and Mental Health Nursing,* 7(1), 15–24. https://doi.org/10.1046/j.1365-2850.2000.00260.x

Evans, S., & Egglestone, C. (2019). *Time for action: Skills for economic growth and social justice.* Learning and Work Institute. https://learningandwork.org.uk/wp-content/uploads/2020/02/Time-for-Action-Skills-for-economic-growth-and-social-justice.pdf

Ferring, D., Balducci, C., Burholt, V., Wenger, C., Thissen, F., Weber, G., & Hallberg, I. (2004). Life satisfaction of older people in six European countries: Findings from the European study on adult well-being. *European Journal of Ageing,* 1, 15–25. https://doi.org/10.1007/s10433-004-0011-4

Ferro, A., Bordin, P., Benacchio, L., Fornasiero, F., Bressan, V., Tralli, V., Moretti, F., & Majori, S. (2020). Influenza vaccination and absenteeism among healthy working adults: A cost-benefit analysis. *Annali di Igiene Medicina Preventiva e di Comunità,* 32(3), 234–244. https://doi.org/10.7416/ai.2020.2346

Findlay, P., Lindsay, C., McIntyre, S., Roy, G., Stewart, R., & Dutton, E. (2021, June). *CIPD Good Work Index 2021: Survey report.* Chartered Institute of Personnel and Development. https://www.cipd.co.uk/Images/good-work-index-survey-report-2021-1_tcm18-96105.pdf

Fitzgerald, S., Murphy, A., Kirby, A., Geaney, F., & Perry, I. J. (2018). Cost-effectiveness of a complex workplace dietary intervention: An economic evaluation of the Food Choice at Work study. *BMJ Open,* 8(3), e019182. http://dx.doi.org/10.1136/bmjopen-2017-019182

Ford, M. T., Cerasoli, C. P., Higgins, J. A., & Decesare, A. L. (2011). Relationships between psychological, physical, and behavioural health and work performance: A review and meta-analysis. *Work & Stress*, **25**(3), 185–204. https://doi.org/10.1080/02678 373.2011.609035

Gazaway, S. B., Schumacher, A. M., & Anderson, L. (2016). Mentoring to retain newly hired nurses. *Nursing Management*, **47**(8), 9–13. https://doi.org/10.1097/01.NUMA.000 0488861.77193.78

Glover, A., Harries, S., Lane, J., & Lewis, S. (2018). *Evaluation of the early implementation of the childcare offer for Wales*. Report no. 61/2018. Welsh Government. Government Social Research. https://www.gov.wales/sites/default/files/statistics-and-research/2019-06/181122-evaluation-early-implementation-childcare-offer-en.pdf

Goodyear, C., & Goodyear, M. (2018). Supporting successful mentoring. *Nursing Management*, **49**(4), 49–53. https://doi.org/10.1097/01.NUMA.0000531173.00718.06

Government Statistical Service. (2019, 25 June). *Measuring disability for the Equality Act 2010 harmonisation guidance*. https://gss.civilservice.gov.uk/policy-store/measuring-disability-for-the-equality-act-2010/

Graham, J., Albery, I. P., Ramirez, A. J., & Richards, M. A. (2001). How hospital consultants cope with stress at work: Implications for their mental health. *Stress and Health: Journal of the International Society for the Investigation of Stress*, **17**(2), 85–89. https://doi.org/10.1002/smi.884

Gritzka, S., MacIntyre, T. E., Dörfel, D., Baker-Blanc, J. L., & Calogiuri, G. (2020). The effects of workplace nature-based interventions on the mental health and well-being of employees: A systematic review. *Frontiers in Psychiatry*, **11**, 323. https://doi.org/10.3389/fpsyt.2020.00323

Gruber-Page, M. (2016). The value of mentoring in nursing: An honor and a gift. *Oncology Nursing Forum*, **43**(4), 420–422. https://doi.org/10.1188/16.ONF.420-422

Gunn, C., Mackus, M., Griffin, C., Munafò, M. R., & Adams, S. (2018). A systematic review of the next-day effects of heavy alcohol consumption on cognitive performance. *Addiction*, **113**(12), 2182–2193. https://doi.org/10.1111/add.14404

Hafner, M., Stepanek, M., Taylor, J., Troxel, W. M., & Van Stolk, C. (2017). Why sleep matters—the economic costs of insufficient sleep: A cross-country comparative analysis. *Rand Health Quarterly*, **6**(4), 11. https://pubmed.ncbi.nlm.nih.gov/28983434/

Hartfiel, N., Burton, C., Rycroft-Malone, J., Clarke, G., Havenhand, J., Khalsa, S. B., & Edwards, R. T. (2012). Yoga for reducing perceived stress and back pain at work. *Occupational Medicine*, **62**(8), 606–612. https://doi.org/10.1093/occmed/kqs168

Hartfiel, N., Clarke, G., Havenhand, J., Phillips, C., & Edwards, R. T. (2017). Cost-effectiveness of yoga for managing musculoskeletal conditions in the workplace. *Occupational Medicine*, **67**(9), 687–695. https://doi.org/10.1093/occmed/kqx161

Hartmann-Boyce, J., McRobbie, H., Butler, A. R., Lindson, N., Bullen, C., Begh, R., Theodoulou, A., Notley, C., Rigotti, N. A., Turner, T., Fanshawe, T. R., & Hajek, P. (2022). Electronic cigarettes for smoking cessation. *Cochrane Database of Systematic Reviews*, **11**, CD010216. https://doi.org/10.1002/14651858.CD010216.pub7

Hatch Regeneris. (2020). *We mind the gap. Social return on investment (SROI) assessment*. https://wemindthegap.org.uk/wp-content/uploads/2021/05/Social-Return-on-Inventm ent-WMTG3.pdf

Haynes, P., Banks, L., & Hill, M. (2014). The relationship between employment and social networks in the older population: A comparative European study. *International Journal of Social Economics*, **41**(4), 321–335. https://doi.org/10.1108/IJSE-10-2012-0201

Health & Her®. (2021). *A fact-based focus on perimenopause and menopause issues faced by women* (MEW0054). https://committees.parliament.uk/writtenevidence/39340/pdf/

Health and Safety Executive. (2019). *Drug misuse at work: A guide for employers.* https://mynl.co.uk/download/54/alcohol-drug-related/2087/drug-misuse-at-work.pdf

Health and Safety Executive. (2021). *Work-related stress, anxiety or depression statistics in Great Britain, 2021.* https://www.hse.gov.uk/statistics/causdis/stress.pdf

Health and Social Care Committee. (2021). *Workforce burnout and resilience in the NHS and social care.* UK Parliament. https://publications.parliament.uk/pa/cm5802/cmselect/cmhealth/22/2202.htm

Heffernan, J., & Pilkington, P. (2011). Supported employment for persons with mental illness: Systematic review of the effectiveness of individual placement and support in the UK. *Journal of Mental Health, 20*(4), 368–380. https://doi.org/10.3109/09638237.2011.556159

Henley, A., & Reuschke, D. (2020). *Covid-19 and self-employment in the UK.* Enterprise Research Centre. https://www.enterpriseresearch.ac.uk/wp-content/uploads/2020/04/ERC-Insight-Covid-19-and-self-employment-in-the-UK.pdf

Hildon, Z., Smith, G., Netuveli, G., & Blane, D. (2008). Understanding adversity and resilience at older ages. *Sociology of Health & Illness, 30*(5), 726–740. https://doi.org/10.1111/j.1467-9566.2008.01087.x

Holmes, J., Meng, Y., Meier, P. S., Brennan, A., Angus, C., Campbell-Burton, A., Guo, Y., Hill-McManus, D., & Purshouse, R. C. (2014). Effects of minimum unit pricing for alcohol on different income and socioeconomic groups: A modelling study. *The Lancet, 383*(9929), 1655–1664. https://doi.org/10.1016/S0140-6736(13)62417-4

Hunter, D. (2010). What makes people healthy and what makes people ill? In F. **Campbell** (Ed.), *The social determinants of health and the role of local government* (pp. 11–15). Improvement and Development Agency. https://www.local.gov.uk/sites/default/files/documents/social-determinants-healt-25f.pdf

Hupkau, C., & Petrongolo, B. (2020). Work, care and gender during the Covid-19 crisis. *Fiscal Studies, 41*(3), 623–651. https://doi.org/10.1111/1475-5890.12245

Imo, U. O. (2017). Burnout and psychiatric morbidity among doctors in the UK: A systematic literature review of prevalence and associated factors. *British Journal of Psychiatry Bulletin, 41*(4), 197–204. https://doi.org/10.1192/pb.bp.116.054247

Impetus—Private Equity Foundation. (2014). *Ready for work. The capabilities young people need to find and jeep work—and the programmes proven to help develop these.* https://www.impetus.org.uk/assets/publications/Report/2014_09-Ready-for-Work.pdf

Inge, N., Ford, R., & Hogan, J. (2012, April). *Social return on investment of Ready for Work.* Business in the community. https://socialvalueuk.org/wp-content/uploads/2016/06/socialreturn.pdf

Institute of Alcohol Studies. (2020, October). *Alcohol in the workplace.* https://www.ias.org.uk/wp-content/uploads/2020/12/Alcohol-in-the-workplace.pdf

International Classification of Diseases-10. (2016). *International statistical classification of diseases and related health problems 10th revision.* https://icd.who.int/browse10/2016/en

IONOS. (2019). *Work-life balance.* https://www.ionos.co.uk/startupguide/productivity/work-life-balance/

Jacob, A., Scott, M., Falkmer, M., & Falkmer, T. (2015). The costs and benefits of employing an adult with autism spectrum disorder: A systematic review. *PLoS One, 10*(10), 1–15. https://doi.org/10.1371/journal.pone.0139896

Keus Van De Poll, M., Bergström, G., Jensen, I., Nybergh, L., Kwak, L., Lornudd, C., & Lohela-Karlsson, M. (2020). Cost-effectiveness of a problem-solving intervention aimed to prevent sickness absence among employees with common mental disorders or occupational stress. *International Journal of Environmental Research and Public Health*, 17(5234), 1–14. https://doi.org/10.3390/ijerph17145234

Kigozi, J., Jowett, S., Lewis, M., Barton, P., & Coast, J. (2017). The estimation and inclusion of presenteeism costs in applied economic evaluation: A systematic review. *Value in Health*, 20(3), 496–506. https://doi.org/10.1016/j.jval.2016.12.006

Kinchin, I., & Doran, C. M. (2017). The economic cost of suicide and non-fatal suicide behavior in the Australian workforce and the potential impact of a workplace suicide prevention strategy. *International Journal of Environmental Research and Public Health*, 14(347), 1–14. https://doi.org/10.3390/ijerph14040347

Knapp, M., Iemmi, V., Tinelli, M., & Guy, D. (2019). *Employment support for autistic adults: economic evidence.* Care Policy and Evaluation Centre, London School of Economics and Political Science. https://essenceproject.uk/wp-content/uploads/2019/08/Essence_14_Employment-support.pdf

Knapp, M., McDaid, D., & Parsonage, M. (2011). *Mental health promotion and mental illness prevention: The economic case.* Department of Health. Personal Social Services Research Unit, London School of Economics and Political Science. http://eprints.lse.ac.uk/32311/1/Knapp_et_al__MHPP_The_Economic_Case.pdf

Knapp, M., Patel, A., Curran, C., Latimer, E., Catty, J., Becker, T., Drake, R.E., Fioritti, A., Kilian, R., Lauber, C., Rössler, W., Tomov, T., van Busschbach, J., Comas-Herrera, A., White, S., Wiersma, D., & Burns, T. (2013). Supported employment: Cost-effectiveness across six European sites. *World Psychiatry*, 12(1), 60–68. https://doi.org/10.1002/wps.20017

Lewis, S. (2020, 19 October). *The rise in entrepreneurialism among older workers post COVID-19.* Centre for Ageing Better. https://ageing-better.org.uk/blogs/rise-entrepreneurialism-among-older-workers-post-covid-19

Lin, L. Y., Wang, J., Ou-Yang, X. Y., Miao, Q., Chen, R., Liang, F. X., Zhang, Y., Tang, Q., & Wang, T. (2021). The immediate impact of the 2019 novel coronavirus (COVID-19) outbreak on subjective sleep status. *Sleep Medicine*, 77, 348–354. https://doi.org/10.1016/j.sleep.2020.05.018

Makanjuola, A., Granger, R., Pisavadia, K., & Edwards, R. T. (2023). Is lifestyle coaching a potential cost-effective intervention to address the backlog for mental health counselling? *medRxiv.* https://doi.org/10.1101/2023.01.20.23284835

Marmot, M., Allen, J., Boyce, T., Goldblatt, P., & Morrison, J. (2020). *Health equity in England: The Marmot review 10 years on.* Institute of Health Equity. https://www.health.org.uk/publications/reports/the-marmot-review-10-years-on

Marmot, M., Allen, J., Goldblatt, P., Boyce, T., McNeish, D., Grady, M., & Geddes, I. (2010). *Fair society, healthy lives: The Marmot review. Strategic review of health inequalities in England post-2010.* https://www.instituteofhealthequity.org/resources-reports/fair-society-healthy-lives-the-marmot-review

Marvell, R., & Cox, A. (2017). *Fulfilling work: What do older workers value about work and why?* Centre for Ageing Better. Institute for Employment Studies. https://ageing-better.org.uk/sites/default/files/2017-12/What-do-older-workers-value.pdf

Maslow, A. H. (1943). A theory of human motivation. *Psychological Review*, 50(4), 370–396. https://doi.org/10.1037/h0054346

Maslow, A. H. (2017). *A theory of human motivation*. BN Publishing.

Matejic, P. (2020, 2 November). *Briefing: Poverty in Wales 2020*. Joseph Rowntree Foundation. https://www.jrf.org.uk/report/poverty-wales-2020

Mavranezouli, I., Megnin-Viggars, O., Cheema, N., Howlin, P., Baron-Cohen, S., & Pilling, S. (2014). The cost-effectiveness of supported employment for adults with autism in the United Kingdom. *Autism*, 18(8), 975–984. https://doi.org/10.1177/13623 61313505720

McKinley, N., McCain, R. S., Convie, L., Clarke, M., Dempster, M., Campbell, W. J., & Kirk, S. J. (2020). Resilience, burnout and coping mechanisms in UK doctors: A cross-sectional study. *BMJ Open*, 10(1), 1–8. https://doi.org/10.1136/bmjopen-2019-031765

Melville, D., Stevens, C., & Vaid, L. (2015). *Access to Work—cost benefit analysis*. Centre for Economic and Social Inclusion. https://www.rnib.org.uk/professionals/knowledge-and-research-hub/research-reports/employment-research/access-work-cost-benefit-analysis

Modini, M., Joyce, S., Mykletun, A., Christensen, H., Bryant, R. A., Mitchell, P. B., & Harvey, S. B. (2016). The mental health benefits of employment: Results of a systematic meta-review. *Australasian Psychiatry*, 24(4), 331–336. https://doi.org/10.1177/10398 56215618523

Mônico-Neto, M., Dos Santos, R. V. T., & Moreira Antunes, H. K. (2020). The world war against the COVID-19 outbreak: Don't forget to sleep! *Journal of Clinical Sleep Medicine*, 16(7), 1215–1215. https://doi.org/10.5664/jcsm.8502

Monteiro, M. G., Rehm, J., & Duennbier, M. (2020). Alcohol policy and coronavirus: An open research Agenda. *Journal of Studies on Alcohol and Drugs*, 81(3), 297–299. https://doi.org/10.15288/jsad.2020.81.297

Nabe-Nielsen, K., Garde, A. H., Albertsen, K., & Diderichsen, F. (2011). The moderating effect of work-time influence on the effect of shift work: A prospective cohort study. *International Archives of Occupational and Environmental Health*, 84(5), 551–559. https://doi.org/10.1007/s00420-010-0592-5

National Autistic Society. (2021). *What is autism?* https://www.autism.org.uk/advice-and-guidance/what-is-autism

National Health Service. (2022, 10 October). *Using e-cigarettes to stop smoking*. https://www.nhs.uk/live-well/quit-smoking/using-e-cigarettes-to-stop-smoking/

National Health Service England. (2017). *The economics of caring: A scoping review*. The Strategy Unit and ICF, NHS Midlands and Lancashire Communication Support Unit. https://www.strategyunitwm.nhs.uk/sites/default/files/2017-12/Caring scoping study - final report.pdf

National Institute for Health and Care Excellence. (2015). *Menopause. Appendix L—Health economics* (Version 1.2). (NG23). https://www.nice.org.uk/guidance/ng23/documents/menopause-appendix-l2

National Institute for Health and Care Excellence. (2021, 30 November). *Tobacco: Preventing uptake, promoting quitting and treating dependence* (NG209). https://www.nice.org.uk/guidance/ng209/resources/tobacco-preventing-uptake-promoting-quitting-and-treating-dependence-pdf-66143723132869

National Institute for Health and Care Excellence. (2022). *Mental wellbeing at work* (NG212). https://www.nice.org.uk/guidance/ng212/resources/mental-wellbeing-at-work-pdf-66143771841733

National Online Manpower Information System. (2018). *Population projections—local authority based by single year of age* [Data set]. https://www.nomisweb.co.uk/datasets/ppsyoala

National Sleep Foundation. (2013). *International bedroom poll.* https://www.thensf.org/wp-content/uploads/2021/03/2013-International-Bedroom-Poll.pdf

New Economics Foundation Consulting. (2022). *NHS England: The socioeconomics of unpaid care.* https://www.nefconsulting.com/our-work/clients/nhs-england-modelling-the-socioeconomics-of-unpaid-care/

Nicholson, P. J., & Mayho, G. (2016). Alcohol, drugs, and the workplace: An update for primary care specialists. *British Journal of General Practice, 66*(652), 556–557. https://doi.org/10.3399/bjgp16X687661

Office for Health Improvement & Disparities. (2022, 29 September). *Nicotine vaping in England: 2022 evidence update main findings.* https://www.gov.uk/government/publications/nicotine-vaping-in-england-2022-evidence-update/nicotine-vaping-in-england-2022-evidence-update-main-findings

Office for Health Improvement & Disparities. (2023, 16 May). *Youth vaping: Call for evidence.* https://www.gov.uk/government/consultations/youth-vaping-call-for-evidence/youth-vaping-call-for-evidence

Office for National Statistics. (2017, 17 March). *Suicide by occupation, England: 2011 to 2015.* https://www.ons.gov.uk/peoplepopulationandcommunity/birthsdeathsandmarriages/deaths/articles/suicidebyoccupation/england2011to2015

Office for National Statistics (2018, 13 August). *Living longer: How our population is changing and why it matters.* https://www.ons.gov.uk/peoplepopulationandcommunity/birthsdeathsandmarriages/ageing/articles/livinglongerhowourpopulationischanging andwhyitmatters/2018-08-13

Office for National Statistics. (2019a, 24 June). *Living longer and old-age dependency—what does the future hold?* https://www.ons.gov.uk/peoplepopulationandcommunity/birthsdeathsandmarriages/ageing/articles/livinglongerandoldagedependencywhatdoesthefuturehold/2019-06-24#the-uks-ageing-population

Office for National Statistics. (2019b, 24 October). *Families and the labour market, UK: 2019.* https://www.ons.gov.uk/releases/familiesandthelabourmarket

Office for National Statistics. (2019c, 3 September). *Number of suicides among health professionals, England and Wales, 2011 to 2018.* https://www.ons.gov.uk/peoplepopulationandcommunity/birthsdeathsandmarriages/deaths/adhocs/10471numberofsuicidesamonghealthprofessionalsenglandandwales2011to2018

Office for National Statistics. (2019d, 2 December). *Disability and employment, UK.* https://www.ons.gov.uk/peoplepopulationandcommunity/healthandsocialcare/disability/bulletins/disabilityandemploymentuk/2019

Office for National Statistics. (2019e, 6 November). *Sickness absence in the UK labour market: 2018.* https://www.ons.gov.uk/employmentandlabourmarket/peopleinwork/labourproductivity/articles/sicknessabsenceinthelabourmarket/2018

Office for National Statistics (2019f, 24 June). *How would you support our ageing population?* https://www.ons.gov.uk/peoplepopulationandcommunity/birthsdeathsandmarriages/ageing/articles/howwouldyousupportourageingpopulation/2019-06-24

Office for National Statistics. (2021, 18 February). *Outcomes for disabled people in the UK: 2020.* https://www.ons.gov.uk/peoplepopulationandcommunity/healthandsocialcare/disability/articles/outcomesfordisabledpeopleintheuk/2020#employment

Office for National Statistics. (2022a, 12 September). *People aged 65 years and over in employment, UK: January to March 2022 to April to June 2022.* https://www.ons.gov.uk/employmentandlabourmarket/peopleinwork/employmentandemployeetypes/articles/peopleaged65yearsandoverinemploymentuk/januarytomarch2022toapriltojune2022

Office for National Statistics. (2022b, 15 December). *Drug misuse in England and Wales: Year ending June 2022.* https://www.ons.gov.uk/peoplepopulationandcommunity/crimeandjustice/articles/drugmisuseinenglandandwales/yearendingjune2022

Office for National Statistics. (2023a, 15 August). *CLA02: Claimant count by age group (experimental statistics).* https://www.ons.gov.uk/employmentandlabourmarket/peoplenotinwork/outofworkbenefits/datasets/cla02claimantcountbyagegroup

Office for National Statistics. (2023b, 19 January). *Unpaid care, England and Wales: Census 2021.* https://www.ons.gov.uk/peoplepopulationandcommunity/healthandsocialcare/healthandwellbeing/bulletins/unpaidcareenglandandwales/census2021

Organisation for Economic Co-operation and Development. (2015). *Government at a glance 2015.* https://doi.org/10.1787/gov_glance-2015-en

Organisation for Economic Co-operation and Development. (2021, 12 May). *Tackling the mental health impact of the COVID-19 crisis: An integrated, whole-of-society response.* https://www.oecd.org/coronavirus/policy-responses/tackling-the-mental-health-impact-of-the-covid-19-crisis-an-integrated-whole-of-society-response-0ccafa0b/

Orme, S., Zarkin, G. A., Luckey, J., Dunlap, L. J., Novak, M. D., Holtyn, A. F., Toegal, F., & Silverman, K. (2023). Cost and cost-effectiveness of abstinence contingent wage supplements. *Drug and Alcohol Dependence, 244,* 109754. doi.org/10.1016/j.drugalcdep.2022.109754

Parsonage, M., & Saini, G. (2017). *Mental health at work: The business costs ten years on.* Centre for Mental Health. https://www.centreformentalhealth.org.uk/publications/mental-health-work-business-costs-ten-years

Patrick, R. (2012). Work as the primary 'duty' of the responsible citizen: A critique of this work-centric approach. *People, Place and Policy Online, 6*(1), 5–16. https://doi.org/10.3351/ppp.0006.0001.0002

Paull, G., La Valle, I., Speight, S., Jones, H., & White, C. (2017). *Evaluation of early implementation of 30 hours free childcare. Research report.* Department for Education. https://assets.publishing.service.gov.uk/government/uploads/system/uploads/attachment_data/file/629460/Evaluation_of_early_implementation_of_30_hours_free_childcare_.pdf

Pickard, L., King, D., Brimblecombe, N., & Knapp, M. (2018). Public expenditure costs of carers leaving employment in England, 2015/2016. *Health & Social Care in the Community, 26*(1), e132–e142. https://doi.org/10.1111/hsc.12486

Pierce, M., Hope, H., Ford, T., Hatch, S., Hotopf, M., John, A., Kontopantelis, E., Webb, R., Wessely, S., McManus, S., & Abel, K. M. (2020). Mental health before and during the COVID-19 pandemic: A longitudinal probability sample survey of the UK population. *The Lancet Psychiatry, 7*(10), 883–892. https://doi.org/10.1016/S2215-0366(20)30308-4

Prospect. (2023, 20 November). *What is the gender pension gap?* https://prospect.org.uk/article/what-is-the-gender-pension-gap/

Public Health England. (2015). *Promoting good quality jobs to reduce health inequalities.* UCL Institute of Health Equity. https://www.gov.uk/government/publications/local-act ion-on-health-inequalities-promoting-good-quality-jobs

Public Health England. (2016a). *Interventions to prevent burnout in high risk individuals: Evidence review.* Leeds Beckett University. https://assets.publishing.service.gov.uk/gov ernment/uploads/system/uploads/attachment_data/file/506777/25022016_Burnout_R apid_Review_2015709.pdf

Public Health England. (2016b). *Briefing for local enterprise partnerships on health and work, worklessness and economic growth.* https://assets.publishing.service.gov.uk/gov ernment/uploads/system/uploads/attachment_data/file/769037/Health_and_work_ local_enterprise_partnerships_April2016.pdf

Public Health England. (2018, 4 October). *Tobacco commissioning support: Principles and indicators.* https://www.gov.uk/government/publications/alcohol-drugs-and-tobacco-commissioning-support-pack/tobacco-commissioning-support-pack-2019-to-2020-pri nciples-and-indicators#workplace-interventions

Public Health England. (2019, 31 January). *Health matters: Health and work.* https://www. gov.uk/government/publications/health-matters-health-and-work/health-matters-hea lth-and-work

Saha, S., Grahn, B., Gerdtham, U. G., Stigmar, K., Holmberg, S., & Jarl, J. (2019). Structured physiotherapy including a work place intervention for patients with neck and/or back pain in primary care: An economic evaluation. *The European Journal of Health Economics,* **20**(2), 317–327. https://doi.org/10.1007/s10198-018-1003-1

Scott, M., Jacob, A., Hendrie, D., Parsons, R., Girdler, S., Falkmer, T., & Falkmer, M. (2017). Employers' perception of the costs and the benefits of hiring individuals with autism spectrum disorder in open employment in Australia. *PLoS One,* **12**(5), 1–16. https://doi.org/10.1371/journal.pone.0177607

Severin, J., Svensson, M., & Akerstrom, M. (2022). Cost-benefit evaluation of an organizational-level intervention program for decreasing sickness absence among public sector employees in Sweden. *International Journal of Environmental Research and Public Health,* **19**(5), 2998. https://doi.org/10.3390/ijerph19052998

Sodexo. (n.d.). *Applying Maslow's hierarchy of needs theory to HR responsibilities.* Sodexo Quality of Life Services. https://www.sodexoengage.com/blog/rewards-recognition/ applying-maslows-hierarchy-of-needs-theory-to-hr-responsibilities

Stevenson, D., & Farmer, P. (2017) *Thriving at work: The Stevenson/Farmer review of mental health and employers.* Department for Work and Pensions and Department of Health and Social Care. https://assets.publishing.service.gov.uk/government/uploads/system/ uploads/attachment_data/file/658145/thriving-at-work-stevenson-farmer-review.pdf

Sutton, B. S., Ottomanelli, L., Njoh, E., Barnett, S., & Goetz, L. (2020). Economic evaluation of a supported employment program for veterans with spinal cord injury. *Disability and Rehabilitation,* **42**(10), 1423–1429. https://doi.org/10.1080/09638 288.2018.1527955

The Sleep Council. (2017). *The Great British bedtime report.* https://www.sleep-hero.co.uk/ the-great-british-bedtime-report

The World Bank. (2012). *Gender equality and development.* https://siteresources.worldb ank.org/INTWDR2012/Resources/7778105-1299699968583/7786210-1315936222006/ Complete-Report.pdf

The World Bank. (2018). *Gender differences in employment and why they matter.* http://sitere sources.worldbank.org/INTWDR2012/Resources/7778105-1299699968583/7786210- 1315936222006/chapter-5.pdf

Thomas, K. H., Dalili, M. N., López-López, J. A., Keeney, E., Phillippo, D., Munafò, M. R., Stevenson, M., Caldwell, D. M., & Welton, N. J. (2021). Smoking cessation medicines and e-cigarettes: A systematic review, network meta-analysis and cost-effectiveness analysis. *Health Technology Assessment*, 25(59), 1–260. http://doi.org/10.3310/hta25590

Trades Union Congress. (2019). *Drug testing in the workplace. Guidance for workplace representatives.* https://www.tuc.org.uk/resource/drug-testing-workplace

United Kingdom Government. (2010, 1 February). *Positive for youth: The statement.* https:// www.gov.uk/government/publications/positive-for-youth-a-new-approach-to-cross- government-policy-for-young-people-aged-13-to-19/positive-for-youth-the-statement

United Kingdom Government. (2021, 27 January). *Funding boost to get more young people into work* [Press release]. Department of Education and HM Treasury. https://www.gov. uk/government/news/funding-boost-to-get-young-people-get-into-work

United Kingdom Government. (2022, 30 June). *Education provision: Childcare under 5 years of age.* https://explore-education-statistics.service.gov.uk/find-statistics/educat ion-provision-children-under-5

United Kingdom Parliament. (2021, 8 June). *Overhaul needed to tackle NHS and social care workforce burnout emergency.* https://committees.parliament.uk/committee/81/hea lth-and-social-care-committee/news/155698/overhaul-needed-to-tackle-nhs-and-soc ial-care-workforce-burnout-emergency/

United Nations Global Compact. (2020). *COVID-19: How business can support women in times of crisis.* https://unglobalcompact.org/academy/how-business-can-support- women-in-times-of-crisis

United Nations Women. (2016, 4 April). *The work that makes work possible.* https://www. unwomen.org/en/news/stories/2016/4/op-ed-the-work-that-makes-work-possible

van den Brand, F. A., Nagelhout, G. E., Winkens, B., Chavannes, N. H., van Schayck, O. C., & Evers, S. M. (2020). Cost-effectiveness and cost–utility analysis of a work-place smoking cessation intervention with and without financial incentives. *Addiction*, 115(3), 534–545. https://doi.org/10.1111/add.14861

van der Noordt, M., IJzelenberg, H., Droomers, M., & Proper, K. I. (2014). Health effects of employment: A systematic review of prospective studies. *Occupational and Environmental Medicine*, 71(10), 730–736. https://doi.org/10.1136/oemed-2013-101891

van de Ven, P., Zwijnenburg, J., & De Queljoe, M. (2018). *Including unpaid household activities: An estimate of its impact on macro-economic indicators in the G7 economies and the way forward* (Working paper no. 91). OECD. https://one.oecd.org/document/ SDD/DOC(2018)4/En/pdf

Van Hasselt, M., Keyes, V., Bray, J., & Miller, T. (2015). Prescription drug abuse and workplace absenteeism: Evidence from the 2008–2012 National Survey on drug use and health. *Journal of Workplace Behavioral Health*, 30(4), 379–392. https://doi.org/10.1080/ 15555240.2015.1047499

Varney, J. (2018, 30 January). Is lack of sleep affecting your work? *UK Health Security Agency Blog.* https://ukhsa.blog.gov.uk/2018/01/30/is-lack-of-sleep-affecting-your-work/

Velentzis, L. S., Salagame, U., & Canfell, K. (2017). Menopausal hormone therapy: A systematic review of cost-effectiveness evaluations. *BMC Health Services Research*, 17(1), 1–17. https://doi.org/10.1186/s12913-017-2227-y

Villar, A., & Strong, M. (2007). Is mentoring worth the money? A benefit-cost analysis and five-year rate of return of a comprehensive mentoring program for beginning teachers. *ERS Spectrum*, 25(3), 1–17. https://eric.ed.gov/?id=EJ795664

Ward, M., Buchanan, I., & Francis-Devine, B. (2023). *Youth unemployment statistics* (Publication no. CBP 5871). House of Commons Library. https://researchbriefings.files.parliament.uk/documents/SN05871/SN05871.pdf

Welsh Government. (2019). *Substance misuse delivery plan 2019–2022*. https://www.gov.wales/sites/default/files/publications/2019-10/substance-misuse-delivery-plan-2019-22.pdf

Wolter, S. C., & Joho, E. (2018). *Apprenticeship training in England—a cost-effective model for firms?* JPMorgan Chase Foundation. Bertelsmann Stiftung. Education Policy Institute. https://epi.org.uk/wp-content/uploads/2018/04/Apprenticeships-in-England_2018.pdf

World Health Organization. (2018). *International classification of diseases for mortality and morbidity statistics* (ICD-11 MMS). https://icd.who.int/browse11/l-m/en

World Health Organization, & Burton, J. (2010). *WHO healthy workplace framework and model: Background and supporting literature and practices*. World Health Organization. https://apps.who.int/iris/handle/10665/113144

Wright, C. J., Livingston, M., Dwyer, R., & Callinan, S. (2021). Second, third, fourth COVID-19 waves and the 'pancession': We need studies that account for the complexities of how the pandemic is affecting alcohol consumption in Australia. *Drug and Alcohol Review*, 40(2), 179–182. https://doi.org/10.1111/dar.13188

Yeandle, S., Bennett, C., Buckner, L., Fry, G., & Price, C. (2014). *Carers, employment and services report series diversity in caring: towards equality for carers*. Carers UK. https://www.wrexham.gov.uk/assets/pdfs/carers/diversity_in_caring_report.pdf

Chapter 6

Living Well for Longer

Carys Stringer, Lucy Bryning,
Llinos H. Spencer, Bethany F. Anthony,
Victory Ezeofor, Catherine L. Lawrence,
and Rhiannon T. Edwards

Introduction

In the United Kingdom (UK), the Office for National Statistics (ONS) uses the age category of over sixty-five years for statistics relating to older people. There are currently over twelve million people aged over sixty-five in the UK (ONS, 2021a), and by 2030, one in five people will be in this age category (ONS, 2022a). As life expectancy has increased, time spent in poor health has also increased (Marmot et al., 2020). The UK has a diverse, multicultural population with people from ethnic minority backgrounds accounting for 14 per cent of the population (Uberoi & Burton, 2022). However, only 8 per cent of people aged over sixty are from ethnic minority backgrounds (ONS, 2018a). One explanatory factor for this difference is that migration to the UK of working-aged people from ethnic minority backgrounds and their families leads to lower average age for this population group. In the UK population as a whole, 55 per cent of people aged over seventy are married or in a civil partnership, whilst 45 per cent are widowed, divorced, or single (ONS, 2020a). Older adults who live alone are more likely to attend accident and emergency (A&E) departments and more likely to visit their general practitioner (GP) than those who live with others (Dreyer et al., 2018).

The social determinants of health are the non-medical factors that influence health outcomes. These factors heavily influence the health that we can achieve at individual and population level. Since the Wanless and colleagues (2006) report into good care for older people, the need to develop integrated approaches to service delivery has been recognized (National Health Service (NHS), 2018). The NHS Long-Term Plan has a goal of Integrated Care Systems (ICSs) being rolled out across England, with a remit of bringing together local organizations

Carys Stringer, Lucy Bryning, Llinos H. Spencer, Bethany F. Anthony, Victory Ezeofor, Catherine L. Lawrence, and Rhiannon T. Edwards, *Living Well for Longer* In: *Health Economics of Well-being and Well-becoming across the Life-course*. Edited by: Rhiannon T. Edwards and Catherine L. Lawrence, Oxford University Press.
© Oxford University Press 2024. DOI: 10.1093/9780191919336.003.0006

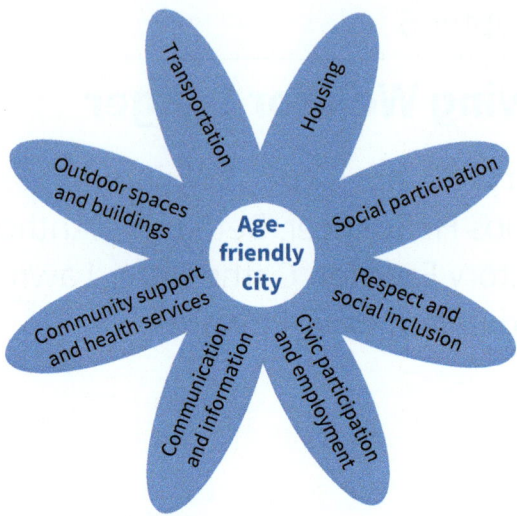

Figure 6.1 Aspects needed to support age-friendly cities, towns, and rural communities
Reproduced with permission from World Health Organization. (2007). *Global age-friendly cities: A guide*. World Health Organization. https://apps.who.int/iris/handle/10665/43755. Copyright © 2007 World Health Organization

across sectors to collaborate on decisions and redesign care services to improve population health (NHS, 2019a). The collective management of resources and performance is a fundamental shift away from the previous model of the NHS and social care services operating as independent silos. For a health and social care system to function well, it needs to take account of the population it serves, its age composition, the most common diseases and conditions, and arrange its services accordingly (NHS, 2019a). In contrast to other chapters in this book, instead of structuring the contents of this chapter on a model of what determines the well-being of older adults, we have focused on how to create an environment in which older adults can flourish. This chapter is organized around the themes identified as important for creating age-friendly environments, as identified in the World Health Organization (WHO; 2007) model shown in Figure 6.1. This model includes the following themes: transportation; housing; social participation; respect and social inclusion; civic participation and employment; communication and information; community support and health services; and outdoor spaces and buildings.

Transportation

Maintaining mobility in older age enables independence, reduces social isolation, and supports continued physical activity levels (Patterson et al., 2018).

Populations in rural areas and by the coast tend to have a higher proportion of older people than urban areas (Department for Environment, Food & Rural Affairs, 2012; ONS, 2020b). Lower population density in rural areas can make it more expensive to create and maintain comprehensive service infrastructures (Age UK, 2019). Rural areas can be disadvantaged in terms of access to services and activities, which can exacerbate risks of social isolation, reduce mobility, and result in older adults lacking adequate support and health care. On average, it takes people living in rural areas over an hour to reach hospital by public transport, compared to thirty-four minutes for people living in urban areas (Department for Transport, 2019). Bus use is associated with a number of benefits such as increased interaction with family, friends, and the community (Donald, 2010; Musselwhite & Shergold, 2013), and a decrease in obesity as buses are a constituent of an active travel system (Laverty et al., 2013). The promotion of active travel, including walking and cycling, has additional advantages such as decreasing air and noise pollution and improving the quality of urban and rural life (Cerin et al., 2017). Town planning modifications to support maintaining mobility in older age include the location of bus stops, transport fares and scheduling, disabled parking, pedestrian infrastructure, and proximity to shops and services (van Leeuwen et al., 2014).

Housing

Since October 2022, 2.8 million (three in ten) older households in England have been living in fuel poverty, exacerbated by rising fuel prices, poor energy efficiency in many homes, the complexity of switching between energy suppliers, and low income (Age UK, 2022a). One-third of older people from ethnic minority backgrounds are living in poverty, compared to 15 per cent of older White people. An economic evidence review developed for the National Institute for Health and Care Excellence (NICE) concluded that, 'rising fuel prices and the transition to a low carbon economy may both contribute to an increase in fuel poverty and, in the current UK policy environment, future energy efficiency programmes will in part be paid for by regressive levies on domestic energy bills which penalise financially disadvantaged households' (NICE, 2015a, p. 28). In response to the energy crisis, 'warm banks' are being offered in communities, giving people a warm space to heat up for free if they cannot afford to turn on the heating in their own home (Birkett, 2022). These publicly accessible spaces (e.g. in libraries and sports centres) have been announced by a number of UK local authorities. Participating local authorities have included a directory on their websites where people can search for specific facilities, such as warm spaces with an accessible entrance, for women or men only, or for people aged fifty years and above (Birmingham City Council, 2022). To help households and businesses manage the rising cost of energy, the Energy Prices Bill was introduced to the UK Parliament in October 2022. This included a £11.7 billion Energy Bills Support Scheme, worth up to £400 each for twenty-eight million households, a £150 disability cost of living payment, and a £650 cost of living payment for households on means-tested benefits (UK Government, 2022).

Deterioration in health is associated with worsening housing conditions (Pevalin et al., 2008). Prior to the coronavirus disease 2019 (COVID-19) pandemic, in 2018/2019 there were 23,200 excess winter deaths in England and Wales, most of which occurred in people aged seventy-five and over (ONS, 2019), 2,060 excess winter deaths in Scotland (National Records of Scotland, 2019), and 560 excess winter deaths in Northern Ireland (Northern Ireland Statistics and Research Agency, 2020). In the 2019 Conservative Party manifesto, the government promised to 'level up our country' to reduce the imbalances between areas and social groups in the UK (The Conservative Party, 2019). However, slow recovery of economies internationally after the pandemic, the war in Ukraine, and the cost of living crisis have led to supply-chain problems, such as fuel, resulting in price increases (McCabe, 2022). For example, the Office of Gas and Electricity Markets (Ofgem) imposed a 54 per cent increase in gas prices from 1 April 2022 (Ofgem, 2022). Age UK (2022b) has called for the UK Government to take immediate action to prevent millions of older people falling into poverty and specifically fuel poverty. The charity warned that many older people will be rationing their heating to afford higher energy bills, particularly those living in older, hard-to-heat homes (Age UK, 2022b). Box 6.1 summarizes cost-effectiveness evidence of cold homes interventions.

The UK has largely had an 'ageing in place' history of housing, with older people choosing to live independently in their own homes for as long as possible (NICE, 2015d; Sixsmith & Sixsmith, 2008). Through providing people with the necessary adaptations and support to live at home, there are potential cost savings to the NHS, for example, a reduction in A&E attendances and length of hospital stays, and savings to local authorities through the avoidance or delay in transition to living in a care home (NICE, 2015d). 'Reablement' is an approach to home care services that supports people to do things for themselves, rather than having things done for them (Francis et al., 2011). There is some evidence that reablement services can provide cost savings through a reduction in care and support needs and prevention of care home admission for older people who are moderately or severely frail (Dixon et al., 2014; Hollinghurst et al., 2020). Integrated care is increasingly promoted as an effective and cost-effective way to support frail older people living with complex needs in the community. A systematic review of preventative, integrated care plans for frail, older people

---

Box 6.1 Summary of cost-effectiveness evidence of cold homes interventions

Most economic evidence relating to reducing winter or cold-related health problems and deaths have focused on household energy efficiency improvements. The National Institute for Health and Care Excellence (NICE; 2015b) modelled the cost-effectiveness of interventions associated with cold homes and found there was some evidence that housing energy efficiency interventions (e.g. roof insulation, double glazing, or boiler replacement) are cost-effective compared with current practice. The highest benefits occur when targeting at-risk groups with health conditions such as chronic obstructive pulmonary disease (COPD) and housing which is of particularly poor standards.

In a review of the public health economic evaluations considered by NICE between 2005 and 2018, there were fifteen economic evaluations identified focusing on cold homes interventions. In addition to housing improvements, these interventions included fuel subsidy programmes, which may help to address fuel poverty. The incremental cost-effectiveness ratio (ICER) of interventions ranged from £28,324 to £509,205 (Owen & Fischer, 2019).

Investments in improving housing energy efficiency would usually not be justified on health grounds alone, however, once a wider range of benefits are considered they appear to be worthwhile investments (NICE, 2015c).

---

living in the community found a lack of cost-effectiveness evidence and generally poor quality of studies (Looman et al., 2018).

Social Participation

'Intergenerational programmes' bring together generations, such as placing preschool centres within care homes for older people and organizing programmes of activities to integrate these bookend generations. These types of programmes are being introduced in Australia, Germany, the UK, and the United States (US). Intergenerational programmes can have bi-directional benefits because older people can gain enjoyment from interaction with children, thereby reducing loneliness, while children can improve their social development and appreciation for older adults (Park, 2015). Figure 6.2 illustrates other potential benefits of such programmes. These include reducing ageism; increasing understanding and sharing of experience between generations; improving mental well-being

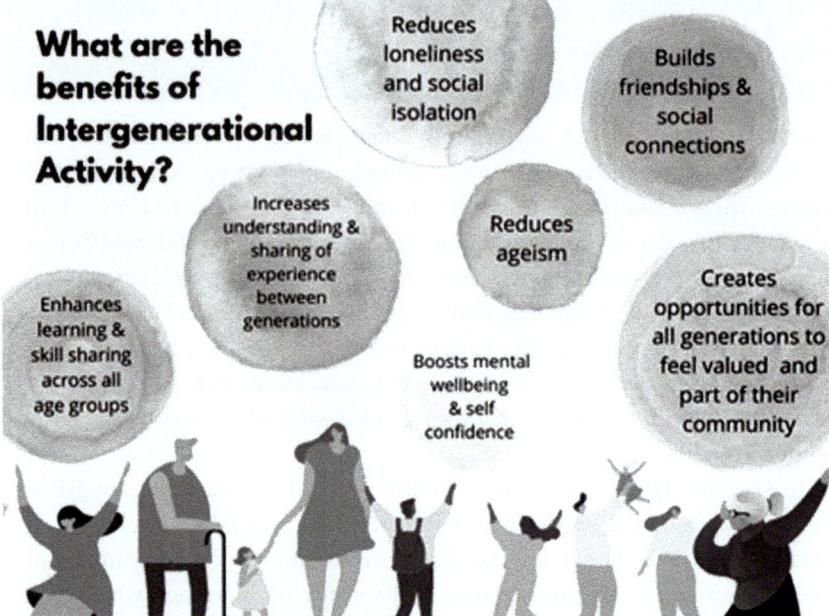

Figure 6.2 Potential benefits of intergenerational living
Reproduced with permission from Linking Generations Northern Ireland. (2021). *Intergenerational practice explained*. https://www.linkinggenerationsni.com/intergenerational-practice-explained. Copyright © 2021 Linking Generations Northern Ireland

and self-confidence; and creating opportunities for all generations to feel valued and part of their community (Linking Generations Northern Ireland, 2021). Sharing facilities and overheads through these types of programmes can also bring financial benefits. However, whilst the psychological outcomes of intergenerational programmes have been widely explored, the economic evidence surrounding these programmes is currently scarce (Vecchio et al., 2020).

Respect and Social Inclusion

In 2022, there were over 2.2 million men aged over sixty-five living alone and over 3.7 million women aged over sixty-five living alone in the UK (Clark, 2023). The health and well-being consequences of social isolation and loneliness in old age are increasingly being recognized (Courtin & Knapp, 2017). Older men are more likely than women to be socially isolated, though women are more likely than men to report feeling lonely (ONS, 2018b). Loneliness can have a considerable impact on demands for public sector services, with significantly higher admission rates to residential care, GP visits, hospital admissions, and A&E visits, compared to older people who self-describe as never feeling lonely (Fulton & Jupp, 2015; Landeiro et al., 2016). Keeping older people independent and mentally well has been found to be beneficial and cost-saving in terms of interventions to prevent loneliness and increase quality of life (Nurse et al., 2014).

Social isolation and loneliness are correlated with poor mental and physical health outcomes (Courtin & Knapp, 2017). Older people who experience loneliness are at an increased risk of depression, cognitive decline, and early death (Cacioppo et al., 2006; Holt-Lunstad et al., 2015; Holwerda et al., 2014; James et al., 2011). There is evidence that loneliness is associated with an increased risk of developing preventable chronic physical conditions such as diabetes, coronary heart disease, and stroke (Valtorta et al., 2016). Poor health can also be an indirect cause of loneliness, particularly when it reduces social interaction and participation (Burholt & Scharf, 2014). Strong social networks are a key factor in protecting cognitive resilience (Kelly et al., 2017) and maintaining individual well-being (Burholt et al., 2020).

There are a wide range of interventions to address social isolation or loneliness, including one-to-one interventions, group-based activities, and wider community engagement (Fakoya et al., 2020). While there is extensive literature highlighting the opportunities for investment in social isolation and loneliness prevention initiatives, such as friendship programmes and social prescribing (discussed in Chapter 2 of this book), the availability of economic evidence of relative cost-effectiveness is limited (Centre for Reviews and Dissemination, 2014; Windle et al., 2011). Evidence from a Finnish study indicated that socially stimulating group activities were cost-effective in reducing isolation and loneliness, improving well-being and improving cognitive function in older people (Pitkala et al., 2009, 2011). Using return on investment (ROI) and social return on investment (SROI) methods, arts and craft activity-based programmes such as Craft Café and the Men-in-Sheds programmes can yield high rates of social value of between £8.27 and £9.77 generated for every £1 invested (Schroeder et al., 2015; Social Value Lab, 2011). The cost savings of reduced service use associated with a reduction in cases of loneliness has been estimated at between £1,700 per person over ten years (McDaid et al., 2016) and £2,040 per person over a lifetime (Fulton & Jupp, 2015). Prevention is key to loneliness and requires joint proactive efforts across agencies and public sectors concerned with the well-being of older people (Jopling, 2015). A systematic review of interventions to improve the health and well-being of people living alone concluded that services that do not address user accessibility in design or evaluation may be limited in their uptake and impact (Johnstone et al., 2021). The researchers recommended that dimensions of access and co-creation principles be integrated into service design processes and be evaluated alongside clinical effectiveness.

Civic Participation and Employment

Even after considering pension costs and increased health and social care costs associated with older age, the annual net contribution of older people to the UK economy is in the region of £796 billion due to their spending, tax contributions, volunteering time, and caring commitments (Iparraguirre, 2017). Spending by older consumers is as high as £319 billion (International Longevity Centre UK, 2019). Additionally, 65 per cent of grandparents in the UK provide some form of childcare and the value of this childcare has been estimated to be worth £7.8 billion per annum (International Longevity Centre UK, 2017; Iparraguirre, 2017).

Length of working life can have a large impact on the overall potential economic contribution of older people. In the UK, 63.4 per cent of people aged fifty-five to sixty-four are in employment. If employment rates for this age group were increased to match Swedish levels of 75.5 per cent, it would boost UK gross domestic product (GDP) by £105 billion each year (Hawksworth et al., 2018). In April to June 2022, there was a record level of 1.468 million people aged sixty-five and over in employment. This increase was driven by rises in part-time work (ONS, 2022b). Strategies to support people to work up to and beyond retirement are needed, particularly creating employment opportunities and environments that are appropriate for an older workforce. Supporting older people to stay in the workforce for longer can also generate productivity gains through retaining large amounts of experience and skills in the workplace (NICE, 2015e). The proportion of older people in the workforce is likely to increase further due to increasing life expectancy, removal of the default retirement age, and changes to the state pension age (see Chapter 5). There is evidence that promoting healthy behaviours at midlife may help extend working life (Hagger-Johnson et al., 2017). Older workers should have the same access to training, progression, mentoring, or leadership as workers of other ages. This includes well-being support and appropriate physical adjustments, appropriate equipment and flexible working arrangements, and all forms of adaptation that are usual in the workplace (Marvell & Cox, 2017). Flexible working arrangements, reduced hours, or the ability to adjust the time and place of work are fundamental to making paid work more age-friendly for those over fifty who may also have caring responsibilities for family or friends (ONS, 2021b).

Older people in a volunteering capacity can act as 'champions', making use of their life experiences in such roles. People aged over sixty-five are the most likely age group to volunteer, with nearly half having done so within the last year (McGarvey et al., 2019). Assigning older people to voluntary, community-based lay public health roles can improve mental and social aspects of their own health as well as give the potential to positively influence the health of others in the community, and provide a positive ROI (Hex & Tatlock, 2011; Woodall et al., 2013). For example, Altogether Better began as a five-year Big Lottery Fund Programme in 2008. The aim of Altogether Better was to build understanding and capacity to empower communities to improve their health and well-being (Hex & Tatlock, 2011). The outcomes of the collaboration were to improve diet and nutrition, increase physical activity, and improve mental health through project activities incorporating a wider set of well-being outcomes. Benefits generated through the projects included a reduction in workplace absence due to stress, increased attendance and participation in social groups, reduced number of people accessing health services, and lower rates of unemployment. An SROI analysis of fifteen case studies from fifteen projects in the Altogether Better programme found that all projects demonstrated a positive ROI of between £0.79 to £112.42 for every £1 invested (Hex & Tatlock, 2011).

Communication and Information

Training on how to use the internet, social media, and other modern communication tools may be a cost-effective way to support older people in maintaining good social links, particularly for those living in rural communities and at a distance from grown-up children and friends (Owen et al., 2015). Online shopping increased during the COVID-19 pandemic national lockdowns, especially for people aged over sixty-five, many of whom were shopping online for the first time (Chevalier, 2021). Box 6.2 summarizes the use of technology-enabled care in health and social care.

Box 6.2 The use of technology-enabled care in health and social care

'Technology-enabled care' is also known as telehealth, tele-medicine, and telecare (Age UK, 2023). It encompasses care relayed through telephone or videocalls, monitoring devices that automatically send readings to health care professionals, and personal alarms that notify a response centre if a person requires assistance. Telehealth has been a focus for the European

Union (EU) since 2018 due to the shift in digitalization of health care and increasing spending on public health care (European Parliament, 2021). However, there are barriers to its implementation including set-up costs, internet connectivity in the recipient's home, the digital competency of the recipient, and their potential preference for face-to-face contact (Scott Kruse et al., 2018).

Telehealth does not replace existing models of care (Stowe & Harding, 2010). It is usually available to people who have been diagnosed with a long-term health condition such as high blood pressure, diabetes, chronic obstructive pulmonary disease (COPD), heart failure, pulmonary rehabilitation, pressure area care, or post-COVID-19 support. Telehealth is of particular potential benefit for people living in remote or rural areas who cannot easily drive to health care services, and it also benefits general practitioners (GPs) and other health care professionals as they have fewer face-to-face appointments and can prioritize the patients who are most in need of medical advice or treatment (Brewster et al., 2014).

Since the early 2000s, there has been a continuing momentum to embed telecare in mainstream care pathways (Morrison et al., 2018). Prior to the COVID-19 pandemic, economic evaluations to explore the impact of telecare and telehealth were limited in number and quality (Bergmo, 2014; Polisena et al., 2009). In a nested economic evaluation in a pragmatic, cluster randomized controlled trial (RCT), Henderson and colleagues (2013) examined the costs and cost-effectiveness of telehealth in addition to standard support and treatment, compared with standard support and treatment alone. They found that the quality-adjusted life year (QALY) gain by patients using telehealth in addition to usual care was similar to that by patients receiving usual care only, and total costs associated with the telehealth intervention were higher. This is an example of evidence that telehealth may not be a cost-effective addition to standard support and treatment. The researchers questioned whether the timeframe of the evaluation was too short to show improvements in health-related quality of life (Henderson et al., 2013).

The COVID-19 pandemic has accelerated the rise of digital health, a broad concept that includes solutions for telemedicine and teleconsultation, remote monitoring, connected devices, digital health platforms, and health apps (European Parliament, 2021). During the pandemic, telehealth provided older people with access to routine primary care while shielding or isolating (Smith et al., 2020). However, while the advancement and application of digital health is building momentum, consideration needs to be taken of the wider social system as people who are most in need of care are least likely to have access to technology (Davies et al., 2021). Without doing so would widen health inequalities and create a digital inverse care law (Davies et al., 2021). Figure 6.3 shows the direct and indirect impacts of digital exclusion on health inequalities.

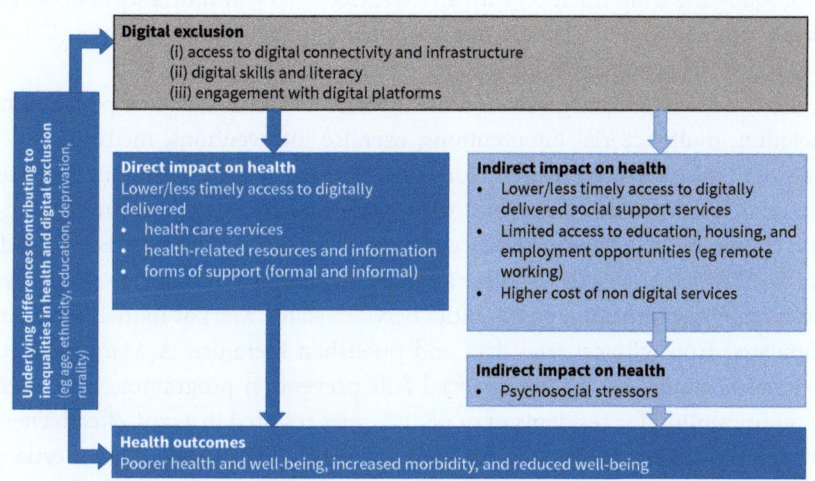

Figure 6.3 The direct and indirect impacts of digital exclusion on health inequalities

Reproduced from Davies, A. R., Honeyman, M., & Gann, B. (2021). Addressing the digital inverse care law in the time of COVID-19: Potential for digital technology to exacerbate or mitigate health inequalities. *Journal of Medical Internet Research*, *23*(4), e21726. https://doi. org/10.2196/21726. Licence: Creative Commons BY 3.0 IGO

Community Support and Health Services

Falls are the second leading cause of accidental or unintentional injury-related death worldwide (WHO, 2021). Older people are at risk of falling due to balance problems, muscle weakness and frailty, poor vision, and acute illness, as well as other environmental hazards (Jin, 2018). Falls and fall-related injuries can have negative effects on the quality of life of older adults, their family, and society. They also impact the functional independence of the individual and are associated with increased morbidity, mortality, and health cost (Montero-Odasso et al., 2021). In the community, the proportion of people who sustain at least one fall over a one-year period varies between 28 per cent and 35 per cent in those aged over sixty-five years; this number rises to 50 per cent of adults over eighty years. Incidence rates in hospitals are higher, and in long-term care settings approximately 30 per cent to 50 per cent of people fall each year, with 40 per cent falling repeatedly (Kenny et al., 2017; NICE, 2017). Around 40 per cent to 60 per cent of falls lead to injuries: they account for 90 per cent of hip and wrist fractures and 60 per cent of head injuries. Injury from a fall is the most common cause of emergency hospital admissions for older people and around 40 per cent of ambulance attendances are related to older people (Mackenzie & McIntrye, 2019). Short and long-term prognoses for patients are generally poor following a hip fracture, with an increased one-year mortality of between 18 per cent and 33 per cent, and negative effects on daily living activities (Office for Health Improvement & Disparities, 2022).

There are several strategies to address the issue of falls in the older population, including multifactorial interventions, exercise interventions, medication reviews and medical interventions, home and environment interventions, feet and footwear interventions, vision and vision aids, and falls detection and prevention technologies. Current evidence on interventions to prevent falls is mixed. Markov models enable us to follow a cohort of patients through various disease states, applying transition probabilities between states. Markov models are often populated from clinical trial data and published literature. A Markov-based simulation model for a multifactorial falls prevention programme compared to no prevention for residents of nursing homes resulted in a cost-effectiveness ratio of £17,014 per quality-adjusted life year (QALY; Müller et al., 2015). Tertiary interventions, such as exercise programmes (Li & Harmer, 2015), can be low cost compared to multi-agency, complex interventions (Hendriks et al., 2008), which involve primary, secondary, and tertiary care. Exercise training in older people has been associated with health benefits such as decreased cardiovascular mortality; benefits for the brain centres that support executive control; maintaining quality of life, health, and physical function, and reducing falls (Langhammer et al., 2018). A physical activity and behaviour maintenance programme, Retirement in Action (REACT), was shown to be cost-effective in comparison to usual care, generating net cost savings and improved health-related quality of life (Snowsill et al., 2022). The REACT randomised controlled trial (RCT) assessed a twelve-month community-based group physical activity and behaviour maintenance intervention to help prevent decline in physical functioning in older adults at increased risk of mobility limitation. Community falls-based interventions for older people can provide positive net benefits. For example, in the Tai Chi: Moving for Better Balance RCT, physically inactive, community dwelling adults aged seventy to ninety-two were randomized to either the Tai Chi programme or a stretching control group (Li et al., 2005). The programme included twenty-four Tai Chi forms that focused on weight shifting, postural alignment, and coordinated movements. The one-hour Tai Chi classes were held three times a week for twenty-six weeks and were delivered by experienced Tai Chi instructors in senior centres, adult activity centres, and community centres.

When compared with the stretching control group, the risk of falling among participants undertaking the Tai Chi intervention was reduced by 55 per cent (Li et al., 2005). The intervention had a net benefit of $529.86 and an ROI of $5.09 for every $1 invested (Carande-Kulis et al., 2015).

Medication reviews should be considered part of a multifactorial assessment in patients at risk of falling (Barker, 2014). NHS Improvement and other bodies are supporting environmental adaptations to hospital wards, such as installing shock-absorbing flooring, which can reduce the cost of falling to £913.51 per patient (NHS Improvement & NHS England, 2019; Latimer et al., 2013), and provide safe and environmentally friendly homes to prevent falls and manage risks in older adults (Bennett et al., 2018). Footwear designed specifically with minimality might be beneficial for stability and physical function in older adults by strengthening muscles and improving postural and dynamic stability than wearing conventional shoes in falls prevention (Cudejko et al., 2019, 2020). Preliminary evidence indicates that such footwear may be cost-effective with incremental cost-effectiveness ratios (ICERs) ranging between £19,494 and £20,593 per additional QALY (Cockayne et al., 2017; Wylie et al., 2017).

Oral Health in Older Adults

Over 400,000 older people live in care homes in the UK. About half of all care home residents have their own natural teeth, but their oral health is much worse than their peers living in the community. The prevalence of caries is 73 per cent in care home residents compared to 40 per cent of community-dwelling older adults (Tsakos et al., 2021). In a survey of care home residents in Wales, it was found that 73 per cent of residents had tooth decay and residents were less likely to brush teeth/dentures twice a day than older people not residing in care homes (Karki et al., 2015). A similar observation was reported by Zander and Boniface (2017) with 58 per cent of patients in residential care found to not brush their teeth. Older people in care homes may have heavily restored teeth and/or need complex and costly restorative treatments such as implants, which need maintenance and care (Patel et al., 2022).

A study by Iliffe and colleagues (2016) showed that the working relationships between the NHS and care homes lack structure and purpose and have generally evolved locally. There are wide variations in the provision of both generalist and specialist health care services to care homes. Larger care home chains may take a systematic approach to both organizing access to NHS generalist and specialist services, and to supplementing gaps with in-house provision. A scoping review by Eow and colleagues (2019) examined the evidence in economic studies of different dental interventions. Of the ninety-one studies identified, thirty-four were preventative dental interventions, fourteen were restorative, thirteen were prosthodontic, and twelve were periodontal interventions. Sixty-eight studies included cost-effectiveness analysis (CEA), seventeen included cost-utility analysis (CUA), and six included cost-benefit analysis (CBA). Most dental interventions in older adults focused on prosthodontics and restorative treatment, though the preventative measures, such as education for nursing home caregivers, showed a reduction in denture plaque scores exceeding those of the control group by 1.15 at one month and by 1.47 at six months. In other preventative interventions, such as providing dental care for elderly nursing home residents compared to dentistry at a fixed clinic, the mean societal cost of domiciliary dental care for elderly nursing home residents was lower than dental care at a fixed clinic, and it was also considered cost-effective (Eow et al., 2019). The result seems to differ when the service offered is upgraded to special care as the cost does not match the benefit.

Phadraig and colleagues (2016) examined the cost-effectiveness of an oral health training intervention introduced into community-based residential settings to improve the oral health of people with intellectual disabilities in Dublin, Ireland. They reported a cost of between €7,000 and €10,000 more to achieve modest improvement scores in comparison to doing nothing in a subsample of care staff. The programme was still a cost-effective means of improving self-reported measures and possibly oral health, relative to doing nothing (Phadraig et al., 2016).

In another study, domiciliary dental care for older persons living in nursing homes in Sweden was found to have a lower societal cost in general and be cost-effective compared to dental care at fixed clinics (Lundqvist et al., 2015). In Germany, Schwendicke and colleagues (2017) examined the cost-effectiveness of professional oral health care versus no professional oral health care in preventing nursing home-acquired pneumonia and the monetary value of eliminating uncertainty. They found that no professional oral health care was less costly (€3,024), but also less effective (0.89 disability-adjusted life years (DALYs)) than professional oral health care (€10,249, 0.55 DALYs). For most presumed payers, professional oral health care was cost-effective. The cost-effectiveness of professional oral health care was higher in smokers and underweight or pulmonary disease patients. Eliminating uncertainty about the nursing home-acquired pneumonia costs, nursing home-acquired pneumonia incidence/mortality, and professional oral health care effectiveness would result in an expected net value of €47 million per year and even higher values at lower GDP thresholds (Schwendicke et al., 2017).

The use of health information technology and telecommunications for oral care to identify high-risk populations, facilitate patient access to dental care, and reduce waiting lists, unnecessary travel, and also inequalities in dental care access and costs for national health systems could be a viable tool for the management of oral care in people who cannot access dental care (Aquilanti et al., 2020). NICE (2016) guidelines support oral health care for adults in care homes and advises that residents have their mouths assessed and care plans put in place, which include daily mouth care. Guidelines call for staff to have the knowledge and skills to support people's oral health and undertake or support daily mouth care (Public Health England, 2020, 2022).

Dementia

'Dementia' is an umbrella term that describes a group of neurodegenerative symptoms that affect memory, thinking and social abilities, emotions, perception, and behaviour. Worldwide, there are more than fifty-five million people living with dementia and there are nearly ten million new cases each year (WHO, 2022). In the UK, the number of people living with dementia is estimated at 850,000 to 885,000, but only around two-thirds of those have been diagnosed (Storey, 2018; Wittenberg et al., 2019). Health care accounts for only 14 per cent of the total costs of dementia, whereas social care (publicly and privately funded) and unpaid care account for 45 per cent and 40 per cent of the total costs, respectively (Wittenberg et al., 2019). Dementia has replaced ischemic heart disease as the leading cause of death in England (125.9 per 100,000 people; ONS, 2022c). As life expectancy increases, the ageing population and changing structure of the population will bring both opportunities and challenges for the economy and health care, especially for people living with dementia (Storey, 2018).

Although no disease-modifying agents capable of reversing the initial pathological changes associated with dementia have yet reached the market, a diagnosis early in the course of the illness provides time to adjust to the diagnosis whilst the person living with dementia can still actively engage, and offers access to advice, financial support, and non-pharmacological and pharmacological treatments (Rasmussen & Langerman, 2019). Though age-specific incidence of dementia has fallen in many countries, probably because of improvements in education, nutrition, health care, and lifestyle changes (Livingston et al., 2020), there is a need to improve detection and recording of dementia in UK general practice and in hospital notes. Public health guidance from NICE (2015f) suggests that taking action in midlife makes it possible to prevent or delay the onset of dementia, frailty, and disability. In Chapter 8 of this book, Table 8.1 shows the modifiable risk factors that have been identified at different life-course stages for dementia (Livingston et al., 2020). Most people with dementia are cared for at home by a family member or friend, referred to as 'informal carers' (Lewis et al., 2014). There is growing literature associated with exercise and lifestyle programmes for people with dementia with mixed effectiveness and cost-effectiveness results (e.g. Harwood et al., 2022; Khan et al., 2019) and interventions to support carers (Vandepitte et al., 2020).

The Role of Informal Carers

Informal care provided by family and friends can include personal care (e.g. helping a person to wash and dress), household activities (e.g. shopping and cooking), or organizational support (e.g. reminding a person when to take their medication or taking them to appointments). Carers can be the key factor that can keep someone living at home or prevent admission to hospital or residential care (Carers UK, 2016). In 2020/2021, there were 4.2 million people providing informal care in the UK (Department for Work and Pensions, 2022). Most of this care is provided to older adults, often by spouses who are an advanced age themselves. Informal care saves the economy £132 billion per year, yet there is a huge financial impact on carers (Buckner & Yeandle, 2015). Over a third of carers are in paid work alongside their caring role, and the impact of caring on physical and mental well-being can be detrimental, with six out of ten carers reporting deteriorated physical health, and seven out of ten carers reporting poorer mental health (Carers UK, 2019). As the effects of caring are considerable, it is necessary to consider the impact of interventions on carers and patients when undertaking economic evaluations. This will potentially reduce the overprovision of services that harm carers. For example, early discharge of a patient from hospital is good for hospital statistics; however, it displaces the burden onto informal carers.

Evidence on the effectiveness and cost-effectiveness of interventions to support carers of people with dementia is mixed. In the Netherlands, Joling and colleagues (2013) evaluated the cost-effectiveness of a family meetings intervention for family carers of people with dementia compared to usual care over a twelve-month period. This type of psychosocial intervention targeted the whole family with the aim to maximize the positive contribution of family members, decrease caregiver burden, and reduce psychological distress. No differences in costs and effects between the intervention and control group were found. Joling and colleagues suggested this could be because of the high level of standard care in the Netherlands. In contrast to these findings, support groups have been shown to have a positive impact on carers' psychological well-being, depression, and social outcomes (Chien et al., 2011; Dahlrup et al., 2014). Educational groups can provide useful information such as caregiving skills, adjusting to the role of carer, information on benefits rights and legal issues, and signposting to resources to reduce carer load.

'Reminiscence therapy' involves discussing thoughts and feelings of lived experiences, using tangible prompts such as photographs or music, to stimulate cognitive activity and evoke memories. There is mixed evidence regarding the effectiveness of this type of therapy. In a multicentre, pragmatic RCT assessing the effectiveness and cost-effectiveness of reminiscence groups (REMCARE) compared to usual care, people with dementia experienced improved autobiographical memory, relationship quality, and overall quality of life following reminiscence sessions. However, their carers reported an increase in anxiety and raised stress levels (Woods et al., 2016). A befriending intervention for carers of people with dementia in the UK found no evidence of effectiveness or cost-effectiveness, and uptake of the scheme was not high (Charlesworth et al., 2008). The STrAtegies for RelaTives (START) manual-based therapy programme to promote the mental health of family carers of people with dementia was found to be cost-effective compared with treatment as usual (Knapp et al., 2013). Evidence from the US suggests that behavioural interventions can help carers of people with dementia manage their time more effectively, with carers in the intervention arm providing significantly lower hours of care than the control group at the end of the intervention (Nichols et al., 2008). A review found that internet-based interventions to support carers of people with dementia may improve carers' depression, perceived stress, and self-efficacy (Leng et al., 2020). WHO (2019) developed 'iSupport', an evidence-informed online training programme to support carers of people with dementia. Windle and colleagues (2022) are currently undertaking the first study in the UK to evaluate the clinical and cost-effectiveness of iSupport for dementia carers. The feasibility study will also work with young carers (aged eleven to seventeen years) to provide information leading to an adapted version of iSupport for young carers.

Respite care can be provided in the home or in the community to give carers a break from their caring role to help carers to manage their own health and well-being. Types of respite care includes: day care centres; homecare from a paid carer; a short stay in a care home; getting support from friends and family members; respite holidays; and sitting services (NHS, 2019b). In the UK, local councils can provide funding support for respite care for the carer or the person being looked after following a needs assessment. Box 6.3 describes an ongoing SROI analysis of a Shared Lives day support service for people living with dementia and their carers (Prendergast et al., 2022, 2023).

A systematic review of the effectiveness and cost-effectiveness of respite for carers of frail older people found mixed results (Mason et al., 2007). More recently, Vandepitte and colleagues (2016) undertook a systematic review of the effectiveness of respite care in supporting informal carers of people with dementia. They found mixed results for the effectiveness of temporary residential

---

Box 6.3 Short breaks for people living with dementia and their carers: Exploring well-being outcomes and informing future practice development through an SROI approach

TRIO is a community-based day support service that provides individualized, person-centred support for people living with mild-to-moderate dementia and their family or friend carers (Prendergast et al., 2022, 2023). In Wales, a social return on investment (SROI) analysis of TRIO is currently underway (Toms et al., 2023). This study is exploring the sustainability and social value generated by a short break provision. Each TRIO companion (a self-employed person who receives training and supervision from the local provider) is matched with and supports a small number of people living with dementia within their community. The companion provides tailored and flexible support based on shared interests with the person living with dementia. This study will evaluate the added social value created by TRIO and identify who benefits from the community-based day support service.

---

admission and unexpected adverse effects on both people with dementia and their carers. Day care services were found to be effective in decreasing carer burden and behavioural problems in people with dementia, but they also accelerated the time to nursing home admission (Vandepitte et al., 2016). Whilst there is some evidence to support respite positively affecting carers, the economic evidence is still limited (Shaw et al., 2009). However, a study of in-home respite to support informal carers of people with dementia was found to be cost-effective with nursing home admittance after five years predicted to be 4 per cent lower in the group receiving respite care, leading to a QALY gain of 0.14 and a cost per QALY gain of €8,690 from a societal perspective (Vandepitte et al., 2020).

Outdoor Space and the Built Environment

A 'whole system' response needs to address the many social engagement barriers older people face, such as issues around accessibility and age-friendly environments, particularly practical aspects including transport and access to toilets (Kinsella, 2015). Continence conditions may limit the amount of time older people can be away from home, and there is a call for public toilets to be designed to be age-friendly, with features such as clear signage and sensor-operated taps (Bichard & Knight, 2010). Box 6.4 discusses public toilets as a health and social care benefit.

Box 6.4 Public toilets as a health and social care benefit

The availability of clean, conveniently located, well-signed, disabled-accessible toilets is generally regarded as an important age-friendly feature of the built environment as it enables older people to get out of their homes and feel less lonely in their day-to-day lives (WHO, 2007). Barriers to the use of public toilets to the older population include heavy doors, heavy toilet seats, and lack of accessibility for people with disabilities (WHO, 2007). Fully emptying the bladder when urinating is an important way for older people to reduce the risk of developing a urinary tract infection (Age UK, 2021). Access to toilets in public spaces can have a major impact on health-related quality of life, particularly for older adults.

During the COVID-19 pandemic, public toilets were closed due to concerns about these spaces acting as a contact hub point for virus transmission due to faecal and urinary derived aerosols (e.g. from toilet flushing) containing the virus, and issues over space, ventilation, and cleaning (Dancer et al., 2021). The pandemic highlighted the fact that many public toilets were closed by local councils due to austerity measures over the past ten years and that there is an unmet need in relation to the provision of public toilets in general.

There is now a greater need than ever to improve parks and green spaces as shared facilities in the UK to address the lack of appropriate facilities for outdoor safety. There is, since the COVID-19 pandemic, a need for public toilets that are cleaned on a regular basis, handwashing facilities, and bins for personal protective equipment (PPE) disposal in parks to enable people of all ages to engage with green spaces in the safest way possible (Freeman & Eykelbosh, 2020; Spencer et al., 2020).

The Impact of the COVID-19 Pandemic on NHS Waiting Lists

Whilst the NHS geared up to deal with the COVID-19 pandemic, routine procedures that could be cancelled or delayed were rescheduled to limit the number of people entering clinical premises, thus minimizing the risk of virus transmission between patients and facilitating the reallocation of resources to manage the pandemic. In addition to the backlog in routine procedures, some people may have delayed seeking treatment as they did not want to attend clinics, thus exacerbating their health condition. For example, age-related macular degeneration is the leading cause of sight loss in the UK, and patients are treated with regular injections. A study found that extending the intervals between injections during the pandemic led to a significant loss in visual acuity compared to patients who maintained their usual treatment schedule (Teo et al., 2020). The long-term impact on the population's health of delayed NHS treatments is likely to be substantial (Charlesworth, 2020). The number of first-time customers purchasing Private Medical Insurance has doubled since the beginning of the COVID-19 pandemic (ActiveQuote, 2020). This includes the number of people taking out private health insurance or paying for procedures such as a cataract operation. Many of these first-time customers are older and very old people who have to consider the impact of the NHS waiting list time on their overall quality of life in their remaining years (Edwards & Davies, 2022). Procedures such as cataract operations have a relatively low cost per QALY and help promote and maintain independence through into very old age.

The Impact of the COVID-19 Pandemic on Charities

Carers receive considerable information and network-based support from charities, social enterprises, and voluntary groups in the third sector. As of 2022, the impact of the COVID-19 pandemic has left many charities under considerable financial strain due to cancelled fundraising events, charity shop closures, and lower cash donations than previous years. This means that the third sector has an uncertain future, compounded now by reduced charitable giving by many people due to the cost of living crisis, and there is a need to reshape the operational model for service provision in order to survive and be sustainable (Chapman, 2020).

Summary

In this chapter, we explored the economic case for investing in older people as assets through appraising the available economic evidence relating to older people (spanning interventions, policies, and practice relevant to the UK), and highlighting the costs of loneliness and the contribution made by informal carers to the economy. The studies presented in this chapter used a wide range of outcome measures, which limits the potential to make direct comparisons across studies. We found programmes that promote independent living and community engagement can reduce loneliness and provide wider economic benefits, such as volunteering and informal caring. Environments and services that promote exercise and active travel can support working for longer and independent living and a healthier old age. There needs to be more recognition of the synergy and interplay between the economic circumstances, the physical environment in which older people live, and access to health and social care services. We do not yet fully understand how to design interventions to support informal carers of people living with dementia at home and must listen to their needs. Many interventions such as falls prevention interventions need to be multi-component and this needs to be taken into account in economic evaluation.

The UK and devolved nations' governments could focus attention on the following key areas:

- Fully integrated health and care services: investing in services to promote prevention, rehabilitation, and reablement, thus reducing the need for hospital admissions, facilitating earlier discharge from hospital, and reducing demands on health and social care services.
- Maintaining physical and mental well-being in older age with a focus on reducing social isolation and loneliness: programmes that promote exercise and improve balance can be cost-effective in terms of improving physical and psychological well-being in older age, reducing falls and the associated need for hospital and community care.
- Keeping older people active and connected in the community: investment in sustainable age-friendly homes, transport, and communities, supporting working for longer, and facilitating volunteering and the care of grandchildren to enable parents to work. Co-production will enable older people to remain active in their community, with bi-directional benefits across the community and public sector services.
- Support for informal carers: many older people are carers, providing substantial support to the detriment of their own health and well-being. Carers can be the key factor in keeping someone living at home or preventing admission to hospital or residential care.

Maintaining mental well-being and independence has been cited as a best-buy for public health (Nurse et al., 2014). Maintaining funding across prevention, rehabilitation, and reablement can generate economic benefits by promoting independent living of older adults, reducing the need for hospital admissions (through initiatives such as Care and Repair), facilitating earlier discharge from hospital, and reducing demands on health and social care services (Edwards et al., 2018, 2019). Supporting older people to safely continue to work, spend in their local economy, and recommence informal care provision with grandchildren could help boost the recovery of the UK economy post-COVID-19 pandemic. In the next chapter we focus on the final life-course stage and explore the economic evidence of effective and cost-effective interventions to support people at the end of life.

Curiosity Questions

- How can qualitative research with carers help design interventions to support informal carers of people living with dementia in their own homes? Many current interventions designed by health services researchers seem to add to the stress of the person with dementia (i.e. someone unknown coming into the home) and thereby add to the stress of the informal carer.

- How can we use online communication to produce effective and cost-effective support, for example, for carers of people living with dementia, in a way that is sufficiently inclusive? This may involve blended support using coaches and alternative access for digitally excluded families.

- In studies of older people, particularly those with cognitive decline (including dementia), how should health economists use and approach the use of proxy versus self-report, preference-based health-related quality of life measures? See Hutchinson et al. (2022) for a systematic review related to this topic.

- What are the most cost-effective interventions that focus on co-production that promote or mitigate barriers to positive well-being for adults in older age?

- What evidence is there that cost-effective interventions in the short run in promoting well-being in older age have a lasting impact and lead eventually to a good death?

References

ActiveQuote. (2020, 2 October). *People buying private healthcare continue to grow younger.* https://www.activequote.com/articles/people-buying-private-healthcare-continue-to-grow-younger/

Age UK. (2019, May). *Later life in the United Kingdom 2019.* https://www.ageuk.org.uk/globalassets/age-uk/documents/reports-and-publications/later_life_uk_factsheet.pdf

Age UK. (2021, 20 April). *Urinary tract infections (UTIs).* https://www.ageuk.org.uk/information-advice/health-wellbeing/conditions-illnesses/urinary-tract-infections-utis/

Age UK. (2022a, 20 September). *2.8m older households will still be living in fuel poverty this winter—despite the Government freezing the energy price cap.* https://www.ageuk.org.uk/latest-press/articles/2022/2.8m-older-households-will-still-be-living-in-fuel-poverty-this-winter---despite-the-government-freezing-the-energy-price-cap/

Age UK. (2022b, 13 January). *Astronomical energy price rises leaving older people in crisis.* https://www.ageuk.org.uk/latest-press/articles/2022/astronomical-energy-price-rises-leaving-older-people-in-crisis/

Age UK. (2023, 10 April). *Telecare and telehealth*. https://www.ageuk.org.uk/information-advice/care/housing-options/adapting-home/telecare/

Aquilanti, L., Santarelli, A., Mascitti, M., Procaccini, M., & Rappelli, G. (2020). Dental care access and the elderly: What is the role of teledentistry? A systematic review. *International Journal of Environmental Research and Public Health, 17*(23), 9053. https://doi.org/10.3390/ijerph17239053

Barker, W. (2014). Assessment and prevention of falls in older people. *Nursing Older People, 26*(6), 18–24. https://doi.org/10.7748/nop.26.6.18.e586

Bennett, L., Honeyman, M., & Bottery, S. (2018, December). *New models of home care*. The King's Fund. https://assets.kingsfund.org.uk/f/256914/x/cb1237e617/new_models_home_care_2018.pdf

Bergmo, T. S. (2014). Using QALYs in telehealth evaluations: A systematic review of methodology and transparency. *BMC Health Services Research, 14*(332), 1–11. https://doi.org/10.1186/1472-6963-14-332

Bichard, J., & Knight, G. (2010, September). *Everybody goes: Designing age friendly public toilet solutions* [Conference presentation abstract]. Cumulus Shanghai 2010 Young Creators for BetterCity Better Life Conference, Shanghai, China.

Birkett, E. (2022). *An emergency response to the energy crises: A five-point plan for the new Prime Minister*. ONWARD. https://www.ukonward.com/wp-content/uploads/2022/09/An-Emergency-Response-to-the-Energy-Crisis.pdf

Birmingham City Council. (2022). *Warm welcome spaces in Birmingham*. https://www.birmingham.gov.uk/directory/73/warm_welcome_spaces_in_birmingham

Brewster, L., Mountain, G., Wessels, B., Kelly, C., & Hawley, M. (2014). Factors affecting front line staff acceptance of telehealth technologies: A mixed-method systematic review. *Journal of Advanced Nursing, 70*(1), 21–33. https://doi.org/10.1111/jan.12196

Buckner, L., & Yeandle, S. (2015). *Valuing carers 2015: The rising value of carer's support*. Carers UK. https://www.sheffield.ac.uk/news/polopoly_fs/1.546409!/file/Valuing-Carers-2015.pdf

Burholt, V., & Scharf, T. (2014). Poor health and loneliness in later life: The role of depressive symptoms, social resources, and rural environments. *Journals of Gerontology: Series B, 69*(2), 311–324. https://doi.org/10.1093/geronb/gbt121

Burholt, V., Winter, B., Aartsen, M., Constantinou, C., Dahlberg, L., Feliciano, V., De Jong Gierveld, J., Van Regenmortel, S., & Waldegrave, C., on behalf of the Working Group on Exclusion from Social Relations. (2020). A critical review and development of a conceptual model of exclusion from social relations for older people. *European Journal of Ageing, 17*, 3–19. https://doi.org/10.1007/s10433-019-00506-0

Cacioppo, J. T., Hughes, M. E., Waite, L. J., Hawkley, L. C., & Thisted, R. A. (2006). Loneliness as a specific risk factor for depressive symptoms: Cross-sectional and longitudinal analyses. *Psychology and Aging, 21*(1), 140–151. https://doi.org/10.1037/0882-7974.21.1.140

Carande-Kulis, V., Stevens, J. A., Florence, C. S., Beattie, B. L., & Arias, I. (2015). A cost–benefit analysis of three older adult fall prevention interventions. *Journal of Safety Research, 52*, 65–70. https://doi.org/10.1016/j.jsr.2014.12.007

Carers UK. (2016). *Pressure points: Carers and the NHS*. https://www.carersuk.org/pressurepoints.bl.uk/collection-items/pressure-points-carers-and-the-nhs

Carers UK. (2019, August). *Facts about carers. Policy briefing.* https://www.carersuk.org/media/5w2h3hn2/facts-about-carers-2019.pdf

Centre for Reviews and Dissemination. (2014). *Interventions for loneliness and social isolation.* NHS NIHR. The University of York Centre for Reviews and Dissemination. https://www.york.ac.uk/media/crd/Loneliness and social isolation.pdf

Cerin, E., Nathan, A., van Cauwenberg, J., Barnett, D. W., & Barnett, A. (2017). The neighbourhood physical environment and active travel in older adults: A systematic review and meta-analysis. *International Journal of Behavioral Nutrition and Physical Activity, 14*(1), 1–23. https://doi.org/10.1186/s12966-017-0471-5

Chapman, T. (2020). *Third sector trends: Covid-19 impact survey.* Community Foundation. https://www.communityfoundation.org.uk/wordpress/wp-content/uploads/2020/08/Third-Sector-Trends-Covid-19-Impact-Survey-August-2020.pdf

Charlesworth, A. (2020). *Shock to the system: COVID-19's long-term impact on the NHS.* The Health Foundation. https://www.health.org.uk/news-and-comment/blogs/shock-to-the-system-covid-19s-long-term-impact-on-the-nhs

Charlesworth, G., Shepstone, L., Wilson, E., Thalanany, M., Mugford, M., & Poland, F. (2008). Does befriending by trained lay workers improve psychological well-being and quality of life for carers of people with dementia, and at what cost? A randomised controlled trial. *Health Technology Assessment, 12*(4), 1–78. https://doi.org/10.3310/hta12040

Chevalier, S. (2021, 7 July). *Coronavirus: First-time online purchases by age group U.S. 2020.* Statista. https://www.statista.com/statistics/1108530/first-time-online-shopping-during-coronavirus-usa-age/

Chien, L.-Y., Chu, H., Guo, J.-L., Liao, Y.-M., Chang, L.-I., Chen, C.-H., & Chou, K.-R. (2011). Caregiver support groups in patients with dementia: A meta-analysis. *International Journal of Geriatric Psychiatry, 26*(10), 1089–1098. https://doi.org/10.1002/gps.2660

Clark, D. (2023, 30 May). *Number of people living alone in the United Kingdom in 2022, by age and gender.* Statista. https://www.statista.com/statistics/531386/people-living-alone-uk-age-and-gender/

Cockayne, S., Rodgers, S., Green, L., Fairhurst, C., Adamson, J., Scantlebury, A., Corbacho, B., Hewitt, C. E., Hicks, K., Hull, R., Keenan, A. M., Lamb, S. E., McIntosh, C., Menz, H. B., Redmond, A., Richardson, Z., Vernon, W., Watson, J., & Torgerson, D. J. (2017). Clinical effectiveness and cost-effectiveness of a multifaceted podiatry intervention for falls prevention in older people: A multicentre cohort randomised controlled trial (the Reducing Falls with Orthoses and a Multifaceted podiatry intervention trial). *Health Technology Assessment, 21*(24), 1–198. https://doi.org/10.3310/hta21240

Courtin, E., & Knapp, M. (2017). Social isolation, loneliness and health in old age: A scoping review. *Health and Social Care in the Community, 25*(3), 799–812. https://doi.org/10.1111/hsc.12311

Cudejko, T., Gardiner, J., Akpan, A., & D'Août, K. (2019). Effects of a systematic exploration of minimal footwear features on physical function, postural and dynamic stability, and perceptions of footwear in healthy older adults. *Footwear Science, 11*(S1), S82–S84. https://doi.org/10.1080/19424280.2019.1606090

Cudejko, T., Gardiner, J., Akpan, A., & D'Août, K. (2020). Minimal footwear improves stability and physical function in middle-aged and older people compared to conventional shoes. *Clinical Biomechanics*, 71, 139–145. https://doi.org/10.1016/j.clin biomech.2019.11.005

Dahlrup, B., Nordell, E., Steen Carlsson, K., & Elmståhl, S. (2014). Health economic analysis on a psychosocial intervention for family caregivers of persons with dementia. *Dementia and Geriatric Cognitive Disorders*, 37(3–4), 181–195. https://doi.org/10.1159/000355365

Dancer, S. J., Li, Y., Hart, A., Tang, J. W., & Jones, D. L. (2021). What is the risk of acquiring SARS-CoV-2 from the use of public toilets? *Science of the Total Environment*, 792, 148341. https://doi.org/10.1016/j.scitotenv.2021.148341

Davies, A. R., Honeyman, M., & Gann, B. (2021). Addressing the digital inverse care law in the time of COVID-19: Potential for digital technology to exacerbate or mitigate health inequalities. *Journal of Medical Internet Research*, 23(4), e21726. https://doi.org/10.2196/21726

Department for Environment, Food & Rural Affairs. (2012). *Rural population and migration*. https://www.gov.uk/government/publications/rural-population-and-migration/rural-population-201415#population-by-age

Department for Transport. (2019). *Journey time statistics: Data tables (JTS)*. https://www.gov.uk/government/statistical-data-sets/journey-time-statistics-data-tables-jts

Department for Work and Pensions. (2022, 31 March). *Family resources survey: Financial year 2020 to 2021*. https://www.gov.uk/government/statistics/family-resources-survey-financial-year-2020-to-2021/family-resources-survey-financial-year-2020-to-2021

Dixon, J., Winterbourne, S., Lombard, D., Watters, S., Trachtenberg, M., Knapp, M., Joy, S., Corral, S., Nzegwu, F., & McNulty, A. (2014). *An analysis of the economic impacts of the British red cross support at home service* [PSSRU Discussion Paper 2869]. Personal Social Services Research Unit, London School of Economics and Political Science. http://eprints.lse.ac.uk/58581/

Donald, N. (2010). *Social return on investment report on dial-a-community bus shopping service*. Buchan Development Partnership. https://socialvalueuk.org/wp-content/uploads/2016/03/dial-a-community-bus-final-sroi-report.pdf

Dreyer, K., Steventon, A., Fisher, R., & Deeny, S. R. (2018). The association between living alone and health care utilisation in older adults: A retrospective cohort study of electronic health records from a London general practice. *BMC Geriatrics*, 18(269), 1–17. https://doi.org/10.1186/s12877-018-0939-4

Edwards, R. T., & Davies, J. (2022, 10 May). *My planned care, your planned care and our planned care in the NHS*. Centre for Health Economics and Medicines Evaluation, Bangor University. https://cheme.bangor.ac.uk/health-blog-3.php.en

Edwards, R. T., Spencer, L. H., Anthony, B., & Bryning, L. (2019). *Wellness in work: The economic arguments for investing in the health and wellbeing of the workforce in Wales*. Centre for Health Economics and Medicines Evaluation, Bangor University. https://cheme.bangor.ac.uk/documents/Wellness-in-Work-Report.pdf

Edwards, R. T., Spencer, L. H., Bryning, L., & Anthony, B. (2018). *Living well for longer: The economic argument for investing in the health and wellbeing of older people in Wales*. Centre for Health Economics and Medicines Evaluation, Bangor University. https://cheme.bangor.ac.uk/documents/livingwell2018.pdf

Eow, J., Duane, B., Solaiman, A., Hussain, U., Lemasney, N., Ang, R., O'Kelly-Lynch, N., Girgis, G., Collazo, L., & Johnston, B. (2019). What evidence do economic evaluations in dental care provide? A scoping review. *Community Dental Health*, **36**(2), 118–125. https://doi.org/10.1922/CDH_4426Eow08

European Parliament. (2021). *The rise of digital health technologies during the pandemic.* https://www.europarl.europa.eu/RegData/etudes/BRIE/2021/690548/EPRS_BRI(2021)690548_EN.pdf

Fakoya, O., McCorry, N., & Donnelly, M. (2020). Loneliness and social isolation interventions for older adults: a scoping review of reviews. *BMC Public Health*, **20**(129), 1–14. https://doi.org/10.1186/s12889-020-8251-6

Francis, J., Fisher, M., & Rutter, D. (2011). *Reablement: A cost-effective route to better outcomes.* Social Care Institute for Excellence. http://hdl.handle.net/10547/594515

Freeman, S., & Eykelbosh, A. (2020). *COVID-19 and outdoor safety: Considerations for use of outdoor recreational spaces.* National Collaborating Centre for Environmental Health. https://ncceh.ca/documents/guide/covid-19-and-outdoor-safety-considerations-use-outdoor-recreational-spaces

Fulton, L., & Jupp, B. (2015, June). *Investing to tackle loneliness: A discussion paper.* Social Finance. Cabinet Office. Calouste Gulbenkian Foundation. Nesta. https://www.social finance.org.uk/assets/documents/investing_to_tackle_loneliness.pdf

Hagger-Johnson, G., Carr, E., Murray, E., Stansfeld, S., Shelton, N., Stafford, M., & Head, J. (2017). Association between midlife health behaviours and transitions out of employment from midlife to early old age: Whitehall II cohort study. *BMC Public Health*, **17**(1), 82. https://doi.org/10.1186/s12889-016-3970-4

Harwood, R. H., Goldberg, S. E., Brand, A., van Der Wardt, V., Booth, V., Di Lorito, C., Hoare, Z., Hancox, J., Bajwa, R., Burgon, C., Howe, L., Cowley, A., Bramley, T., Long, A., Lock, J., Tucker, R., Adams, E., O'Brien, R., Kearney, F. . . . Masud, T. (2022). Promoting activity, independence and stability in early dementia and mild cognitive impairment (PrAISED): A randomised controlled trial. *medRxiv*. https://doi.org/10.1101/2022.12.20.22283699

Hawksworth, J., Stubbings, C., Cheung, C., Utkarshini, S., & Saloni, G. (2018). *PwC Golden Age index—unlocking a potential $3.5 trillion prize from longer working lives.* https://www.pwc.co.uk/economic-services/golden-age/golden-age-index-2018-final-sanitised.pdf

Henderson, C., Knapp, M., Fernandez, J.-L., Beecham, J., Hirani, S. P., Cartwright, M., Rixon, L., Beynon, M., Rogers, A., Bower, P., Doll, H., Fitzpatrick, R., Steventon, A., Bardsley, M., Hendy, J., & Newman, S. P. (2013). Cost effectiveness of telehealth for patients with long term conditions (Whole Systems Demonstrator telehealth questionnaire study): Nested economic evaluation in a pragmatic, cluster randomised controlled trial. *BMJ*, **346**, f1035. https://doi.org/10.1136/bmj.f1035

Hendriks, M. R., Evers, S. M., Bleijlevens, M. H., van Haastregt, J. C., Crebolder, H. F., & van Eijk, J. T. M. (2008). Cost-effectiveness of a multidisciplinary fall prevention program in community-dwelling elderly people: A randomized controlled trial (ISRCTN 64716113). *International Journal of Technology Assessment in Health Care*, **24**(2), 193–202. https://doi.org/10.1017/S0266462308080276

Hex, N., & Tatlock, S. (2011). *Altogether Better social return on investment case studies.* https://static1.squarespace.com/static/5ad4879c5cfd798df87393cd/t/5c052bc84fa51a1085249672/1543842760685/AB-Social-Return-on-Investment-Case-Studies.pdf

Hollinghurst, J., Fry, R., Akbari, A., Watkins, A., Williams, N., Hillcoat-Nallétamby, S., Lyons, R. A., Clegg, A., & Rodgers, S. E. (2020). Do home modifications reduce care home admissions for older people? A matched control evaluation of the Care & Repair Cymru service in Wales. *Age and Ageing*, 49(6), 1056–1061. https://doi.org/10.1093/age ing/afaa158

Holt-Lunstad, J., Smith, T. B., Baker, M., Harris, T., & Stephenson, D. (2015). Loneliness and social isolation as risk factors for mortality: A meta-analytic review. *Perspectives on Psychological Science*, 10(2), 227–237. https://doi.org/10.1177/1745691614568352

Holwerda, T. J., Deeg, D. J. H., Beekman, A. T. F., van Tilburg, T. G., Stek, M. L., Jonker, C., & Schoevers, R. A. (2014). Feelings of loneliness, but not social isolation, predict dementia onset: Results from the Amsterdam Study of the Elderly (AMSTEL). *Journal of Neurology, Neurosurgery and Psychiatry*, 85(2), 135–142.

Hutchinson, C., Worley, A., Khadka, J., Milte, R., Cleland, J., & Ratcliffe, J. (2022). Do we agree or disagree? A systematic review of the application of preference-based instruments in self and proxy reporting of quality of life in older people. *Social Science & Medicine*, 305(115046). https://doi.org/10.1016/j.socscimed.2022.115046

Iliffe, S., Davies, S. L., Gordon, A. L., Schneider, J., Dening, T., Bowman, C., Gage, H., Martin, F. C., Gladman, J. R., Victor, C., Meyer, J., & Goodman, C. (2016). Provision of NHS generalist and specialist services to care homes in England: Review of surveys. *Primary Health Care Research & Development*, 17(2), 122–137. https://doi.org/10.1017/S1463423615000250

International Longevity Centre UK. (2017). *Grandparent army report*. https://ilcuk.org.uk/wp-content/uploads/2018/10/The-Grandparent-Army.pdf

International Longevity Centre UK. (2019). *Maximising the longevity dividend*. https://ilcuk.org.uk/wp-content/uploads/2019/12/Maximising-the-longevity-dividend.pdf

Iparraguirre, J. (2017). *The economic contribution of older people in the United Kingdom—an update to 2017*. https://www.ageuk.org.uk/globalassets/age-uk/documents/reports-and-publications/reports-and-briefings/active-communities/the_economic_contribution_of_older_-people_-update_-to_-2017.pdf

James, B. D., Wilson, R. S., Barnes, L. L., & Bennett, D. A. (2011). Late-life social activity and cognitive decline in old age. *Journal of the International Neuropsychological Society*, 17(6), 998–1005. https://doi.org/10.1017/S1355617711000531

Jin, J. (2018). Prevention of falls in older adults. *JAMA*, 319(16), 1734–1734. https://doi.org/10.1001/jama.2018.4396

Johnstone, G., Dickins, M., Lowthian, J., Renehan, E., Enticott, J., Mortimer, D., & Ogrin, R. (2021). Interventions to improve the health and wellbeing of older people living alone: A mixed-methods systematic review of effectiveness and accessibility. *Ageing & Society*, 41(7), 1587–1636. https://doi.org/10.1017/S0144686X19001818

Joling, K. J., Bosmans, J. E., van Marwijk, H. W., van der Horst, H. E., Scheltens, P., Vroomen, J. L., & van Hout, H. P. (2013). The cost-effectiveness of a family meetings intervention to prevent depression and anxiety in family caregivers of patients with dementia: A randomized trial. *Trials*, 14(1). https://doi.org/10.1186/1745-6215-14-305

Jopling, K. (2015). *Promising approaches to reducing loneliness and isolation in later life*. Campaign to End Loneliness. Age UK. https://www.campaigntoendloneliness.org/wp-content/uploads/Promising-approaches-to-reducing-loneliness-and-isolation-in-later-life.pdf

Karki, A., Monaghan, N., & Morgan, M. (2015). Oral health status of older people living in care homes in Wales. *British Dental Journal, 219*(7), 331–334. https://doi.org/10.1038/sj.bdj.2015.756

Kelly, M. E., Duff, H., Kelly, S., McHugh Power, J. E., Brennan, S., Lawlor, B. A., & Loughrey, D. G. (2017). The impact of social activities, social networks, social support and social relationships on the cognitive functioning of healthy older adults: A systematic review. *Systematic Reviews, 6*(259), 1–18. https://doi.org/10.1186/s13643-017-0632-2

Kenny, R. A., Romero-Ortuno, R., & Kumar, P. (2017). Falls in older adults. *Medicine, 45*(1), 28–33. https://doi.org/10.1016/j.mpmed.2016.10.007

Khan, I., Petrou, S., Khan, K., Mistry, D., Lall, R., Sheehan, B., & Lamb, S. (2019). Does structured exercise improve cognitive impairment in people with mild to moderate dementia? A cost-effectiveness analysis from a confirmatory randomised controlled trial: The dementia and physical activity (DAPA) trial. *PharmacoEconomics-Open, 3*, 215–227. https://doi.org/10.1007/s41669-018-0097-9

Kinsella, S. (2015). *Older people and social isolation evidence: A review of the evidence.* Wirral Council Business & Public Health Intelligence Team. https://www.wirralintellig enceservice.org/media/1081/older_people__social_isolation_2015_final.pdf

Knapp, M., King, D., Romeo, R., Schehl, B., Barber, J., Griffin, M., Rapaport, P., Livingston, D., Mummery, C., Walker, Z., Hoe, J., Sampson, E. L., Cooper, C., & Livingston, G. (2013). Cost effectiveness of a manual based coping strategy programme in promoting the mental health of family carers of people with dementia (the START (STrAtegies for RelaTives) study): a pragmatic randomised controlled trial. *BMJ, 347*, f6342. https://doi.org/10.1136/bmj.f6342

Landeiro, F., Leal, J., & Gray, A. M. (2016). The impact of social isolation on delayed hospital discharges of older hip fracture patients and associated costs. *Osteoporosis International, 27*(2), 737–745. https://doi.org/10.1007/s00198-015-3293-9

Langhammer, B., Bergland, A., & Rydwik, E. (2018). The importance of physical activity exercise among older people. *BioMed Research International, 2018*, 7856823. https://doi.org/10.1155/2018/7856823

Latimer, N., Dixon, S., Drahota, A. K., & Severs, M. (2013). Cost–utility analysis of a shock-absorbing floor intervention to prevent injuries from falls in hospital wards for older people. *Age and Ageing, 42*(5), 641–645. https://doi.org/10.1093/ageing/aft076

Laverty, A. A., Mindell, J. S., Webb, E. A., & Millett, C. (2013). Active travel to work and cardiovascular risk factors in the United Kingdom. *American Journal of Preventive Medicine, 45*(3), 282–288. https://doi.org/10.1016/j.amepre.2013.04.012

Leng, M., Zhao, Y., Xiao, H., Li, C., & Wang, Z. (2020). Internet-based supportive interventions for family caregivers of people with dementia: Systematic review and meta-analysis. *Journal of Medical Internet Research, 22*(9), e19468. https://doi.org/10.2196/19468

Lewis, F., Karlsberg Schaffer, S., Sussex, J., O'Neill, P., & Cockcroft, L. (2014, 1 June). *The trajectory of dementia in the UK-making a difference.* Office of Health Economics Consulting Reports. https://www.ohe.org/publications/trajectory-dementia-uk-mak ing-difference/

Li, F., & Harmer, P. (2015). Economic evaluation of a Tai Ji Quan intervention to reduce falls in people with Parkinson disease, Oregon, 2008–2011. *Preventing Chronic Disease, 12*, e120. https://doi.org/10.5888/pcd12.140413

Li, F., Harmer, P., Fisher, K. J., McAuley, E., Chaumeton, N., Eckstrom, E., & Wilson, N. L. (2005). Tai Chi and fall reductions in older adults: A randomized controlled trial. *The Journals of Gerontology Series A: Biological Sciences and Medical Sciences*, 60(2), 187–194. https://doi.org/10.1093/gerona/60.2.187

Linking Generations Northern Ireland. (2021). *Intergenerational practice explained*. https://www.linkinggenerationsni.com/intergenerational-practice-explained

Livingston, G., Huntley, J., Sommerlad, A., Ames, D., Ballard, C., Banerjee, S., Brayne, C., Burns, A., Cohen-Mansfield, J., Cooper, C., Costafreda, S. G., Dias, A., Fox, N., Gitlin, L. N., Howard, R., Kales, H. C., Kivimäki, M., Larson, E. B., Ogunniyi, A., . . . Mukadam, N. (2020). Dementia prevention, intervention, and care: 2020 report of the Lancet Commission. *The Lancet*, 396(10248). https://doi.org/10.1016/S0140-6736(20)30367-6

Looman, W. M., Huijsman, R., & Fabbricotti, I. N. (2018). The (cost-) effectiveness of preventive, integrated care for community-dwelling frail older people: A systematic review. *Health & Social Care in the Community*, 27(1), 1–30. https://doi.org/10.1111/hsc.12571

Lundqvist, M., Davidson, T., Ordell, S., Sjöström, O., Zimmerman, M., & Sjögren, P. (2015). Health economic analyses of domiciliary dental care and care at fixed clinics for elderly nursing home residents in Sweden. *Community Dental Health*, 32(1), 39–43. https://doi.org/10.1922/CDH_3407Lundqvist05

Mackenzie, L., & McIntyre, A. (2019). How do general practitioners (GPs) engage in falls prevention with older people? A pilot survey of GPs in NHS England suggests a gap in routine practice to address falls prevention. *Frontiers in Public Health*, 7(32), 1–10. https://doi.org/10.1001/10.3389/fpubh.2019.00032

Marmot, M., Allen, J., Boyce, T., Goldblatt, P., & Morrison, J. (2020). *Health equity in England: The Marmot review 10 years on*. Institute of Health Equity. https://www.health.org.uk/publications/reports/the-marmot-review-10-years-on

Marvell, R., & Cox, A. (2017). *What do older workers value about work and why?* Centre for Ageing Better. https://www.ageing-better.org.uk/sites/default/files/2017-12/What-do-older-workers-value.pdf

Mason, A., Weatherly, H., Spilsbury, K., Golder, S., Arksey, H., Adamson, J., & Drummond, M. (2007). The effectiveness and cost-effectiveness of respite for caregivers of frail older people. *Journal of the American Geriatrics Society*, 55(2), 290–299. https://doi.org/10.1111/j.1532-5415.2006.01037.x

McCabe, S. (2022). *Examining the evolving cost-of-living crisis*. https://www.open-access.bcu.ac.uk/12951/1/Examining%20the%20Evolving%20Cost-of-Living%20Crisis.pdf

McDaid, D., Park, A., & Fernandez, J. (2016). *Reconnections evaluation interim report*. Personal Social Services Research Unit, London School of Economics and Political Science. https://s3.eu-west-2.amazonaws.com/golab.prod/documents/McDaid_et_al._2016.pdf

McGarvey, A., Jochum, V., Davies, J., Dobbs, J., & Hornung, L. (2019, 1 January). *Time well spent: A national survey on the volunteer experience*. https://www.ncvo.org.uk/news-and-insights/news-index/time-well-spent-national-survey-volunteer-experience/#/

Montero-Odasso, M., Van Der Velde, N., Alexander, N. B., Becker, C., Blain, H., Camicioli, R., Close, J., Duan, L., Duque, G., Ganz, D.A., Gómez, F., Hausdorff, J. M., Hogan, D. B., Jauregui, J. R., Kenny, R. A., Lipsitx, L. A., Logan, P. A., Lord, A.

R., Mallet, L., . . . Masud, T. Task force on global guidelines for falls in older adults. (2021). New horizons in falls prevention and management for older adults: A global initiative. *Age and Ageing*, **50**(5), 1499–1507. https://doi.org/10.1093/ageing/afab076

Morrison, V., Spencer, L. H., Totton, N., Pye, K., Yeo, S. T., Butterworth, C., Hall, L., Whitaker, R., Edwards, R. T., Timmis, L. J., Hoare, Z., Neal, R. D., Wilkinson, C., & Leeson, S. (2018). Trial of optimal personalised care after treatment—gynaecological cancer (TOPCAT-G). *International Journal of Gynecological Cancer*, **28**(2), 401–411. https://doi.org/10.1097/IGC.0000000000001179

Müller, D., Borsi, L., Stracke, C., Stock, S., & Stollenwerk, B. (2015). Cost-effectiveness of a multifactorial fracture prevention program for elderly people admitted to nursing homes. *The European Journal of Health Economics*, **16**, 517–527. https://doi.org/10.1007/s10198-014-0605-5

Musselwhite, C. B. A., & Shergold, I. (2013). Examining the process of driving cessation in later life. *European Journal of Ageing*, **10**(2), 89–100. https://doi.org/10.1007/s10433-012-0252-6

National Health Service. (2018). *Breaking down barriers to better health and care*. https://www.england.nhs.uk/publication/breaking-down-barriers-to-better-health-and-care/

National Health Service. (2019a). *The NHS Long Term Plan* (v.1.2). https://www.longtermplan.nhs.uk/wp-content/uploads/2019/08/nhs-long-term-plan-version-1.2.pdf

National Health Service. (2019b). *Carers' breaks and respite care*. https://www.nhs.uk/conditions/social-care-and-support-guide/support-and-benefits-for-carers/carer-breaks-and-respite-care/

National Health Service Improvement & NHS England (2019). *The NHS patient safety strategy. Safer culture, safer systems, safer patients*. https://www.england.nhs.uk/wp-content/uploads/2020/08/190708_Patient_Safety_Strategy_for_website_v4.pdf

National Institute for Health and Care Excellence. (2015a). *Evidence review & economic analysis of excess winter deaths for the National Institute for Health and Care Excellence (NICE). Review 3 Delivery and implementation of approaches for the prevention of excess winter deaths and morbidity* (NG6). London School of Hygiene & Tropical Medicine. Public Health England. https://www.nice.org.uk/guidance/ng6/evidence/evidence-review-3-delivery-and-implementation-of-approaches-for-the-prevention-of-excess-winter-deaths-and-morbidity-pdf-544621935

National Institute for Health and Care Excellence. (2015b). *Excess winter deaths and illness and the health risks associated with cold homes* (NG6). https://www.nice.org.uk/guidance/ng6

National Institute for Health and Care Excellence. (2015c). *Evidence review & economic analysis of excess winter deaths for the National Institute for Health and Care Excellence (NICE). Review 2. Interventions and economic studies* (NG6). London School of Hygiene & Tropical Medicine. Public Health England. University College London. https://www.nice.org.uk/guidance/ng6/evidence/evidence-review-2-interventions-and-economic-studies-pdf-544621934

National Institute for Health and Care Excellence. (2015d). *Home care: Delivering personal care and practical support to older people living in their own homes* (NG21). https://www.nice.org.uk/guidance/ng21

National Institute for Health and Care Excellence. (2015e). *Workplace health: Management practices* (NG13). https://www.nice.org.uk/guidance/ng13/resources/workplace-health-management-practices-pdf-1837269751237

National Institute for Health and Care Excellence. (2015f). *Dementia, disability and frailty in later life—mid-life approaches to delay or prevent onset* (NG16). https://www.nice.org. uk/guidance/ng16

National Institute for Health and Care Excellence. (2016). *Oral health for adults in care homes* (NG48). https://www.nice.org.uk/guidance/ng48

National Institute for Health and Care Excellence. (2017). *Falls in older people: Prevention NICE quality standard* (QS86). https://www.nice.org.uk/guidance/qs86/documents/ draft-quality-standard-2

National Records of Scotland. (2019). *Winter mortality in Scotland 2018/19*. https://www. nrscotland.gov.uk/files/statistics/winter-mortality/2019/winter-mortality-18-19- pub.pdf

Nichols, L. O., Chang, C., Lummus, A., Burns, R., Martindale-Adams, J., Graney, M. J., Coon, D. W., & Czaja, S. (2008). The cost-effectiveness of a behavior intervention with caregivers of patients with Alzheimer's disease. *Journal of the American Geriatrics Society, 56*(3), 413–420. https://doi.org/10.1111/j.1532-5415.2007.01569.x

Northern Ireland Statistics and Research Agency. (2020). *Excess winter mortality in Northern Ireland*. https://www.nisra.gov.uk/sites/nisra.gov.uk/files/publications/Exc ess%20Winter%20Mortality%20NI%20Report%20201920.pdf

Nurse, J., Dorey, S., Yao, L., Sigfrid, L., Yfantopolous, P., McDaid, D., & Moreno, J. M. (2014). *The case for investing in public health. A public health summary report for EPHO 8*. WHO Regional Office for Europe. https://apps.who.int/iris/bitstream/handle/10665/ 351406/WHO-EURO-2014-2581-42337-58615-eng.pdf

Office for Health Improvement & Disparities. (2022, 25 February). *Falls: Applying all our health*. https://www.gov.uk/government/publications/falls-applying-all-our-health

Office for National Statistics. (2018a). *Ethnicity facts and figures*. https://www.ethnicity- facts-figures.service.gov.uk/british-population/national-and-regional-populations/pop ulation-of-england-and-wales/latest

Office for National Statistics. (2018b, 10 April). *Loneliness—what characteristics and circumstances are associated with feeling lonely?* https://www.ons.gov.uk/peoplepopulat ionandcommunity/wellbeing/articles/lonelinesswhatcharacteristicsandcircumstances areassociatedwithfeelinglonely/2018-04-10

Office for National Statistics. (2019, 27 November). *Excess winter mortality in England and Wales: 2018 to 2019 (provisional) and 2017 to 2018 (final)*. https://www.ons.gov. uk/peoplepopulationandcommunity/birthsdeathsandmarriages/deaths/bulletins/ excesswintermortalityinenglandandwales/2018to2019provisionaland2017to2018final

Office for National Statistics. (2020a, 24 March). *Coronavirus and employment for those aged 70 years and over in the UK: October 2018 to September 2019*. https://www.gov.uk/ government/statistics/coronavirus-and-employment-for-those-aged-70-years-and- over-in-the-uk-october-2018-to-september-2019

Office for National Statistics. (2020b, 20 July). *Living longer: Trends in subnational ageing across the UK*. https://www.ons.gov.uk/peoplepopulationandcommunity/birthsdea thsandmarriages/ageing/articles/livinglongertrendsinsubnationalageingacrosstheuk/ 2020-07-20

Office for National Statistics. (2021a). *Estimates of the population for the UK, England and Wales, Scotland and Northern Ireland*. https://www.ons.gov.uk/peoplepopulationandco

mmunity/populationandmigration/populationestimates/datasets/populationestimatesf
orukenglandandwalesscotlandandnorthernireland

Office for National Statistics. (2021b, 25 August). *Living longer: Impact of working from home on older workers*. https://www.ons.gov.uk/peoplepopulationandcommunity/birth sdeathsandmarriages/ageing/articles/livinglongerimpactofworkingfromhomeonolder workers/2021-08-25

Office for National Statistics. (2022a, 12 January). *2020-based interim national population projections*. https://www.ons.gov.uk/peoplepopulationandcommunity/populationandmi gration/populationprojections/datasets/tablea21principalprojectionukpopulationinag egroups

Office for National Statistics. (2022b, 12 September). *People aged 65 years and over in employment, UK: January to March 2022 to April to June 2022*. https://www.ons.gov.uk/ employmentandlabourmarket/peopleinwork/employmentandemployeetypes/articles/ peopleaged65yearsandoverinemploymentuk/januarytomarch2022toapriltojune2022

Office for National Statistics. (2022c, 27 April). *Monthly mortality analysis, England and Wales: March 2022*. https://www.ons.gov.uk/peoplepopulationandcommunity/birthsdea thsandmarriages/deaths/bulletins/monthlymortalityanalysisenglandandwales/march2 022#leading-causes-of-death

Office of Gas and Electricity Markets. (2022, 3 February). *Price cap to increase by £693 from April*. https://www.ofgem.gov.uk/publications/price-cap-increase-ps693-april

Owen, L., & Fischer, A. (2019). The cost-effectiveness of public health interventions examined by the National Institute for Health and Care Excellence from 2005 to 2018. *Public Health*, **169**, 151–162. https://doi.org/10.1016/j.puhe.2019.02.011

Owen, L., Tierney, R., Rtveladze, K., Pritchard, C., & Nolan, K. (2015). Cost-utility analysis of an internet and computer training intervention to improve independence and mental wellbeing of older people. *The Lancet*, **386**(S2), 62. https://doi.org/10.1016/ S0140-6736(15)00900-9

Park, A.-L. (2015). The effects of intergenerational programmes on children and young people. *International Journal of School and Cognitive Psychology*, **2**(1), 1–5. http://epri nts.lse.ac.uk/62083/1/the-effects-of-intergenerational-programmes-on-children-and-young-people.pdf

Patel, R., Fitzgerald, R., Warburton, F., Robertson, C., Pitts, N. B., & Gallagher, J. E. (2022). Refocusing dental care: A risk-based preventative oral health programme for dentate older people in UK care homes. *Gerodontology*, **39**(2), 131–138. https://doi.org/ 10.1111/ger.12543

Patterson, R., Webb, E., Millett, C., & Laverty, A. A. (2018). Physical activity accrued as part of public transport use in England. *Journal of Public Health*, **41**(2), 222–230. https:// doi.org/10.1093/pubmed/fdy099

Pevalin, D. J., Taylor, M. P., & Todd, J. (2008). The dynamics of unhealthy housing in the UK: A panel data analysis. *Housing Studies*, **23**(5). 679–695. https://doi.org/10.1080/ 02673030802253848

Phadraig, C. M. G., Nunn, J., Guerin, S., & Normand, C. (2016). Should we provide oral health training for staff caring for people with intellectual disabilities in community based residential care? A cost-effectiveness analysis. *Evaluation and Program Planning*, **55**, 46–54. https://doi.org/10.1016/j.evalprogplan.2015.12.003

Pitkala, K. H., Routasalo, P., Kautiainen, H., Sintonen, H., & Tilvis, R. S. (2011). Effects of socially stimulating group intervention on lonely, older people's cognition: A randomized, controlled trial. *The American Journal of Geriatric Psychiatry*, **19**(7), 654–663. https://doi.org/10.1097/JGP.0b013e3181f7d8b0

Pitkala, K. H., Routasalo, P., Kautiainen, H., & Tilvis, R. S. (2009). Effects of psychosocial group rehabilitation on health, use of health care services, and mortality of older persons suffering from loneliness: A randomized, controlled trial. *Journals of Gerontology—Series A Biological Sciences and Medical Sciences*, **64**(7), 792–800. https://doi.org/10.1093/gerona/glp011

Polisena, J., Coyle, D., Coyle, K., & McGill, S. (2009). Home telehealth for chronic disease management: A systematic review and an analysis of economic evaluations. *International Journal of Technology Assessment in Health Care*, **25**(3), 339–349. https://doi.org/10.1017/S0266462309990201

Prendergast, L., Toms, G., Seddon, D., Edwards, R. T., Anthony, B., & Jones, C. (2022). 'It was just—everything was normal': Outcomes for people living with dementia, their unpaid carers, and paid carers in a Shared Lives day support service. *Aging & Mental Health*, **18**, 1–9. https://doi.org/10.1080/13607863.2022.2098921

Prendergast, L. M., Toms, G., Seddon, D., Jones, C., Anthony, B. F., & Edwards, R. T. (2023). Supporting social connection for people living with dementia: Lessons from the findings of the TRIO study. *Working with Older People* **28**(1). https://doi.org/10.1108/WWOP-10-2022-0050

Public Health England. (2020, 27 November). *Oral health toolkit for adults in care homes*. Public Health England Guidance. https://www.gov.uk/government/publications/adult-oral-health-in-care-homes-toolkit/oral-health-toolkit-for-adults-in-care-homes

Public Health England. (2022, 4 April). *Adult oral health: applying All Our Health*. Public Health England Guidance. https://www.gov.uk/government/publications/adult-oral-health-applying-all-our-health/adult-oral-health-applying-all-our-health

Rasmussen, J., & Langerman, H. (2019). Alzheimer's disease—why we need early diagnosis. *Degenerative Neurological and Neuromuscular Disease*, **9**, 123–130. https://doi.org/10.2147/DNND.S228939

Schroeder, J., Sowden, J., & Watt, J. (2015). *Social return on investment: The Westhill and District Men's Shed Scotland*. Scottish Men's Sheds Association. https://scottishmsa.org.uk/wp-content/uploads/2016/05/Social-Return-on-Investment-Final-SMSA-Acrobat-9-V1.7.pdf

Schwendicke, F., Stolpe, M., & Müller, F. (2017). Professional oral health care for preventing nursing home-acquired pneumonia: A cost-effectiveness and value of information analysis. *Journal of Clinical Periodontology*, **44**(12), 1236–1244. https://doi.org/10.1111/jcpe.12775

Scott Kruse, C., Karem, P., Shifflett, K., Vegi, L., Ravi, K., & Brooks, M. (2018). Evaluating barriers to adopting telemedicine worldwide: A systematic review. *Journal of Telemedicine and Telecare*, **24**(1), 4–12. https://doi.org/10.1177/1357633X16674087

Shaw, C., McNamara, R., Abrams, K., Cannings-John, R., Hood, K., Longo, M., Myles, S., O'Mahony, S., Roe, B., & Williams, K. (2009). Systematic review of respite care in the frail elderly. *Health Technology Assessment*, **13**(20), 1–246. https://doi.org/10.3310/hta13200

Sixsmith, A., & Sixsmith, J. (2008). Ageing in Place in the United Kingdom. *Ageing International*, 32(3), 219–235. https://doi.org/10.1007/s12126-008-9019-y

Smith, A. C., Thomas, E., Snoswell, C. L., Haydon, H., Mehrotra, A., Clemensen, J., & Caffery, L. J. (2020). Telehealth for global emergencies: Implications for coronavirus disease 2019 (COVID-19). *Journal of Telemedicine and Telecare*, 26(5), 309–313. https://doi.org/10.1177/1357633X20916567

Snowsill, T. M., Stathi, A., Green, C., Withall, J., Greaves, C. J., Thompson, J. L., Taylor, G., Gray, S., Johansen-Berg, H., Bilzon, J.L., de Koning, J. L., Bollen, J, C., Moorlock, S. J., Western, M. J., Guralnik, J. M., Rejeski, W. J., Fox, K. R., & Medina-Lara, A. (2022). Cost-effectiveness of a physical activity and behaviour maintenance programme on functional mobility decline in older adults: An economic evaluation of the REACT (Retirement in Action) trial. *The Lancet Public Health*, 7(4), e327–e334. https://doi.org/10.1016/S2468-2667(22)00030-5

Social Value Lab. (2011, August). *Craft Cafe: Creative solutions to isolation and loneliness. Social return on investment evaluation.* http://www.socialvaluelab.org.uk/wp-content/uploads/2013/05/CraftCafeSROI.pdf

Spencer, L. H., Lynch, M., Lawrence, C. L., & Edwards, R. T. (2020). A scoping review of how income affects accessing local green space to engage in outdoor physical activity to improve well-being: Implications for post COVID-19. *International Journal of Environmental Research and Public Health*, 17, 9313. https://doi.org/10.3390/ijerph17249313

Storey, A. (2018, 13 August). *Living longer: How our population is changing and why it matters.* Office for National Statistics. https://www.ons.gov.uk/peoplepopulationandcommunity/birthsdeathsandmarriages/ageing/articles/livinglongerhowourpopulationischangingandwhyitmatters/2018-08-13

Stowe, S., & Harding, S. (2010). Telecare, telehealth and telemedicine. *European Geriatric Medicine*, 1(3), 193–197. https://doi.org/10.1016/j.eurger.2010.04.002

Teo, K. Y. C., Nguyen, V., Barthelmes, D., Arnold, J. J., Gillies, M. C., & Cheung, C. M. G. (2020). Extended intervals for wet AMD patients with high retreatment needs: Informing the risk during COVID-19, data from real-world evidence. *Eye*, 35(10), 2793–2801. https://doi.org/10.1038/s41433-020-01315-x

The Conservative Party. (2019). *The Conservative and Unionist Party Manifesto 2019.* https://www.conservatives.com/our-plan/conservative-party-manifesto-2019

Toms, G. R., Stringer, C. L., Prendergast, L. M., Seddon, D., Anthony, B. F., & Edwards, R. T. (2023). A study to explore the feasibility of using a social return on investment approach to evaluate short breaks. *Health & Social Care in the Community*, 2023, 4699751. https://doi.org/10.1155/2023/4699751

Tsakos, G., Brocklehurst, P. R., Watson, S., Verey, A., Goulden, N., Jenkins, A., Hoare, Z., Pye, K., Wassall, R. R., Sherriff, A., Heilmann, A., O'Neill, C., Smith, C. J., Langley, J., Venturelli, R., Cairns, P., Lievesley, N., Watt, R. G., Kee, F., & McKenna, G. (2021). Improving the oral health of older people in care homes (TOPIC): A protocol for a feasibility study. *Pilot and Feasibility Studies*, 7(1), 138. https://doi.10.1186/s40814-021-00872-6

Uberoi, E., & Burton, M. (2022). *Ethnic diversity in politics and public life.* https://researchbriefings.files.parliament.uk/documents/SN01156/SN01156.pdf

United Kingdom Government. (2022, 21 October). *How households and businesses will be supported by the Energy Prices Bill.* https://www.gov.uk/government/publications/ene rgy-prices-bill-how-households-and-businesses-will-be-supported/how-households-and-businesses-will-be-supported-by-the-energy-prices-bill

Valtorta, N. K., Kanaan, M., Gilbody, S., Ronzi, S., & Hanratty, B. (2016). Loneliness and social isolation as risk factors for coronary heart disease and stroke: Systematic review and meta-analysis of longitudinal observational studies. *Heart (British Cardiac Society),* 102(13), 1009–1016. https://doi.org/10.1136/heartjnl-2015-308790

van Leeuwen, K. M., Malley, J., Bosmans, J. E., Jansen, A. P. D., Ostelo, R. W., van der Horst, H. E., & Netten, A. (2014). What can local authorities do to improve the social care-related quality of life of older adults living at home? Evidence from the Adult Social Care Survey. *Health & Place,* 29, 104–113. https://doi.org/10.1016/j.healthpl ace.2014.06.004

Vandepitte, S., Putman, K., Van Den Noortgate, N., Verhaeghe, N., & Annemans, L. (2020). Cost-effectiveness of an in-home respite care program to support informal caregivers of persons with dementia: A model-based analysis. *International Journal of Geriatric Psychiatry,* 35(6), 601–609. https://doi.org/10.1002/gps.5276

Vandepitte, S., Van Den Noortgate, N., Putman, K., Verhaeghe, S., Verdonck, C., & Annemans, L. (2016). Effectiveness of respite care in supporting informal caregivers of persons with dementia: A systematic review. *International Journal of Geriatric Psychiatry,* 31(12), 1277–1288. https://doi.org/10.1002/gps.4504

Vecchio, N., Comans, T., Harris, P., Graham, V., Cully, A., Harris, N., Fitzgerald, J., Cartmel, J., Golenko, X., & Radford, K. (2020). Economic evaluation of intergenerational programs: Suggested measures and design. *Journal of Intergenerational Relationships,* 19(4), 421–440. https://doi.org/10.1080/15350 770.2020.1810194

Wanless, D., Forder, J., Fernández, J., Poole, T., Beesley, L., Henwood, M., & Mosconne, F. (2006). *Wanless social care review: Securing good care for older people, taking a long-term view.* The King's Fund. https://www.kingsfund.org.uk/sites/default/files/field/field_publi cation_file/securing-good-care-for-older-people-wanless-2006.pdf

Windle, G., Flynn, G., Hoare, Z., Masterson-Algar, P., Egan, K., Edwards, R. T., Jones, C., Spector, A., Algar-Skaife, K., Hughes, G., Brocklehurst, P., Goulden, N., Skelhorn, D., & Stott, J. (2022). Effects of an e-health intervention 'iSupport' for reducing distress of dementia carers: Protocol for a randomised controlled trial and feasibility study. *BMJ Open,* 12(9), e064314. http://dx.doi.org/10.1136/bmjopen-2022-064314

Windle, K., Francis, J., & Coomber, C. (2011, October). *SCIE Research briefing 39: Preventing loneliness and social isolation: Interventions and outcomes.* Social Care Institute for Excellence. https://www.scie.org.uk/prevention/connecting/loneliness-soc ial-isolation-research-2011

Wittenberg, R., Hu, B., Barraza-Araiza, L., & Rehill, A. (2019). *Projections of older people with dementia and costs of dementia care in the United Kingdom, 2019–2040.* Care Policy and Evaluation Centre, London School of Economics and Political Science. https:// www.alzheimers.org.uk/sites/default/files/2019-11/cpec_report_november_2019.pdf

Woodall, J., White, J., & South, J. (2013). Improving health and well-being through community health champions: A thematic evaluation of a programme in Yorkshire and

Humber. *Perspectives in Public Health*, **133**(2), 96–103. https://doi.org/10.1177/17579 13912453669

Woods, R. T., Orrell, M., Bruce, E., Edwards, R. T., Hoare, Z., Hounsome, B., Keady, J., Moniz-Cook, E., Orgeta, V., Rees, J., & Russell, I. (2016). REMCARE: Pragmatic multi-centre randomised trial of reminiscence groups for people with dementia and their family carers: Effectiveness and economic analysis. *PLoS One*, **11**(4), 1–116. https://doi.org/10.1371/journal.pone.0152843

World Health Organization. (2007). *Global age-friendly cities: A guide.* https://apps.who.int/iris/handle/10665/43755

World Health Organization. (2019, 9 May). *iSupport for dementia.* https://www.who.int/publications/i/item/9789241515863

World Health Organization. (2021, 26 April). *Falls fact sheet.* http://www.who.int/mediacen tre/factsheets/fs344/en/

World Health Organization. (2022). *Dementia: Key facts.* https://www.who.int/health-top ics/dementia

Wylie, G., Menz, H.B., McFarlane, S., Ogston, S., Sullivan, F., Williams, B., Young, Z., & Morris, J. (2017). Podiatry intervention versus usual care to prevent falls in care homes: pilot randomised controlled trial (the PIRFECT study). *BMC Geriatrics*, **17**, 1–13. https://doi.org/10.1186/s12877-017-0541-1

Zander, A., & Boniface, D. (2017). Directly observed daily mouth care provided to care home residents in one area of Kent, UK. *Community Dental Health*, **34**(1), 32–36. https://doi.org/10.1922/CDH_3956Zander05

Chapter 7

Dying Well

Carys Stringer, Eira Winrow, Kalpa Pisavadia,
Catherine L. Lawrence, and
Rhiannon T. Edwards

Introduction

Throughout this book we focus on how we can stay healthy and well across the life-course and how our health and lifestyle choices at one life-course stage can shape our experiences in the future. Ultimately, however, the time comes for death, and it is important to consider the factors that we can influence to ensure that we have a 'good death'. Campbell (2020) offered a model of factors that can influence what might be considered a good death:

- place of death;
- one's company in death;
- cause of death; and
- one's manner of facing death.

As health economists, we focus this chapter on health economics and end of life care; palliative care and advance care planning; place of death; the role of care homes; and globalization of end of life carer support in rare dementia. Finally, we present some examples of economic evidence of effective and cost-effective interventions to support people at the end of life.

In 2021, there were 667,479 registered deaths in the United Kingdom (UK), a decrease from 689,629 deaths in the previous year, which saw the most deaths in a single year since 1918 (when there were 715,000 deaths; Clark, 2023). The proportion of avoidable deaths, which means those that were considered preventable or treatable for people aged under seventy-five years, had been trending downwards in the UK for over twenty years. However, in 2020 the coronavirus disease 2019 (COVID-19) pandemic led to a statistically significant rise in avoidable deaths similar to the levels last seen in 2010 of roughly one in five deaths being avoidable (Office for National Statistics (ONS), 2022a). Avoidable mortality includes deaths caused by alcohol-related or drug-related disorders,

Carys Stringer, Eira Winrow, Kalpa Pisavadia, Catherine L. Lawrence, and Rhiannon T. Edwards, *Dying Well* In: *Health Economics of Well-being and Well-becoming across the Life-course*. Edited by: Rhiannon T. Edwards and Catherine L. Lawrence, Oxford University Press. © Oxford University Press 2024. DOI: 10.1093/9780191919336.003.0007

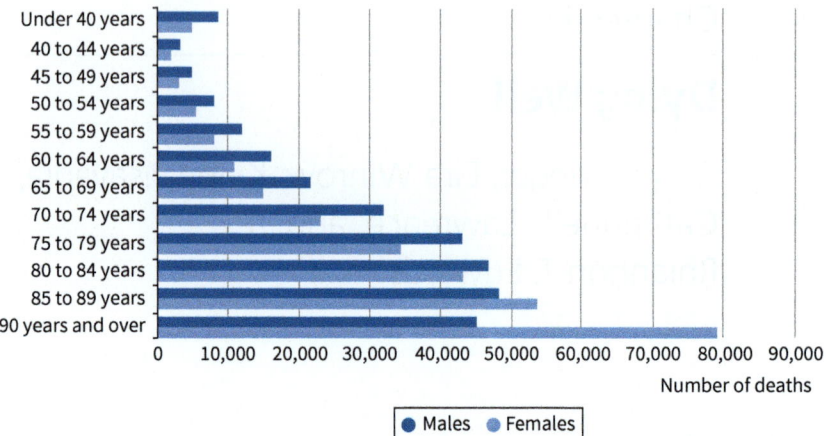

Figure 7.1 Number of registered deaths by sex and age group in England and Wales in 2022

Reproduced from Office for National Statistics. (2023, 11 April). *Death registration summary statistics, England and Wales: 2022.* https://www.ons.gov.uk/peoplepopulationandcommunity/birthsdeathsandmarriages/deaths/articles/deathregistrationsummarystatisticsenglandandwales/2022. Copyright © 2023 Office for National Statistics. Reproduced under the Open Government License 3.0

neoplasms (cancers), and more recently, COVID-19 (ONS, 2022a). There have been over 229,000 deaths with COVID-19 recorded on the death certificate in the UK (UK Government, 2023). Excess deaths are those that occur above the expected number observed during a given time period. Between March 2020 and December 2021 there were 133,623 excess deaths in England and Wales, most due to or involving COVID-19 (ONS, 2022b). When deaths due to COVID-19 were excluded, the leading causes of excess death were old age and frailty, cirrhosis and other diseases of the liver, and diabetes.

The proportion of avoidable deaths is higher in more deprived areas, for example, 40 per cent of male deaths in the most deprived areas of England are avoidable, compared to 18 per cent in the least deprived areas (ONS, 2022c). A United States (US) study into the preventable factors of deaths found that the main risk factors were smoking, high blood pressure, obesity, physical inactivity, high blood glucose, high low-density lipoprotein (LDL) cholesterol, high dietary sodium, low dietary omega-3 fatty acids, high dietary trans fatty acids, excessive alcohol consumption, and low intake of fruits and vegetables (Danaei et al., 2009). Pre-COVID-19 pandemic, the leading cause of male deaths in the UK was ischaemic heart disease (15 per cent of deaths in males aged sixty-five to seventy-nine, and 17 per cent in males aged fifty to sixty-four). In females, the leading cause of death was malignant neoplasm of the trachea, bronchus, or lung (10 per cent of deaths in females aged sixty-five to seventy-nine, and 10 per cent of deaths in females aged fifty to sixty-four). In adults aged forty-nine and below, the leading causes of death included suicide and injury or poisoning of undetermined intent (ONS, 2020a). Figure 7.1 illustrates the number of registered deaths in England and Wales in 2022 by sex and age group, and as might be expected, most deaths occur in older people (ONS, 2023). The figure shows that the number of deaths was higher for males than females for the majority of age groups.

Health Economics and End of Life Care

Medical and technological advances have led to increased treatment options for people in later life; however, the UK National Health Service (NHS) budget is under increasing pressure and does not stretch to offering all treatments to all people, so choices have to be made about what to fund. This is the rationale for health economics as a sub-discipline of economics. The standard approach of cost-effectiveness analysis is to compare the costs and outcomes, often in terms of quality-adjusted life year (QALY) gains and costs of competing treatment options. This approach can be problematic for interventions involving end of life care for three reasons:

1. A significant proportion of costs are borne outside the NHS (e.g. by the third sector, social care sector, and individuals and their families).
2. The QALY is a composite measure of quality of life and quantity of life—improvements in length of life are rarely possible at the end of life stage.
3. The quality of life component of the QALY does not always capture aspects of quality of life that are important to people at the end of life and often it is the family carer who may be the beneficiary of any formal care support or third sector support, for example, Macmillan nurses may support the family carer as much as the person dying (Diernberger et al., 2021).

Health economics and economic evaluation have very much been focused on capturing the cost-effectiveness of the production of health gain in terms of quality-adjusted life expectancy. There has been much less focus on the process of the very end of life. This has been addressed more in the capability paradigm. Researchers from the University of Birmingham and now at the University of Bristol, in collaboration with Marie Curie Cancer Care and researchers at the University of South Australia, have been developing capability measures relating to care at the end of life (Kinghorn & Coast, 2018; Sutton & Coast, 2014). In a European Research Council-funded project, these researchers argued that an imperative to assess the economic impact of care at the end of life is emerging in response to national policy developments in a number of settings. Current focus on health benefits in economic evaluation, that is, through the National Institute for Health and Care Excellence (NICE) reference case (NICE, 2013, 2022) may not appropriately capture benefits of interventions at the end of life (Sutton & Coast, 2014). Though NICE has a range of guidance relating to the death of adults (NICE, 2015, 2019a), adolescents, and infants (NICE, 2019b), this is a challenging area for health economists.

Within the capability paradigm, as an alternative to the QALY paradigm (i.e. length and quality of life) in end of life research, other attributes may be more relevant. The EconEndLife project explored how to assess end of life outcomes and developed two outcome measures: the ICECAP Supportive Care Measure (ICECAP-SCM) and the ICECAP Close Person Measure (ICECAP-CPM; Canaway et al., 2017; Sutton & Coast, 2014). These two measures were developed from a capability approach and include attributes such as choice, love and affection, physical suffering, emotional suffering, dignity, being supported, and preparation. Both the ICECAP-SCM and ICECAP-CPM are suitable for use in palliative care settings.

Palliative Care and Advance Care Planning

Palliative care has been put forward as a Human Right on the basis that humans should have the right to health and the right to be free from cruel, inhuman, and degrading treatment (Brennan, 2007). The World Health Organization (WHO, 2020) defines palliative care as: 'an approach that improves the quality of life of patients (adults and children) and their families who are facing problems associated with life-threatening illness. It prevents and relieves suffering through the early identification, correct assessment and treatment of pain and other problems, whether physical, psychosocial or spiritual.'

Although we have chosen to include the topic of palliative care in this final life-course stage chapter of the book, it is important to acknowledge that it has relevance across all life-course stages where life-limiting illness, which can be genetic, may affect children and adults of all ages.

Whilst palliative care adopts a holistic approach, covering the whole spectrum of a person's remaining lifespan of their illness, end of life care is solely focused on the last months of life (Krau, 2016). The NICE guidelines for the care of adults in the last two to three days of life aims to improve end of life care through involving patients in decision-making and maintaining their comfort and dignity (NICE, 2015). In the UK, people can receive palliative care, in theory at least, in hospices, hospitals, care homes, or at home, depending on the individual's needs and preferences. Availability of these services and hence choices for the individual and their family will vary across the UK. Place of death, whether this is in the deceased person's place of residence or care home, is considered a key performance indicator (KPI) for quality in end of life care (Department of Health, 2012). Identifying and supporting people's preferences to be cared for and die in their place of choice are promoted in the UK Government's 'Our commitment to you for end of life care' document (Department of Health, 2016).

'Advance care planning' is the process of offering people the opportunity to discuss their future care needs and preferences, while they still have the capacity to do so. It is particularly relevant for people who risk losing mental capacity (e.g. through dementia or other progressively degenerative conditions), and for people whose mental capacity fluctuates (e.g. through poor mental health). People can undertake advance care planning independently without a health care professional. However, input from a professional may help individuals consider relevant matters for their plan, such as advance refusal of treatment or proxy decision-making (NICE, 2018). Advance care planning has been found to significantly reduce depression and anxiety of carers and improve their quality of life (Brinkman-Stoppelenburg et al., 2014; Detering et al., 2010). Moreover, it may also be cost-effective (Bauer et al., 2021). In this economic modelling study, the cost-effectiveness of advance care planning offered systematically to older people at the end of life was compared with standard care, from a health and social care perspective with a one-year time horizon. The total mean cost per person in the advance care planning group was £3,739 and in the standard care group the mean cost was £3,069. The QALY gain to carers was 0.03 for the intervention group in comparison with the standard care group. Based on a carer's health-related quality of life, the average cost per QALY was £18,965, below the NICE threshold of £20,000. Advance care planning has been associated with health care savings in a number of studies, especially those involving people living in nursing homes, people with high support needs, and people living with dementia in the community (Dixon et al., 2019). It can significantly increase the possibility of dying at home or in a care home compared to the hospital. People who recorded a preference for place of death were also more likely to be rated by their family members as receiving 'outstanding' or 'excellent' care than those without expressed preferences (Dixon et al., 2019).

Where We Want to Die and Where We Actually Die

In the UK, most deaths occur in hospital (241,219; 44.0 per cent), followed by at home (157,312; 28.7 per cent), in a care home (110,563; 20.2 per cent), in a hospice (23,882; 4.4 per cent), or elsewhere (14,672; 2.7 per cent; Office for Health

Improvement and Disparities, 2022). Research in England, and more recently in Wales, shows that the deprivation level of a person's residence affects the place of death and the quality of care received at the end of life. Long hospital stays are driven by patient attributes (such as age, sex, and health status); availability of community services; access to hospital services; the way in which hospital services are managed; deprivation; and geographical access to a hospital over a more preferred place (Imison et al., 2012). More recently, in Wales, Ziwary and colleagues (2017) combined mortality statistics from 2005 to 2014 and Welsh Index of Multiple Deprivation rankings for each lower super output area (small areas of the country specifically devised to improve the reporting and comparison of local statistics). The study found that the distribution of place of death was concentrated in three places: hospital (60 per cent), home (21 per cent), and care home (13 per cent). Other places of death included hospice (3 per cent), elsewhere (2 per cent), and psychiatric units (<1 per cent). Despite the high number of hospital deaths, especially for more deprived areas, this was the least preferred place of death (Ziwary et al., 2017). During the COVID-19 pandemic, there was a significant shift in where people die. During 2020 to 2022, there were more than 105,000 extra deaths occurring at home in the UK (Keeble et al., 2022).

As shown in Figure 7.2, there is a contrast between actual place of death and preference for place of death (Shucksmith et al., 2013; ONS, 2020b). The British

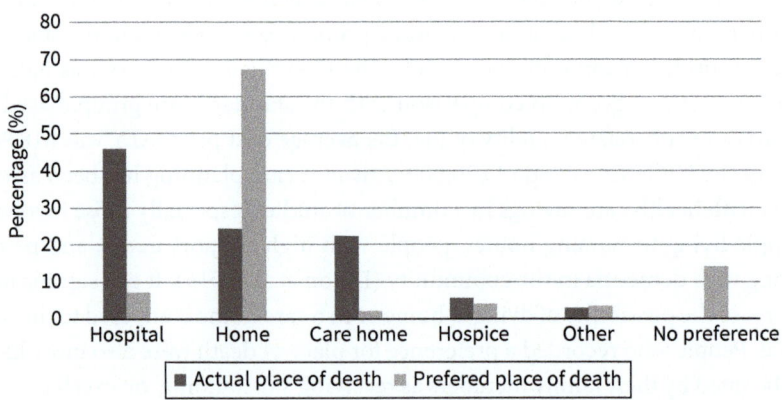

Figure 7.2 Comparison of actual place of death to preferred place of death
Sources: Shucksmith, J., Carlebach, S., & Whittaker, V. (2013). *British Social Attitudes 30 survey module on attitudes to end of life care and dying.* National Centre Social Research. www.dying matters.org/sites/default/files/BSA30_Full_Report.pdf
Office for National Statistics. (2020b). *Deaths registered in England and Wales.* https://www. ons.gov.uk/peoplepopulationandcommunity/birthsdeathsandmarriages/deaths/datasets/ deathsregisteredinenglandandwalesseriesdrreferencetables. Copyright © 2020 Office for National Statistics

Social Attitudes survey of preferences around dying and place of death found that 67 per cent of people would prefer to die at home; 7 per cent of people would choose to die in hospital; 4 per cent would choose to die in a hospice; 8 per cent would choose to die elsewhere; and 14 per cent had no preference about place of death (Shucksmith et al., 2013). However, 60 per cent of the people who stated that they would prefer to die at home changed their response when asked if they would still prefer to die at home if there was insufficient support from family, friends, or health and social care professionals (Shucksmith et al., 2013). A 2017 study found that people aged over sixty-five and receiving palliative care services would prefer a home death (56 per cent of participants), which mirrors the general population's preference. In contrast to the hospital being the second most preferred place of death for the general population, a palliative care or hospice unit was the second most preferred place of death (22 per cent of participants), and hospital was third (4 per cent) (Higginson et al., 2017).

Palliative Care, Hospices, and Hospice at Home

WHO has developed a public health strategy for integrating palliative care into a country's health care service. The four pillars of the public health strategy are: 1) appropriate government policies; 2) adequate medication availability; 3) education of policy decision-makers, health care professionals, and the public; and 4) the implementation of palliative care services at all levels of society (Stjernswärd et al., 2007). Whilst the UK arguably meets the criterion of the first three pillars, there is room for improvement in achieving equitable access to services. Individuals with lower socioeconomic status are less likely to access services (Buck et al., 2020; Sleeman et al., 2016). However, it is important to acknowledge that individuals have different preferences. The British Social Attitudes survey on dying found that people from lower socioeconomic groups were less likely to have a preference for dying at home and were more likely than those of a higher socioeconomic status to prefer to die in a hospital (Shucksmith et al., 2013).

Each year, hospices provide care for 225,000 people in the UK with terminal or life-limiting illnesses (Hospice UK, 2020). Hospices aim to provide holistic care, which encompasses a person's medical, emotional, social, practical, psychological, and spiritual needs, along with the needs of their family (NHS, 2018). Care is provided by a multidisciplinary team that includes paid staff and volunteers. The services are typically free in the UK and patients are referred by a General Practitioner (GP), hospital professional, or community nurse.

There are three main types of hospice service provision: inpatient, day therapy, and hospice at home. Inpatient units provide care for patients whilst also offering respite to carers. Patients may be admitted for ongoing care or short spells and subsequently return to their usual place of residence if their condition has improved. Day therapy services may include physiotherapy, complementary therapies, rehabilitation, respite for carers, spiritual help, or signposting towards information for financial support. Day therapy also provides a social setting for patients to meet others with a life-limiting illness and participate in supervised activities. Hospice at home services aim to enable patients with a terminal illness to be cared for and die at home if they so wish (National Association for Hospice at Home, 2020). The value of hospice at home services to patients includes avoiding hospital admissions, giving carers brief respite, knowledgeable staff who can manage patient symptoms, and communication with health care professionals who were able to sensitively handle difficult discussions about dying (Jack et al., 2016). A study of hospice at home service provision found that there was an unmet need as demand outstripped supply. There were also inequalities in access to services related to socioeconomic status, with more affluent patients more likely to receive services (Buck et al., 2020). This is known as the 'inverse care law'. The inverse care law is a concept proposed by Julian Tudor Hart in 1971 in an attempt to explore the relationship between the need for health care and the efficiency of the distribution of health care (Hart, 1971). Hart's commentary on the provision of health care through the NHS identified research conducted within the relatively new all-inclusive health system in the UK which described disparities between the rich and the poor, even under this universal system. It was believed that these disparities stemmed from the fact that richer individuals with a better education knew how the system worked and knew what to ask for (Titmuss & Seldon, 1968). Health inequality was already an issue just fifteen years into the delivery of services by the NHS. Hart wrote: 'The availability of good medical care tends to vary inversely with the need for it in the population served. This inverse care law operates more completely where medical care is most exposed to market forces, and less so where such exposure is reduced' (Hart, 1971, p. 405). As nations deal with ageing populations, appropriate services must be developed to care for them.

People with cancer make up the majority of people who die in hospices, with nine out of ten hospice deaths in England having a recorded cause of cancer (Public Health England, 2018). A study of changing demographics of hospice patients over time found that the average age of hospice users between 1993 and 2012 was over sixty-five years, with 30 per cent of hospice patients below sixty-five years old (Sleeman et al., 2016). As with the socioeconomic profile of hospice at home patients, Sleeman and colleagues (2016) found that there has been a shift in the patients' socioeconomic status over time. Twenty-two per cent of patients were in the most deprived quintile in 1993 to 1997, yet only 18 per cent were in the least deprived quintile in 2008 to 2012. People living in the least deprived areas are more likely to die in inpatient hospices than people living in the most deprived areas. This gap has increased over time (Sleeman et al., 2016). Whilst the main role of hospices is to provide support to patients, they also provide support to patients' families. In 2018/2019, over 72,000 people received bereavement support from hospices (Hospice UK, 2020). Provision of bereavement support services was found to be an attribute of hospice service provision that family members valued; however, hospice support post-bereavement was often reactive rather than proactive (Hughes et al., 2019).

Most UK adult and children hospice income (72 per cent) comes via community fundraising, donations, legacies, corporate supporters, and trading activities (Hospice UK, 2018). The government tops up the remaining funds of £350 million per year (price year 2017). However, the level of government funding that hospices receive varies by region (28 per cent in Wales through to 38 per cent in Scotland). Hospice volunteers contribute £200 million of support each year (Hospice UK, 2020). The COVID-19 pandemic and subsequent economic crisis meant that although the hospice sector overall generated surplus on their core activities of £36 million, this was wiped out by a £44 million reduction in the value of their investments. This meant the sector recorded a collective loss of £9 million in the year to 31 March 2020 (Hospice UK, 2021). The cost of living crisis continues to dampen the ability of the population to make charitable gifts (Salutin, 2023).

Compared to adult hospices, children's hospices have a greater dependence on donations: donations account for 56 per cent of income in children's hospices, and only 31 per cent of income in adult hospices. The proportion of government funding received by children's hospices is comparatively lower, with only 15 per cent of their income accruing from government funding (Hospice UK, 2018). In 2017, nearly a third of hospices had an annual expenditure of £8 million. The main expenditure categories for hospices are the provision of hospice services (mainly staffing costs), costs for their retail outlets, fundraising expenditure, and lottery expenditure. The proportion of spending for each category is relatively consistent across different hospice sizes (Hospice UK, 2018).

Hospitals

The majority of deaths in hospitals are in adults, with 67 per cent of hospital deaths occurring in adults aged seventy-five and older (Public Health England,

2018). An observational study of adults aged over eighty-five found that adults classified as frail spent more time in hospital than non-frail adults over seven years. Frail adults had more than a two-fold increased mortality risk than non-frail adults (Keeble et al., 2019). As well as age, factors associated with a higher risk of dying in hospital include gender, social deprivation, ethnicity, and marital status (Public Health England, 2018). The National Audit Office (2008) found that a lack of prompt access to community-based services such as advice and medication can lead to people being unnecessarily admitted to hospital near the end of their life. The National Audit Office also found that lack of information sharing between services could lead to inappropriate hospital admissions if 'do not attempt resuscitation' notices on a patient's file were not known about.

Care Homes

Although the UK has an ageing population, data from the 2021 census shows that the number of people residing in care homes has decreased since 2011. In 2021, there were 33,353 adult residents in care homes in Scotland, 11 per cent fewer than in 2011 (Public Health Scotland, 2022). Ninety-one per cent of residents in care homes were older people. In 2021, there were 29,317 long stay residents in care homes for older people, a reduction of 10 per cent since 2011 (Public Health Scotland, 2022). In England, from March 2021 to February 2022, there were 360,792 care home residents, a 7.9 per cent fall from before the COVID-19 pandemic. Of these, 34.9 per cent were self-funded residents, a 12.4 per cent fall since pre-pandemic (ONS, 2022d). Care homes located in the least deprived areas of England had a statistically significantly higher proportion of self-funders (52.5 per cent) than care homes in the most deprived areas (18.7 per cent; ONS, 2022d). In 2020, in Wales, there were 24,178 people living in care homes, 8.5 per cent were aged sixty-five to seventy-four years, and 26.7 per cent were aged over seventy-five years (ONS, 2020c). In 2020, in Northern Ireland, there were 16,080 care home beds registered. There was a similar number of residential and nursing care homes registered in 2020 compared to 2016 (Kinghan et al., 2020).

The NICE guidance on the care of dying adults recognizes the importance of communication, individualized care, and shared decision-making at the end of life (NICE, 2015). The Six Steps to Success in End of Life Care pathway (Six Steps programme) aims to enhance end of life care provision in care homes through staff education and organizational change (see Figure 7.3). This pathway was set out in the national End of Life Care Strategy (Department of Health and Social Care, 2008). The programme consists

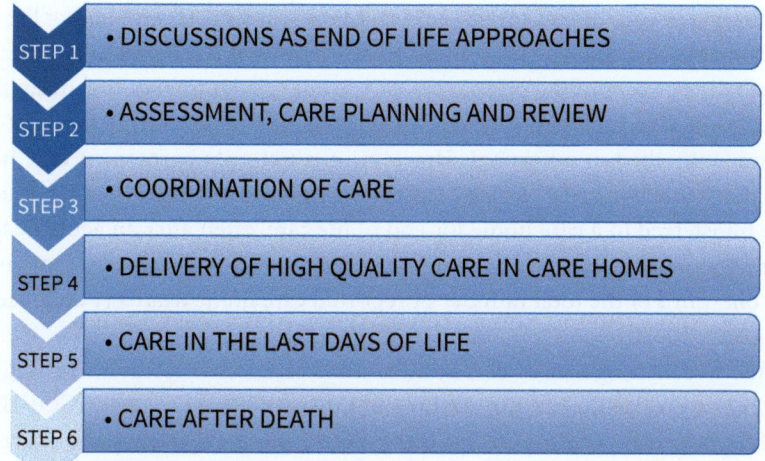

Figure 7.3 The Six Steps to Success in End of Life Care

of an initial discussion about death and future care, assessment and provision of coordinated care, support in the resident's final days, and care after death (Springett, 2017). Initially introduced in North West England, the Six Steps programme has been adapted and implemented in Betsi Cadwaladr University Health Board (BCUHB) in North Wales (Royal College of Nursing Wales, 2021). Following an evaluation of the eight-month programme, findings showed a reduction in the incidence of unplanned admissions to hospital, an increase in the documentation of preferred place of death, and an increase from 83.7 per cent to 93.0 per cent of care home staff perceiving that they 'always' or 'often' discussed wishes and preference for end of life care with residents. Residents were also more likely to die in their preferred place. Advance care planning in nursing homes increased from 31.3 per cent to 87.3 per cent following the programme, and from 32 per cent to 83.3 per cent in residential homes. Confidence levels in nursing and care home staff all increased (Royal College of Nursing Wales, 2021). In an economic analysis of the provision of the Six Steps+ End of Life Care Programme (which was developed to include addressing care for people with dementia) across ten care homes, Springett (2015) found that the cost of providing the programme is met by contributing to averting six avoidable hospital admissions or a 6.8 per cent reduction in avoidable hospital admissions.

There are over 460,000 care home beds in England, of which almost half are allocated for residents needing nursing care (Public Health England, 2017a). Care homes are a large provider of end of life care, with over a fifth of all deaths occurring in care homes (ONS, 2021a). Many residents receive end of life care in the days and months leading up to a final hospital admission resulting in death, 71 per cent of the permanent care home residents who died in England in 2015 died in their place of residence, whilst the remaining 29 per cent predominantly died in a hospital. However, it is not only permanent care home residents that live in care homes. People who usually live in their own home but are transferred to a care home for end of life care, often after an acute hospital admission, are referred to as temporary residents. Temporary residents make up one-third of the total number of reported care home deaths (Public Health England, 2017b).

The five leading causes of deaths of male care home residents in England in 2021 were: dementia and Alzheimer's disease (26.4 per cent); COVID-19 (11.5 per cent); cerebrovascular diseases (5.5 per cent); ischaemic heart diseases (5.3 per cent); and malignant neoplasm of prostate (4.1 per cent; ONS, 2022e). In female care home residents, dementia and Alzheimer's disease (34 per cent) and COVID-19 (10.8) were also the top two leading causes of death, followed by symptoms, signs, and ill-defined conditions (8 per cent), cerebrovascular diseases (6.1 per cent), and ischaemic heart diseases (4.0 per cent). A similar pattern was found in Wales, with dementia and Alzheimer's disease (28.3 per cent); COVID-19 (12.9 per cent); cerebrovascular diseases (7.6 per cent); ischaemic heart diseases (5.8 per cent); and symptoms, signs, and ill-defined conditions (3.7 per cent) being the top five leading causes of death in male care home residents. In females residing in care homes in Wales, the top five causes were: dementia and Alzheimer's disease (36.2 per cent); COVID-19 (11.1 per cent); symptoms, signs, and ill-defined conditions (7.3 per cent); cerebrovascular diseases (6.7 per cent); and ischaemic heart disease (4 per cent) (ONS, 2022e).

Globalization of End of Life Carer Support in Rare Dementia

The globalization of communication via online platforms such as Zoom and Teams, which grew exponentially through necessity during the COVID-19 pandemic, has given rise to some interesting service developments. For example, in the case of the provision of online support to carers of rare dementias, such as: familial Alzheimer's disease (FAD), frontotemporal dementia (FTD), familial frontotemporal dementia (fFTD), posterior cortical atrophy (PCA), primary progressive aphasia (PPA), Lewy body dementia (LBD), and young-onset Alzheimer's disease (YOAD). The Rare Dementia Support (RDS) group led by University College London is now offering online support internationally to carers worldwide (https://www.raredementiasupport.org). The RDS Impact study is currently underway and will be the first major study of the value of multicomponent support groups for people living with or supporting someone with a rare dementia (Brotherhood et al., 2019).

The specific challenges posed to informal carers of people with rare and sometimes early-onset dementia, which are life-limiting, mean that there are unlikely to be sources of specialized support locally or even within that country's health or social care system. For the health economist, this poses interesting challenges of what perspective of analysis to adopt when identifying, measuring, and valuing costs and outcomes in the evaluation of such international online support services for informal carers of people living with rare dementias. The costs of running the online support service may be accrued in London, where UK NHS cost tariffs are appropriate. However, if the recipients of this service live in other European countries, North America, or the Middle East, any implications for the use of wider health or social care services would involve identifying, measuring, and valuing service use in those countries' systems and presumably at local costs. We are faced with asking: when does a societal perspective move from being the society of a single country to an international or global society perspective?

Economic Evidence of Effective and Cost-effective Interventions to Support People at the End of Life

A review of international evidence on the costs and cost-effectiveness of palliative care interventions in any setting, including hospital-based, home-based, and hospice care settings, identified forty-six relevant papers (Smith et al., 2014). In two out of six studies that included cost data, the costs of the palliative care intervention were significantly lower than the costs for the control group (Brumley et al., 2007; Gade et al., 2008). Three other studies reported lower costs for the palliative care intervention, although this was not significantly different, or no statistical significance was reported. One study evaluated the cost-effectiveness of a new palliative care service for people with multiple sclerosis (Higginson et al., 2009). Patients were either randomly allocated to a multidisciplinary palliative care team immediately (fast track) or the control group who continued best usual care for three months and then met with the palliative care team. Findings varied by outcome measure used to assess effectiveness. The fast track intervention group had lower costs and worse outcomes when using the Palliative Care Outcome Scale (POS-8), which measures anxiety, patient and carer concerns, and practical needs. When using the Zarit Burden Inventory (ZBI), which measures carer burden, the fast track intervention group had higher costs and better outcomes (Higginson et al., 2009). A more recent systematic review of the cost-effectiveness of out of hours palliative care found no eligible papers, indicating a lack of available evidence (Johnston et al., 2020). A Cochrane review of hospital-based specialist palliative care services for adults with advanced illnesses and their caregivers found thirteen studies with economic evidence; however, this evidence was inconsistent (Bajwah et al., 2020).

Due to the ageing population of the UK, there is a need to identify sustainable interventions to support people at the end of life and their families; however, conducting research in palliative care settings can be challenging. A survey of researchers working in palliative care identified five barriers that they faced: 1) lack of funding and limited expertise on grant review panels; 2) limited institutional capacity of palliative care service providers to support research; 3) lack of trained researchers and mentoring opportunities; 4) issues surrounding the study population (e.g. participants' ability to take part in research) and attrition in longitudinal studies; and 5) public and professionals' perceptions and discomfort with research in palliative care (Chen et al., 2014). 'Gatekeeping' refers to when an individual or organization takes it upon themselves to decide who has access rights to a community. A systematic review of reasons for gatekeeping in palliative care research identified that gatekeeping barriers could be applied by health care professionals, research ethics committees, service provider management, family members of patients, and researchers themselves (Kars et al., 2016). The most reported reason for gatekeeping from research was the fear of burdening participants. Karlawish (2003) set out the conditions in which it is deemed acceptable to include participants in end of life research when an intervention is not intended to benefit the participant directly but to generate knowledge that will benefit future patients or carers. These conditions include an acceptable risk level of burden or discomfort, availability of a proxy for decision-making, respecting participants' assent or dissent, and obtaining advance consent from participants. The Methods of Researching End of Life Care (MORECare) project developed a thirty-six item good practice standard for evaluating interventions in end of life care (Higginson et al., 2013). The good practice standard included recommendations for ethics, minimizing the burden for staff participants, selecting appropriate outcome measures, and handling attrition and missing data. A review of research priorities in palliative care found seven key priority areas: 1) service models; 2) continuity of care; 3) training and education for palliative care specialists and non-specialists; 4) inequality of access; 5) communication; 6) patient preferences and experiences;

and 7) recognizing family needs (Hasson et al., 2020). Methodological challenges in conducting research in patients at the end of life (e.g. measuring and valuing outcomes) from a health economics perspective is discussed further by Round (2016).

Assisted Dying

It is very difficult to write about the cost-effectiveness of the huge ethical challenge of the issue of permitting assisted dying. Societies in different countries have taken different approaches, with the most liberal approaches taken in countries such as Switzerland, the Netherlands, and Canada. One paper of interest in this area is by Shaw and Morton (2020) who argued that consideration of economic factors should not provide the rationale for assisted dying, but rather should be a secondary societal consideration in relation to the small population that seeks assisted suicide or euthanasia. They proffered three arguments for consideration:

1. That permitting assisted dying allows consenting patients to avoid negative QALYs, enabling avoidance of suffering.

2. At a societal level, that the resources consumed by patients who are denied assisted dying could instead be used to provide additional (positive) QALYs for patients elsewhere in the health care system who wish to continue living and to improve their quality of life.

3. That organ donation may be an additional potential source of QALYs in this context.

These authors argued that denying assisted dying is a lose-lose situation for all patients (Shaw & Morton, 2020).

Early Lessons from the COVID-19 Pandemic

Between February 2020 and March 2022, the UK Government announced spending of £376 billion on the COVID-19 pandemic, including £147 billion in support for business, £89 billion in support for health and social care, £75 billion in support for other public services and emergency responses, £60 billion in support for individuals, and £5 billion for other support and operational expenditure (National Audit Office, 2022). Pre-vaccination roll-out, over 90 per cent of COVID-19-related deaths in England and Wales were in people with at least one pre-existing health condition. Mortality rates were higher in older people (ONS, 2020d). For example, the mortality rate from COVID-19 was four times higher for people aged seventy-five to seventy-nine than people aged sixty-five to sixty-nine and sixteen times higher for people aged eighty-five to eighty-nine compared to sixty-five to sixty-nine-year-olds (ONS, 2020d). Across all age groups, males had a higher risk of dying from COVID-19 than females, and this increased risk was estimated to be 70 per cent (Spiegelhalter, 2020).

The restrictions associated with the COVID-19 pandemic had a negative impact on the cognition, mental well-being and behaviour of residents in care homes (Wales COVID-19 Evidence Centre, 2021). Increased infection and prevention control procedures during the pandemic increased stress and burden among care staff as a result of increased workload and dilemmas between adhering well to infection and prevention control procedures and providing the best care for the care recipients (Wales COVID-19 Evidence Centre, 2021). During the pandemic, reduced service provision for people with dementia was a concern for dementia care professionals and people with dementia were more advanced in their symptoms once services reopened (Wales COVID-19 Evidence Centre, 2022).

The COVID-19 pandemic had a significant impact on care home residents, with 23 per cent of care home residents' deaths in England and Wales being attributed to COVID-19 between 17th March and 11th September 2020, and 26 per cent of deaths between 12th September 2020 and 2nd April 2021 (ONS, 2021b). The UK Government's early response to the pandemic was to discharge COVID-19 patients from hospitals to care homes to free up NHS capacity. The guidance for care homes was to manage residents in their rooms as much as possible as a shielding measure (British Geriatrics Society, 2020). This represented a loss of autonomy for residents and a challenge to staff to monitor residents effectively (Gordon et al., 2020). Furthermore, isolation of residents from each other and from visitors increased the risk of cognitive or functional decline (British Geriatrics Society, 2020).

A qualitative exploratory study found that at the beginning of the COVID-19 pandemic (during April to May 2020), elderly care practitioners observed loneliness, depressive symptoms, decreased food intake, increased somatic symptoms (i.e. pain), physical deterioration and, in psychogeriatric residents, rapid cognitive decline and changes in neuropsychiatric symptoms (including agitation and aggression) as a result of the restrictions in visitations (Sizoo et al., 2020). In the study of residents in a Canadian care home by Iaboni and colleagues (2020), reduced visitation and isolation measures were associated with increased levels of agitation and aggression resulting in increased drug prescriptions. In June 2021, still within the pandemic period, the UK Government updated its guidance on care home visits in England. They recommended that each resident nominate up to five named visitors for indoor visits with physical contact, with other visitors allowed for outdoor visits or visits behind windows (Department of Health and Social Care, 2021). A Belgian qualitative study by Kaelen and colleagues (2021) found that nursing home residents experienced losses of freedom, social life, autonomy, and recreational activities that deprived them of their basic psychological needs following the introduction of infection and prevention control measures such as isolation, social distancing, and reduced or paused visitation.

Summary

Factors such as place of death, company in death, cause of death, and manner of facing death play a role in determining a good death (Campbell, 2020). There is a contrast between actual place of death and expressed preference for place of death. For example, in the UK, 44 per cent of deaths occur in hospital and 29 per cent occur at home, however, only 7 per cent of people said they would choose to die in hospital and 67 per cent said they would prefer to die at home (Office for Health Improvement and Disparities, 2022; Shucksmith et al., 2013). People from lower socioeconomic groups are less likely to have a preference for dying at home and are more likely than those of a higher socioeconomic status to prefer to die in a hospital (Shucksmith et al., 2013). Advance care planning has been shown to be cost-effective and so it is important to understand the preferences of individuals while they have the capacity to make informed choices. With an ageing population, there is a need for appropriate health and social care services to be available to support people at the end of life. Research with people and their families at the end of life is challenging but can inform choice and better ways to provide such support. In the final chapter of this book we return to the concepts of well-being and well-becoming through the life-course. We reflect the content of the book and set out an agenda for diversifying health economics to provide a life-course lens on health, well-being, and well-becoming.

Curiosity Questions

- How would a shift in social norms of where we die affect the costs of the last year of life, maintaining a good quality to the care received?
- What are the most cost-effective interventions, programmes, and policies to promote or mitigate barriers to a good death for the individual and their family left behind?

References

Bajwah, S., Oluyase, A. O., Yi, D., Gao, W., Evans, C. J., Grande, G., Todd, C., Costantini, M., Murtagh, F. E., & Higginson, I. J. (2020). The effectiveness and cost-effectiveness of hospital-based specialist palliative care for adults with advanced illness and their caregivers. *Cochrane Database of Systematic Reviews*, **9**, CD012780. https://doi.org/10.1002/14651858.CD012780.pub2

Bauer, A., Dixon, J., Knapp, M., & Wittenberg, R. (2021). Exploring the cost-effectiveness of advance care planning (by taking a family carer perspective): Findings of an economic modelling study. *Health & Social Care in the Community*, **29**(4), 967–981. https://doi.org/10.1111/hsc.13131

Brennan, F. (2007). Palliative care as an international human right. *Journal of Pain and Symptom Management*, **33**(5), 494–499. https://doi.org/10.1016/j.jpainsymman.2007.02.022

Brinkman-Stoppelenburg, A., Rietjens, J. A., & Van der Heide, A. (2014). The effects of advance care planning on end-of-life care: A systematic review. *Palliative Medicine*, **28**(8), 1000–1025. https://doi.org/10.1177/0269216314526272

British Geriatrics Society. (2020, 30 March). *COVID-19: Managing the COVID-19 pandemic in care homes for older people.* https://www.bgs.org.uk/resources/covid-19-managing-the-covid-19-pandemic-in-care-homes

Brotherhood, E. V., Stott, J., Windle, G., Barker, S., Culley, S., Harding, E., Camic, P.M., Caufield, M., Ezeofor, V., Hoare, Z., McKee-Jackson, R., Roberts, J., Sharp, R., Suarez-Gonzalez, A., Sullivan, M. P., Edwards, R. T., Walton, J., Waddington, C., Winrow, E., & Crutch, S. J. (2019). Protocol for the rare dementia support impact study: RDS impact. *International Journal of Geriatric Psychiatry*, **35**(8), 833–841. https://doi.org/10.1002/gps.5253

Brumley, R., Enguidanos, S., Jamison, P., Seitz, R., Morgenstern, N., Saito, S., McIlwane, J., Hillary, K., & Gonzalez, J. (2007). Increased satisfaction with care and lower costs: Results of a randomized trial of in-home palliative care. *Journal of the American Geriatrics Society*, **55**(7), 993–1000. https://doi.org/10.1111/j.1532-5415.2007.01234.x

Buck, J., Webb, L., Moth, L., Morgan, L., & Barclay, S. (2020). Persistent inequalities in Hospice at Home provision. *BMJ Supportive and Palliative Care*, **10**(3), e23. https://doi.org/10.1136/bmjspcare-2017-001367

Campbell, S. M. (2020). Well-being and the good death. *Ethical Theory and Moral Practice*, **23**(3), 607–623. https://doi.org/10.1007/s10677-020-10101-3

Canaway, A., Al-Janabi, H., Kinghorn, P., Bailey, C., & Coast, J. (2017). Development of a measure (ICECAP-Close Person Measure) through qualitative methods to capture the benefits of end-of-life care to those close to the dying for use in economic evaluation. *Palliative Medicine*, **31**(1), 53–62. https://doi.org/10.1177/0269216316650616

Chen, E. K., Riffin, C., Reid, M. C., Adelman, R., Warmington, M., Mehta, S. S., & Pillemer, K. (2014). Why is high-quality research on palliative care so hard to do? Barriers to improved research from a survey of palliative care researchers. *Journal of Palliative Medicine*, **17**(7), 782–787. https://doi.org/10.1089/jpm.2013.0589

Clark, D. (2023, 12 May). *Death in the UK—statistics & facts.* Statista. https://www.statista.com/topics/6656/death-in-the-uk/#topicOverview

Danaei, G., Ding, E. L., Mozaffarian, D., Taylor, B., Rehm, J., Murray, C. J. L., & Ezzati, M. (2009). The preventable causes of death in the United States: Comparative risk assessment of dietary, lifestyle, and metabolic risk factors. *PLoS Medicine*, 6(4), e1000058. https://doi.org/10.1371/journal.pmed.1000058

Department of Health. (2012). *End of life care strategy fourth annual report.* https://www.gov.uk/government/publications/end-of-life-care-strategy-fourth-annual-report

Department of Health. (2016). *Our commitment to you for end of life care: The government response to the review of choice in end of life care.* https://assets.publishing.service.gov.uk/government/uploads/system/uploads/attachment_data/file/536326/choice-respo nse.pdf

Department of Health and Social Care. (2008). *End of life care strategy: Promoting high quality care for adults at the end of their life.* https://www.gov.uk/governm ent/publications/end-of-life-care-strategy-promoting-high-quality-care-for-adu lts-at-the-end-of-their-life

Department of Health and Social Care. (2021). *Guidance on care home visiting.* https://www.gov.uk/government/publications/visiting-care-homes-during-coronavirus/upd ate-on-policies-for-visiting-arrangements-in-care-homes

Detering, K. M., Hancock, A. D., Reade, M. C., & Silvester, W. (2010). The impact of advance care planning on end of life care in elderly patients: Randomised controlled trial. *BMJ*, 340, 1–9. https://doi.org/10.1136/bmj.c1345

Diernberger, K., Shinkins, B., Hall, P., Kaasa, S., & Fallon, M. (2021). Incompatible: End-of-life care and health economics. *BMJ Supportive & Palliative Care*, 11(3), 296–298. https://doi.org/10.1136/bmjspcare-2020-002388

Dixon, J., King, D., & Knapp, M. (2019). Advance care planning in England: Is there an association with place of death? Secondary analysis of data from the National Survey of Bereaved People. *BMJ Supportive and Palliative Care*, 9(3), 316–325. https://doi.org/10.1136/bmjspcare-2015-000971

Gade, G., Venohr, I., Conner, D., McGrady, K., Beane, J., Richardson, R. H., Williams, M.P., Liberson, M., Blum, M., & Penna, R. D. (2008). Impact of an inpatient palliative care team: A randomized controlled trial. *Journal of Palliative Medicine*, 11(2), 180–190. doi.org/10.1089/jpm.2007.0055

Gordon, A. L., Goodman, C., Achterberg, W., Barker, R. O., Burns, E., Hanratty, B., Martin, F. C., Meyer, J., O'Neill, D., Schols, J., & Spilsbury, K. (2020). Commentary: COVID in care homes—challenges and dilemmas in healthcare delivery. *Age and Ageing*, 49(5), 701–705. https://doi.org/10.1093/ageing/afaa113

Hart, J. T. (1971). The inverse care law. *The Lancet*, 297(7696), 405–412. https://doi.org/10.1016/S0140-6736(71)92410-X

Hasson, F., Nicholson, E., Muldrew, D., Bamidele, O., Payne, S., & McIlfatrick, S. (2020). International palliative care research priorities: A systematic review. *BMC Palliative Care*, 19(1), 1–16. https://doi.org/10.1186/s12904-020-0520-8

Higginson, I. J., Daveson, B. A., Morrison, R. S., Yi, D., Meier, D., Smith, M., Ryan, K., McQuillan, R., Johnston, B. M., Normand, C., on behalf of BuildCARE. (2017). Social and clinical determinants of preferences and their achievement at the end of life: Prospective cohort study of older adults receiving palliative care in three countries. *BMC Geriatrics*, 17(1), 1–14. https://doi.org/10.1186/s12877-017-0648-4

Higginson, I. J., Evans, C. J., Grande, G., Preston, N., Morgan, M., McCrone, P., Lewis, P., Fayers, P., Harding, R., Hotopf, M., Murray, S. A., Benalia, H., Gysels, M., Farquhar, M., & Todd, C. (2013). Evaluating complex interventions in end of life care: The

MORECare Statement on good practice generated by a synthesis of transparent expert consultations and systematic reviews. *BMC Medicine*, **11**(1), 1–11. https://doi.org/10.1186/1741-7015-11-111

Higginson, I. J., McCrone, P., Hart, S. R., Burman, R., Silber, E., & Edmonds, P. M. (2009). Is short-term palliative care cost-effective in multiple sclerosis? A randomized phase II trial. *Journal of Pain and Symptom Management*, **38**(6), 816–826. https://doi.org/10.1016/j.jpainsymman.2009.07.002

Hospice UK. (2018). *Hospice accounts: Analysis of the accounts of UK charitable hospices for the year ended 31 March 2017*. https://hukstage-bucket.s3.eu-west-2.amazonaws.com/s3fs-public/2022-06/hospice-accounts-report-2018_web.pdf

Hospice UK. (2020). *Hospice UK facts and figures*. https://www.hospiceuk.org/about-hospice-care/media-centre/facts-and-figures

Hospice UK. (2021). *Hospice accounts: Analysis of the accounts of UK charitable hospices for the year ended 31 March 2020*. https://hukstage-bucket.s3.eu-west-2.amazonaws.com/s3fs-public/2022-05/hospice-accounts-report-2021.pdf

Hughes, N. M., Noyes, J., Eckley, L., & Pritchard, T. (2019). What do patients and family-caregivers value from hospice care? A systematic mixed studies review. *BMC Palliative Care*, **18**(1), 1–13. https://doi.org/10.1186/s12904-019-0401-1

Iaboni, A., Cockburn, A., Marcil, M., Rodrigues, K., Marshall, C., Garcia, M. A., Quirt, H., Reynolds, K.B., Keren, R., & Flint, A. J. (2020). Achieving safe, effective, and compassionate quarantine or isolation of older adults with dementia in nursing homes. *The American Journal of Geriatric Psychiatry*, **28**(8), 835–838. https://doi.10.1016/j.jagp.2020.04.025

Imison, C., Poteliakhoff, E., & Thompson, J. (2012). *Older people and emergency bed use. Exploring variation*. The King's Fund. https://www.kingsfund.org.uk/sites/default/files/field/field_publication_file/older-people-and-emergency-bed-use-aug-2012.pdf

Jack, B. A., Mitchell, T. K., Cope, L. C., & O'Brien, M. R. (2016). Supporting older people with cancer and life-limiting conditions dying at home: A qualitative study of patient and family caregiver experiences of Hospice at Home care. *Journal of Advanced Nursing*, **72**(9), 2162–2172. https://doi.org/10.1111/jan.12983

Johnston, B. M., McCauley, R., McQuillan, R., Rabbitte, M., Honohan, C., Mockler, D., Thomas, S., & May, P. (2020). Effectiveness and cost-effectiveness of out-of-hours palliative care: A systematic review. *HRB Open Research*, **3**(9), 1–13. https://doi.org/10.12688/hrbopenres.13006.1

Kaelen, S., van den Boogaard, W., Pellecchia, U., Spiers, S., De Cramer, C., Demaegd, G., Fouqueray, E., Van den Bergh, R., Goublomme, S., Decroo, T., Quinet, M., Van Hoof, E., & Draguez, B. (2021). How to bring residents' psychosocial well-being to the heart of the fight against Covid-19 in Belgian nursing homes—a qualitative study. *PLoS One*, **16**(3), e0249098. https://doi.org/10.1371/journal.pone.0249098

Karlawish, J. H. T. (2003). Conducting research that involves subjects at the end of life who are unable to give consent. *Journal of Pain and Symptom Management*, **25**(4), S14–S24. https://doi.org/10.1016/S0885-3924(03)00098-8

Kars, M. C., Van Thiel, G. J. M. W., Van Der Graaf, R., Moors, M., De Graeff, A., & Van Delden, J. J. M. (2016). A systematic review of reasons for gatekeeping in palliative care research. *Palliative Medicine*, **30**(6), 533–548. https://doi.org/10.1177/0269216315616759

Keeble, E., Parker, S. G., Arora, S., Neuburger, J., Duncan, R., Kingston, A., Hanratty, B., Jagger, C., Robinson, L., & Kirkwood, T. (2019). Frailty, hospital use and mortality in the older population: Findings from the Newcastle 85+ study. *Age and Ageing*, **48**(6), 797–802. https://doi.org/10.1093/ageing/afz094

Keeble, E., Scobie, S., & Hutchings, R. (2022). *Support at the end of life: The role of hospice services across the UK*. Nuffield Trust. https://www.nuffieldtrust.org.uk/files/2022-06/hospice-services-web-1-.pdf

Kinghan, D., Carson, P. S., Flanagan, A., & Megaw, M. (2020). *Statistics on community care for adults in Northern Ireland*. https://www.health-ni.gov.uk/sites/default/files/publications/health/cc-adults-ni-19-20_0.pdf

Kinghorn, P., & Coast, J. (2018) Assessing the capability to experience a 'good death': A qualitative study to directly elicit expert views on a new supportive care measure grounded in Sen's capability approach. *PLoS One*, **13**(2), e0193181. https://doi.org/10.1371/journal.pone.0193181

Krau, S. D. (2016). The difference between palliative care and end of life care: More than semantics. *Nursing Clinics of North America*, **51**(3). https://doi.org/10.1016/j.cnur.2016.07.002

National Association for Hospice at Home. (2020). *What is hospice at home?* https://www.nahh.org.uk/about-hospice-care/what-is-hospice-at-home

National Audit Office. (2008, 26 November). *End of life care*. https://www.nao.org.uk/reports/end-of-life-care/

National Audit Office. (2022, 23 June). *COVID-19 cost tracker*. https://www.nao.org.uk/covid-19/cost-tracker/

National Health Service. (2018). *Hospice care*. https://www.nhs.uk/conditions/end-of-life-care/hospice-care/

National Institute for Health and Care Excellence (2013). *Guide to the methods of technology appraisal 2013* (PMG9). https://www.nice.org.uk/process/pmg9/chapter/foreword

National Institute for Health and Care Excellence. (2015). *Care of dying adults in the last days of life* (NG31). https://www.nice.org.uk/guidance/ng31

National Institute for Health and Care Excellence. (2018). *Decision-making and mental capacity* (NG108). https://www.nice.org.uk/guidance/ng108

National Institute for Health and Care Excellence. (2019a). *End of life care for adults: Service delivery* (NG142). https://www.nice.org.uk/guidance/ng142

National Institute for Health and Care Excellence. (2019b). *End of life care for infants, children and young people with life-limiting conditions: Planning and management* (NG61). https://www.nice.org.uk/guidance/ng61

National Institute for Health and Care Excellence. (2022). *NICE health technology evaluations: The manual* (PMG36). https://www.nice.org.uk/process/pmg36

Office for Health Improvement and Disparities. (2022). *Palliative and end of life care profiles*. https://fingertips.phe.org.uk/profile/end-of-life/data#page/1

Office for National Statistics. (2020a, 27 March). *Leading causes of death, UK: 2001 to 2018*. https://www.ons.gov.uk/peoplepopulationandcommunity/healthandsocialcare/causesofdeath/articles/leadingcausesofdeathuk/2001to2018

Office for National Statistics. (2020b). *Deaths registered in England and Wales*. https://www.ons.gov.uk/peoplepopulationandcommunity/birthsdeathsandmarriages/deaths/datasets/deathsregisteredinenglandandwalesseriesdrreferencetables

Office for National Statistics. (2020c, 8 September). *Care home and non-care home populations used in the Deaths involving COVID-19 in the care sector article, England and Wales*. https://www.ons.gov.uk/peoplepopulationandcommunity/birthsdeathsandmarriages/deaths/adhocs/12215carehomeandnoncarehomepopulationsusedinthedeathsinvolvingcovid19inthecaresectorarticleenglandandwales

Office for National Statistics. (2020d, 17 July). *Deaths involving COVID-19, England and Wales: Deaths occurring in June 2020*. https://www.ons.gov.uk/peoplepopulationandcommunity/birthsdeathsandmarriages/deaths/bulletins/deathsinvolvingcovid19englandandwales/deathsoccurringinjune2020

Office for National Statistics. (2021a). *Deaths registered in England and Wales*. https://www.ons.gov.uk/peoplepopulationandcommunity/birthsdeathsandmarriages/deaths/datasets/deathsregisteredinenglandandwalesseriesdrreferencetables

Office for National Statistics. (2021b, 11 May). *Deaths involving COVID-19 in the care sector, England and Wales: Deaths registered between week ending 20 March 2020 and week ending 2 April 2021*. https://www.ons.gov.uk/peoplepopulationandcommunity/birthsdeathsandmarriages/deaths/articles/deathsinvolvingcovid19inthecaresectorenglandandwales/deathsregisteredbetweenweekending20march2020andweekending2april2021

Office for National Statistics. (2022a, 7 March). *Avoidable mortality in the UK: 2020*. https://www.ons.gov.uk/peoplepopulationandcommunity/healthandsocialcare/causesofdeath/bulletins/avoidablemortalityinenglandandwales/2020

Office for National Statistics. (2022b, 22 March). *Excess deaths in England and Wales: March 2020 to December 2021*. https://www.ons.gov.uk/peoplepopulationandcommunity/birthsdeathsandmarriages/deaths/articles/excessdeathsinenglandandwales/march2020todecember2021

Office for National Statistics. (2022c, 28 March). *Socioeconomic inequalities in avoidable mortality in England: 2020*. https://www.ons.gov.uk/peoplepopulationandcommunity/birthsdeathsandmarriages/deaths/bulletins/socioeconomicinequalitiesinavoidablemortalityinengland/2020

Office for National Statistics. (2022d, 30 May). *Care homes and estimating the self-funding population, England: 2021 to 2022*. https://www.ons.gov.uk/peoplepopulationandcommunity/healthandsocialcare/socialcare/articles/carehomesandestimatingtheselffundingpopulationengland/2021to2022

Office for National Statistics. (2022e, 22 November). *Deaths of care home residents, England and Wales: 2021*. https://www.ons.gov.uk/peoplepopulationandcommunity/birthsdeathsandmarriages/deaths/bulletins/deathsinthecaresectorenglandandwales/2021

Office for National Statistics. (2023, 11 April). *Death registration summary statistics, England and Wales: 2022*. https://www.ons.gov.uk/peoplepopulationandcommunity/birthsdeathsandmarriages/deaths/articles/deathregistrationsummarystatisticsenglandandwales/2022

Public Health England. (2017a). *The role of care homes in end of life care briefing 1: Care home bed provision and potential end of life care need in people aged 75 or older in England*. https://assets.publishing.service.gov.uk/government/uploads/system/uploads/

attachment_data/file/828120/Briefing_1_Care_home_provision_and_potential_end_o
f_life_care.pdf

Public Health England. (2017b). *The role of care homes in end of life care briefing 2: Place
and cause of death for permanent and temporary residents of care homes.* https://assets.
publishing.service.gov.uk/government/uploads/system/uploads/attachment_data/file/
828122/Briefing_2_Place_and_cause_of_death_for_permanent_and_temporary_resi
dents_of_care_homes.pdf

Public Health England. (2018). *Atlas of variation for palliative and end of life care in
England.* https://fingertips.phe.org.uk/profile/atlas-of-variation

Public Health Scotland. (2022, 9 November). *Care home census far adults in
Scotland: Statistics for 2011 to 2021.* https://www.publichealthscotland.scot/publicati
ons/care-home-census-for-adults-in-scotland/care-home-census-for-adults-in-scotl
and-statistics-for-2011-to-2021-part-1/

Round, J. (Ed.). (2016). *Care at the end of life: An economic perspective.* Springer. https://doi.
org/10.1007/978-3-319-28267-1

Royal College of Nursing Wales. (2021). *Nursing in care homes.* https://www.rcn.org.uk/-/
media/royal-college-of-nursing/documents/countries-and-regions/wales/2021/care-
home-report.pdf

Salutin, G. (2023). *Giving back: How to foster a stronger and more resilient charity sector.*
Social Market Foundation. https://www.smf.co.uk/wp-content/uploads/2023/04/Giv
ing-back-April-2023.pdf

Shaw, D., & Morton, A. (2020). Counting the cost of denying assisted dying. *Clinical Ethics,*
15(2), 65–70. https://doi.org/https://doi.org/10.1177/1477750920907996

Shucksmith, J., Carlebach, S., & Whittaker, V. (2013). *British Social Attitudes 30 survey
module on attitudes to end of life care and dying.* National Centre Social Research. www.
dyingmatters.org/sites/default/files/BSA30_Full_Report.pdf

Sizoo, E. M., Monnier, A. A., Bloemen, M., Hertogh, C. M., & Smalbrugge, M. (2020).
Dilemmas with restrictive visiting policies in Dutch nursing homes during the COVID-
19 pandemic: A qualitative analysis of an open-ended questionnaire with elderly care
physicians. *Journal of the American Medical Directors Association,* 21(12), 1774–1781.
https://doi.org/10.1016/j.jamda.2020.10.024

Sleeman, K. E., Davies, J. M., Verne, J., Gao, W., & Higginson, I. J. (2016). The changing
demographics of inpatient hospice death: Population-based cross-sectional study in
England, 1993–2012. *Palliative Medicine,* 30(1), 45–53. https://doi.org/10.1177/02692
16315585064

Smith, S., Brick, A., O'Hara, S., & Normand, C. (2014). Evidence on the cost and cost-
effectiveness of palliative care: A literature review. *Palliative Medicine,* 28(2), 130–150.
https://doi.org/10.1177/0269216313493466

Spiegelhalter, D. (2020). Use of 'normal' risk to improve understanding of dangers of covid-
19. *BMJ,* 370, m3259. https://doi.org/10.1136/bmj.m3259

Springett. A. (2015, October). *Economic assessment for the Six Steps+ End of Life Care
Programme.* St Wilfrid's Hospice, Chichester, West Sussex. https://www.rcn.org.uk/-/
media/royal-college-of-nursing/documents/professional-development/research/inno
vations/burdetters-case-studies/angela-springett-case-study.pdf

Springett, A. (2017). Practice improvement as a result of an end of life care programme for
care homes. *Nursing Older People,* 29(3), 23–27. https://doi.org/10.7748/nop.2017.e890

Stjernswärd, J., Foley, K. M., & Ferris, F. D. (2007). The public health strategy for palliative care. *Journal of Pain and Symptom Management*, 33(5), 486–493. https://doi.org/10.1016/j.jpainsymman.2007.02.016

Sutton, E. J., & Coast, J. (2014). Development of a supportive care measure for economic evaluation of end-of-life care using qualitative methods. *Palliative Medicine*, 28(2), 151–157. https://doi.org/10.1177/0269216313489368

Titmuss, R. M., & Seldon, A. (1968). Commitment to welfare. *Social Policy & Administration*, 2(3), 196–200. https://doi.org/10.1111/j.1467-9515.1968.tb00093.x

United Kingdom Government. (2023, 17 August). *Deaths in the United Kingdom*. https://coronavirus.data.gov.uk/details/deaths

Wales COVID-19 Evidence Centre. (2021). *Have infection control and prevention measures resulted in any adverse outcomes for care home and domiciliary care residents and staff?* (RR_00018). http://www.primecentre.wales/resources/RR/Clean/RR00018_Wales_COVID-19_Evidence_Centre_Rapid_Review_Infection_control_and_prevention_measures_care_homes_November-2021.pdf

Wales COVID-19 Evidence Centre. (2022). *A rapid evidence summary indicating the evidence of the inverse care law in social care in Wales and has this been exacerbated by the COVID-19 pandemic?* (RES00019). http://www.primecentre.wales/resources/RES/RES00019-Wales_COVID-19_Evidence_Centre-Inverse_Care_Law_in_Social_Care-February_2022.pdf

World Health Organization. (2020, 5 August). *Palliative care fact sheet*. https://www.who.int/news-room/fact-sheets/detail/palliative-care

Ziwary, S. R., Samad, D., Johnson, C. D., & Edwards, R. T. (2017). Impact of place of residence on place of death in Wales: An observational study. *BMC Palliative Care*, 16(72), 1–16. https://doi.org/10.1186/s12904-017-0261-5

Chapter 8

Diversifying Health Economics to Provide a Life-course Lens on Health, Well-being, and Well-becoming

Rhiannon T. Edwards, Catherine L. Lawrence, and Abraham Makanjuola

Introduction

This final chapter of the book revisits concepts of well-being and well-becoming, how they are beginning to be used in health economics, and puts forward a range of ideas for future research and policy support. The author of *Doughnut economics*, Kate Raworth (2017), has argued that a picture is worth a thousand words. To this end, we draw the reader's attention to 'The well-being and well-becoming wheel' infographic (see Figure 8.1) (Edwards, 2022). This infographic widens the evaluative space, both in terms of breadth and time horizon, in the design, conduct, and reporting of economic evaluations, particularly of public health and preventative interventions.

We were struck listening to the Minister for Health and Social Care in Wales say that they would like to shift the emphasis of the National Health Service (NHS) and social care policy from treatment to prevention, but that there is 'no money' to do so. In order to unleash the power of prevention to support well-being and well-becoming across the life-course, there is a necessary step for health economists to provide evidence of where rational disinvestment could take place across health and social care (Donaldson et al., 2010). This may seem an impossibility at a time when health and social care systems are overstretched. However, systems thinking may help to release such resources. In England, savings of £500 million annually have been identified through managed reduction of dependency-forming medicines (e.g. antidepressants, painkillers, and sleeping pills; Davies et al., 2022). Though services to support patients through this process would incur costs themselves, this provides an example of where it

Rhiannon T. Edwards, Catherine L. Lawrence, and Abraham Makanjuola, *Diversifying Health Economics to Provide a Life-course Lens on Health, Well-being, and Well-becoming* In: *Health Economics of Well-being and Well-becoming across the Life-course*. Edited by: Rhiannon T. Edwards and Catherine L. Lawrence, Oxford University Press.

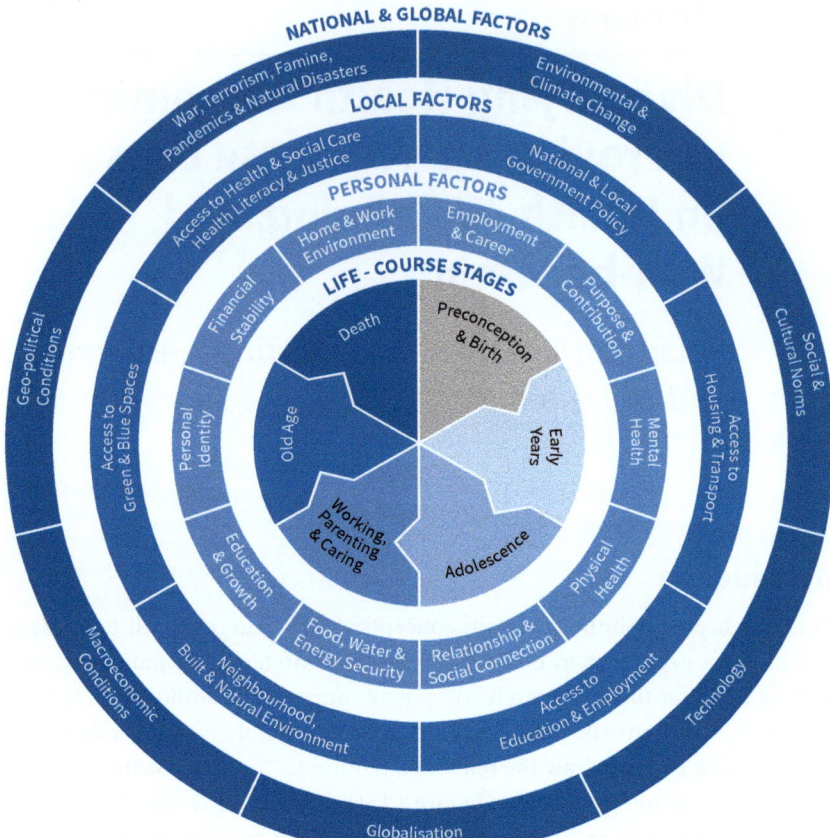

Figure 8.1 The well-being and well-becoming wheel
Reproduced from Edwards, R. T. (2022). Well-being and well-becoming through the life-course in public health economics research and policy: A new infographic. *Frontiers in Public Health, 10*, 1–8. https://doi.org/10.3389/fpubh.2022.1035260. Licence: Creative Commons BY 3.0 IGO.

may be possible to release resources to be moved into prevention. Along with this is the realization that health economists are probably more in the business of providing evidence that is relevant to the redistribution of health than the maximization of health. This is against the backdrop that the NHS itself has, since 1948, been probably the largest in-kind redistributor of benefits from the wealthy to those worse-off in society. There is no doubt that this redistribution is currently threatened with ever-shrinking government services and more and more responsibility is shifted to individuals, families, and communities.

Where the fiscal space (i.e. what countries are able or politically prepared to spend on health and social care) is limited, there is little chance of making the paradigm shift from 'cure' to 'prevention' led by central services. There is a role for health economists to show the potential benefits of 'disinvestment' in low value care, however it is defined (i.e. care that is not cost-effective). More seriously is the need to be open about where medicine actually does harm, known as 'iatrogenesis' (Illich, 1982). These two actions could help show where resources could be freed up for investment in prevention through the life-course to promote better health and well-being, and well-becoming.

Some Reflections on This Book

'Well-being' in the concept of population health can be thought of as 'the balance point between an individual's resource pool and the challenges faced' (Dodge et al., 2012, p. 230). The World Health Organization (WHO) has promoted the concept of well-being since 1948 (Almond & Currie, 2011). There is still little consensus as to how it should be measured across many academic disciplines, including health economics, behavioural economics, and psychology, and the term is often used interchangeably with terms like 'happiness' and 'health-related quality of life' (Medvedev & Landhuis, 2018). Notably, however, HM Treasury's 'Wellbeing guidance for appraisal: Supplementary Green Book guidance' (Green Book), updated in 2021, has introduced the use of 'well-being adjusted life years' (WELLBYs) based on life satisfaction measurement (HM Treasury, 2021). In psychology and behavioural economics research, there is a distinction made between 'hedonic well-being' and 'eudaimonic well-being' (Ryan & Deci, 2001). The hedonic viewpoint is based on the notion that increased pleasure and avoidance of pain leads to happiness (Kahneman et al., 1999). The eudaimonic viewpoint is defined more broadly to incorporate dynamic processes such as self-actualization and the degree to which a person is fully functioning in society (Martela & Sheldon, 2019; Ryff & Singer, 1998). Well-being is often made up of multiple components and is normative or subjective.

'Well-becoming' can be thought of as 'our multitude of life-journeys towards meaning and purposefulness, not some steady-state of managed contentment' (Kane, 2007). As discussed in Chapter 1, the term well-becoming is not new, but is not a term we routinely use in our everyday language or in research in public health and health economics. Where it has appeared, it has predominantly been in early years research, for example, in research surrounding child development (Cassidy, 2017; Nsamenang, 2010). In an education context, it has been used to carefully distinguish between how we help children in 'being well' in the present and in well-becoming in shaping their future 'being' and hence opportunities. For example, 'in contrast to the immediacy of well-being, well-becoming describes a future focus (i.e. preparing children to be productive and happy adults, and to avoid social exclusion)' (Ben-Arieh & Frønes, 2011, p. 470). Biggeri and Santi (2012) discussed the concept of well-becoming in terms of system change in education to promote flourishing through a capability model aimed to support creativity, critical thinking, and care. In the field of health economics, the only place we have found reference to it is in the development of capability measures through the life-course (Mitchell et al., 2021; see Table 1.4, Chapter 1, in this book). In mainstream economics, the financial benefits of investing in well-becoming are found in the work of James Heckman, a Chicago Nobel Prize-winning economist (Heckman, 2008). Heckman demonstrated the lifetime benefits of investing in high-quality preschool care and the mitigating influence this can have on those with the worst start in life. Heckman has re-vised downwards some of his original estimates, but his arguments are still very powerful. Well-becoming is based on the concept of assets-based public health, which is concerned with identifying protective factors that support health and well-being in communities (Morgan & Ziglio, 2007).

It has been argued that concern for well-becoming should reach as far as fu-ture generations (Falkenberg, 2015). This links the concern for well-being with the concern for sustainable development and sustainable living (Falkenberg, 2015). For policymakers and public health economists here in the United Kingdom (UK), this attunes closely to the Well-being of Future Generations Act passed in Wales in 2015 (Welsh Government, 2015). In a later paper, Falkenberg (2019) introduced the WB2-Framework for well-being and well-becoming and posited five components of well-being and well-becoming in an educational setting: 1) having agentic capabilities linked to human needs; 2) experiencing situational opportunities to engage one's agentic capabilities; 3) enjoying life; 4) living a meaningful life; and 5) experiencing personal and communal con-nections that contribute to one's well-being and well-becoming. Agentic refers to an individual's power to control his or her own goals, actions, and destiny. In the United States (US) in 2021, the Youth Transition Funders Group made re-commendations for investing in the well-being and well-becoming of America's young people (defined as the onset of puberty to the mid-twenties; Langford et al., 2021). They referred to well-being and well-becoming of young people in an equitable, inclusive, and holistic (whole person, whole life) context and offered a series of recommendations to transform public systems and commu-nities to nurture and enhance lifelong well-being for vulnerable young people as they make the transition into adulthood. Again, from a UK public health economics perspective, this echoes emerging work on adverse childhood ex-periences (ACEs) and their lifetime costs to both the individual and society (Bellis et al., 2019). The ethos of health economics is predicated on a societal goal of health gain, which implies health gain or reducing health losses from where we are now. In the same way, the concept of well-becoming is predicated on a goal of improving well-being (or minimizing potential well-being losses) in future life-course stages. It is up to societies at a systems level to take an instrumental approach to enabling good life-course health and well-being opportunity architecture.

The Well-being and Well-becoming Wheel Infographic

In Chapter 2, we looked at Maslow's (1943, 2017) hierarchy of needs model (see Figure 2.1) and the Dahlgren-Whitehead (2006) rainbow model of health determinants (see Figure 2.2). These models appear as very static representations of human need and the wider determinants of health. They do not show any movement through the life-course. 'The well-being and well-becoming wheel' infographic (see Figure 8.1), designed by the lead author of this chapter (Rhiannon T. Edwards), is a more recent infographic which redefines well-being as a process of growth through life, articulated as well-becoming (Edwards, 2022). This infographic shows movement through the life-course at its centre, with concentric rings summarizing personal, local, and national and global factors that have an impact on well-being and well-becoming of individuals through the life-course. Of note is the inclusion of death, which is a topic often avoided. The infographic reflects an underlying concept of 'the wheel of life', a cyclic representation of life found on the walls of Tibetan Buddhist temples and monasteries (Dalai Lama XIV Bstan-'dzin-rgya-mtsho, 2015). The choice of the life stages in the infographic came from a review of existing models in the literature (Bibby & Lovell, 2018; Campbell, 2020; Findlay et al., 2021; Ross et al., 2020; United Nations Children's Fund (UNICEF), 2007; WHO, 2011). This infographic complements the work of Raworth who developed the concept of doughnut economics, a model of human well-being which recognizes that well-being depends on enabling every person to lead a life of dignity and opportunity, while safeguarding the integrity of Earth's life-supporting systems (Raworth, 2017).

In 2018, The Health Foundation put forward a 'road map' of what makes us healthy, referring to factors such as: good work; our surroundings; money and resources; housing; education and skills; the food we eat; transport; and family, friends, and communities (Bibby & Lovell, 2018). This road map helped shape the inner ring, labelled 'personal factors', in 'The well-being and well-becoming wheel' infographic (see Figure 8.1). The second concentric ring on the infographic, labelled as 'local factors', was informed by a number of models of the factors that influence well-being (e.g. Campbell, 2020; Findlay et al., 2021; Ross, 2020; UNICEF, 2007; WHO, 2011). This infographic also reflects the work of Paul Dolan (2014) who described happiness as experiences of pleasure and purpose over time. Neighbourhoods are explicitly mentioned in the infographic to reflect the emphasis placed on neighbourhood environments as key determinants of the health and life expectancy gradient by Michael Marmot and colleagues in the reports 'Fair society, healthy lives: The Marmot review' and 'Health equity in England: The Marmot review 10 years on' (Marmot et al., 2010, 2020). The third concentric ring in the infographic reflects national and global factors that determine or have an impact on well-being and well-becoming through the life-course. These are: environmental and climate change; social and cultural norms; technology; globalization; macroeconomic conditions; geo-political conditions; and war, terrorism, famine, pandemics, and natural disasters.

Health economists in the field of public health have a crucial role given the relatively short time horizon of politics and local planning to provide evidence of both short-term and longer-term costs and outcomes of using resources in different ways to address population health priorities (Edwards & McIntosh, 2019). A life-course lens on well-being and well-becoming applied to health economics research routinely may in time help to shift the focus of policy further towards commitment to a prevention agenda. It is hoped that 'The well-being and well-becoming wheel' infographic can be a useful addition to emerging debate. The infographic does not attempt to convey directions of causality or feedback loops, whilst it recognizes that these are complex and many. Neither does it attempt to convey the fact that the central life-course stages can sometimes be overlapping and are very different from individual to individual. Instead, it attempts to convey the concepts of flow, growth, and well-becoming through life as a basis for how we approach the design of public health interventions, evaluate their effectiveness and cost-effectiveness, and set overarching priorities for public spending (Edwards & McIntosh, 2019).

Some Reflections on the Current Use of a Life-course Approach to Well-being and Well-becoming in Health Economics

Health economics has evolved over the last sixty years within a medical, evidence-based model of health. Within this medical model of health, the National Institute for Health and Care Excellence (NICE; 2013, 2022) has promoted the use of a lifetime horizon in health technology assessment in its reference case for the evaluation of cost-effectiveness. Most economic evaluation studies are of single interventions which form part of pathways of care for patients and are treatment or cure focused. The application of health economics to public health requires a far broader perspective of analysis with which to view costs and outcomes, and a far more diverse toolbox of methods of analysis spanning cost-benefit analysis (CBA) and social return on investment (SROI) analysis through to econometric modelling at a population level. Hence, just as there has been a move to a more socioeconomic conceptualization of health, we are amongst other health economists who have aligned themselves with such a paradigm shift in health economics (Edwards, 2001). This has been in terms of public health economics (Edwards & McIntosh, 2019) and in terms of addressing equity considerations in cost-effectiveness analysis (CEA) (Cookson et al., 2020).

As a challenge to the quality-adjusted life year (QALY) used by NICE, there is a programme of work developing in the capability paradigm of outcome measurement in health economics. This centres around a framework based on conceiving capabilities as evolving across the life-course (Mitchell et al., 2021). Concerning children and young people, the term 'well-being capability' is used. There is definitely a synergy of ideas evolving and the need for expanding the evaluative space beyond health functioning towards broader capabilities is very relevant to our understanding of well-being and well-becoming. The capability movement in outcome measurement in health economics is addressing the challenge of measuring outcomes within a life-course model. This approach allows for the development of an economic evaluation framework that places different capabilities at the centre of attention depending on where an individual is at in their life-course trajectory (Mitchell et al., 2021). Deidda and colleagues (2022) provided a useful example of a CEA of a public health prevention intervention which used both QALYs and well-being capabilities in the area of reducing sedentary behaviour across four European countries. It is still useful to have evidence of the cost per QALY of preventative interventions as this allows for comparison with the cost per QALY of new medicines routinely funded by the UK NHS.

At a policy level, the life-course approach to dynamic microsimulation modelling can support long-term thinking in the development and evaluation of government policy particularly with respect to the early years. Skarda and colleagues (2021) presented such an example of a dynamic microsimulation model for childhood policy analysis that models developmental, economic, social, and health outcomes from birth to death for each child in the Millennium Cohort Study (MCS) in England, together with public costs and a summary well-being measure. The model draws on observational data from the MCS focusing on health, conduct disorder, mortality, health-related quality of life, public costs, and a general well-being metric. The paper includes a discussion of the shortcomings of unweighted benefit cost analysis and alternatives including utilitarian and prioritarian approaches to economic evaluation based on explicitly individual well-being and social welfare functions (Cookson et al., 2020).

It may be that it is not single cost-effectiveness studies that have the biggest impact on shifting emphasis from 'cure to prevention', but rather the availability of a growing body of evidence on cost-effectiveness and return on investment (ROI) that effectively shifts thinking in political circles towards a longer time horizon for policy. This was perhaps encapsulated as far back as 1977 when Carol Weiss, an American scholar of education and policy analysis, wrote:

> the major use of social research is not the application of specific data to specific decisions. Rather, government decision-makers tend to use research indirectly, as a source of ideas, information, and orientations to the world. Although the process is not easily discernible, over time it may have profound effects on policy. Even research that challenges current values and political feasibilities is judged useful by decision makers. (Weiss, 1977, p. 531)

Another approach in health economics which could be characterized by a life-course approach is the calculation of costs of 'late intervention' in childhood problems. Chowdry and Fitzsimons (2016) estimated the financial sum spent at local authority level across England and Wales as a result of late intervention in early childhood problems. Of the total annual spend of £16.6 billion in 2016/2017 prices, £6.4 billion was spent by local government (39 per cent); £3.7 billion was spent by the NHS (22 per cent); £2.7 billion was spent by the Department for Work and Pensions (16 per cent); £1.6 billion was spent by the police (10 per cent); £1.5 billion was spent by the criminal justice system (9 per cent); and £655 million was spent by education (4 per cent).

Marmot has argued that: 'Given the attack on science by politicians of bad faith, it is important to recognize that epidemiology and public health have a crucial role to play in providing evidence to improve health of society and reduce inequalities' (Marmot, 2017, p. 537). In the same spirit, health economists in the field of public health have an equally crucial role, given the relatively short time horizon of politics and local planning, to provide evidence of both short-term and longer-term costs and outcomes of using resources in different ways to address population health priorities (Edwards & McIntosh, 2019). The need for balanced evidence on the likely costs and benefits of precision public health is an example of where health economists can take a population view of where scarce resources could and should be targeted. The use of data to guide interventions that benefit populations more efficiently is a strategy we call precision public health (Dowell et al., 2016). There is a growing interest in the use of biomarkers, genetics, and epigenetics at a population level in order to stratify the population as to who could benefit from which preventative interventions in order to, for example, delay dementia and other conditions that affect health-related quality of life and premature mortality. On the one hand, there is a danger that we are returning to a medical model of health; on the other hand, if such targeting can support public policy and co-production of prevention and lifestyle choices, precision public health may have a lot to offer. A report by the Organisation for Economic Co-operation and Development (OECD) called for an increase proportion internationally of gross domestic product (GDP) of around 1.4 per cent to be directed to funding prevention over and above treatment in health systems (Morgan & James, 2022). This is as a precaution of readiness in the event of a further pandemic and in recognition of 80 per cent of chronic health problems, such as premature heart disease, stroke, and diabetes, being largely preventable (WHO, 2005). A life-course lens on well-being and well-becoming may in time help to shift the focus of policy further towards commitment to a prevention agenda.

Example of a Life-course Stage Approach to Public Health Prevention—Dementia

Livingston and colleagues (2020), in a Lancet Commission report, set out twelve potentially modifiable risk factors for dementia. Table 8.1 shows what percentage of prevalence of dementia could be reduced by eliminating twelve risk factors across the life-course. These risk factors are: limited or less education; hearing loss; traumatic brain injury; hypertension; alcohol (>21 units per week); obesity; smoking; depression; social isolation; physical inactivity; air pollution; and diabetes. This report used three life-course stages and relates the above risk factors to life, midlife, and later life. Overall, Livingston and colleagues concluded that 40 per cent of risk factors may be modifiable earlier in the life-course, while 60 per cent are at present unknown.

Table 8.1 Modifiable risk factors for dementia by life stage

Life stage	Risk factor	Percentage reduction in dementia prevalence if risk factor is eliminated (%)
Early life	Less education	7
Midlife	Hearing loss	8
	Traumatic brain injury	3
	Hypertension	2
	Alcohol >21 units per week	1
	Obesity	1
Later life	Smoking	5
	Depression	4
	Social isolation	4
	Physical inactivity	2
	Air pollution	2
	Diabetes	1
Sum of potentially modifiable risk factors		40
Unknown risk factors		60

Adapted from Livingston, G., Huntley, J., Sommerlad, A., Ames, D., Ballard, C., Banerjee, S., Brayne, C., Burns, A., Cohen-Mansfield, J., Cooper, C., Costafreda, S. G., Dias, A., Fox, N., Gitlin, L. N., Howard, R., Kales, H. C., Kivimäki, M., Larson, E. B., Ogunniyi, A., . . . Mukadam, N. (2020). Dementia prevention, intervention, and care: 2020 report of the Lancet Commission. *The Lancet*, *396*(10248), 413–446. https://doi.org/10.1016/S0140-6736(20)30367-6 Copyright © 2020, with permission from Elsevier.

The Advent of Personalized Prevention, Precision Public Health, and Population Pharmacogenomics

The next twenty years will see the roll-out of scientific advance in the adoption of routine testing for biomarkers that make it possible to predict which people are at risk of developing future diseases and disabilities with associated premature mortality (e.g. dementia). Developments in pharmacogenomics mean we will know which patients will respond positively or negatively to which medicines (Magavern et al., 2021). What does all this mean for health economists working in the field of prevention, public health, and well-being economics? The premise of health economics, developed in the UK, has been one of producing evidence on cost-effectiveness to support policy and commissioning in a predominantly publicly financed health care system. Personalized medicine is likely to be high cost, involving testing to find biomarkers for risk factors at a population level. Proponents argue that it may save money, reducing wastage of ineffective medicines in people who cannot benefit from them. There are many medicines used in preventing or slowing down conditions or are used side by side with lifestyle modifications. In addition to genetic data, precision medicine research gathers information about three factors that modulate gene expression: lifestyles, environments, and communities (Meagher et al., 2017; Zhou & Lauschke, 2022). There are major systems level considerations relating to the future use of big data and artificial intelligence (AI) with associated ethical issues moving towards precision prevention. These relate to medicines and encouraging behaviour-based modifiable risk factors. In terms of well-being and well-becoming, society needs to ask, 'just because we can in future predict who is likely to experience chronic disease, disability, and premature death later at future stages of their life-course, is it the right thing to tell patients and how can we protect patient choice?'.

Pushing the Boundaries of Health Economics towards Health and Well-being Economics

Health economists need to broaden their evaluative space when addressing the evaluation of interventions, including public health and prevention interventions to improve well-being and well-becoming. In 2015, Brazier and Tsuchiya categorized ongoing attempts to broaden evaluative frameworks to take into account cross-sector comparisons (Brazier & Tsuchiya, 2015). We summarize their findings in Table 8.2. This provides an extremely helpful starting point for future research in this field.

Table 8.2 Categories of approaches used to broaden the evaluative space to facilitate cross-sector comparison in health economics

Extending the QALY beyond health	Using well-being to value outcomes	Using money to value outcomes
Statistical mapping to EQ-5D Bolting on to EQ-5D Valuing on a common scale using preferences	Valuing by association with well-being, including capabilities Developing a WELLBY Direct valuation of own health or well-being states	Public sector implied WTP Contingent valuation using WTP (welfarist) Societal WTP (non-welfarist) Monetarize health and other outcomes using experience

EQ-5D = EuroQol five-dimensional questionnaire

QALY = quality-adjusted life year

WELLBY = well-being-adjusted life year

WTP = willingness-to-pay

Source: Brazier, J., & Tsuchiya, A. (2015). Improving cross-sector comparisons: Going beyond the health-related QALY. *Applied Health Economics and Health Policy*, *13*(6), 557–565. https://doi.org/10.1007/s40258-015-0194-1. Copyright © 2023 Springer Nature

Methodological Framing Issues and Horizon Scanning in the Health Economics of Well-being and Well-becoming

In this section, we first address what we see as future developments in the framing of economic evaluation in health, well-being, and well-becoming. We then go on to present some overarching horizon scanning of developments in the field. We recognize well the challenges of applying health economics in the field of public health. These were originally summarized as: attribute of effects; measuring and valuing outcomes; identifying intersectoral costs and consequences; and incorporating equity considerations (Weatherly et al., 2009). Today, given limited fiscal space for public spending on prevention, the policy challenge is now on how public, private, and combinations of public and private 'money' can be put to work within the economy as a lever to engage effective and cost-effective interventions to promote well-being and well-becoming. We can think of this as 'smart capacitating investment' (EuroHealthNet, 2023).

Systems thinking and complexity health economics to support well-being and well-becoming across the life-course

Perhaps there is much to be learned by health economists from the sub-specialty of economics known as 'complexity economics' (Sweeney & Griffiths, 2002). Just as an economy can be viewed as a complex system of stocks and flows with feedback loops, so the NHS and social care systems need to be viewed in terms of stocks and flows of patients with complex feedback loops. 'Much of medicine and organizational theory is built upon the foundation of the classic scientific model . . . could it be that we have now solved most of the problems where this model of the world is most useful?' (Plsek, 2002, p. v). The model we bring with us may not be the most useful for the complex challenges we now face. Moore and colleagues (2019) set out a research agenda for how within public health science the evaluation of complex interventions can be framed using a complex systems lens, and to this we would add economic evaluation should run alongside such studies.

The importance of 'place' and place-based evaluation

Austerity in government funding and public service reform have placed pressure and expectations on UK communities to develop activities and resources supportive of population health (Lee et al., 2020). Methodologies for capturing impacts have in the past been insufficiently robust to inform policy requirements and economic assessment. Health economists are making progress here, for example, place-based studies to evaluate interventions to promote physical activity and reduce sedentary behaviour in the Midlands (Gokal et al., 2022; The Health Foundation, 2020) and the use of health economics to impact local obesity policy (Frew et al., 2022). There is a strong argument for deeper investigation of 'programme theories' underpinning such activities to better understand what needs to be in place to trigger their potential for generating positive health and well-being outcomes, and their cost-effectiveness (Lee et al., 2020).

A greater focus on implementation for health and well-being economics in the future

There is a growing recognition that to fulfil potential impact in decision-making and resource allocation in health economics, and in the context of this book, in prevention policy, there is a need for health economists to build into the latter phases of their analysis a focus on implementation (Heggie et al., 2023). This could be addressed through extended sensitivity analysis of uptake, compliance, and budget impact analysis with a focus on the implementation and scalability of, for example, complex interventions in different settings.

Social return on investment analysis alongside randomized controlled trials and other study designs

Confidence in SROI methodology could be increased if, as well as traditional economic evaluation and process evaluation alongside clinical trials, it was possible to conduct SROI analysis alongside randomized controlled trials (RCTs) or other study designs, such as natural experiments in public health and prevention. Guidelines for reporting SROIs could emphasize the benefits of stating if future SROIs have been 'RCT informed', which might help with the inevitable value judgements required with respect to estimating deadweight loss, attribution, and displacement needed to give confidence to the realistic impact of an intervention in the absence of a control group in SROI analysis (Doungsong et al., 2023). It is important to remember that CBA also requires value judgements in the range of costs and benefits considered.

Greater use of logic models and wider use of realist evaluation and realist review/synthesis methods in the economic evaluation of complex interventions

The Medical Research Council (MRC) guidance for the development and evaluation of complex interventions (Skivington et al., 2021) and other commentators undertaking economic evaluation of public health interventions (e.g. Edwards & McIntosh, 2019) advocate the regular use of logic models, or theory of change models, in health economics analysis plans (HEAPs). Logic models may also be useful in grant applications when seeking funding to indicate how and why certain measures are being included in data collection in a trial or other study design. While the gold standard systematic review can assess whether or not an intervention works, they can fail to suggest reasons for the efficacy of complex interventions, meaning that practitioners can struggle to successfully implement research findings in real-world settings (Hunter et al., 2022). Realist research approaches (realist evaluation or realist review/synthesis) can help make sense of complex interventions. 'Realist evaluation' aims to identify the mechanisms responsible for the observed outcomes following an intervention and the contextual conditions that facilitated this (Public Health England, 2021). The focus is on 'what works, for whom, under what circumstances and how' (Wong et al., 2016, p. 1). A 'realist review' is 'a type of literature review that seeks to explain why programmes work the way they do, who they work for and in what circumstances they work. It is characterized by its theory led approach and its generative understanding of causation' (Hunter et al., 2022, p. 244). The difference between the two approaches is that in a realist evaluation the researcher undertakes primary research by collecting data, whereas in a realist review/synthesis the researcher undertakes secondary research by examining primary data sourced from documents (e.g. studies and policy documents).

Developments in Well-being and Well-becoming across the Life-course as the Unit of Outcome for Policy

In Chapter 1, we highlighted the work of the Well-being Movement which proposes routine use of WELLBYs as a measure of societal well-being based on subjective evaluation of life satisfaction (Dolan et al., 2021). In the HM Treasury's (2021) Green Book, the above principles are operationalized, going so far as to attach a monetary value to a WELLBY of £13,000. This is the recommended standard value of one WELLBY—a one-point change in life satisfaction for one year at 2019 prices. The HM Treasury guidance warns of the danger of double-counting if using WELLBYs and QALYs in the same evaluation of a programme. Box 8.1 shows a simplified version of the well-being measurement checklist included in the Green Book (HM Treasury, 2021).

The checklist in Box 8.1 probably has wider application across a range of approaches measuring health, well-being, and well-becoming across the life-course broader than that proposed by the HM Treasury's Green Book. It is for this reason we have included it here.

Box 8.1 A checklist for analysts assessing well-being across the policy development process

- At an early stage of the policy cycle, are you familiar with the relevant well-being research, including the well-being implications of related policy interventions?
- Have you considered well-being impacts in your critical success factors, at longlist appraisal stage?
- Have you developed a theory of change to consider well-being impacts for the proposed way forward?
- Have you considered unintended consequences, including well-being externalities and relative well-being effects?
- Have you considered setting an appropriate timeframe over which to appraise well-being impacts? Have you given regard to the duration of impact and the potential for adaption to a change of state?
- In your shortlist appraisal, have you weighed the relative merits of cost benefit analysis, cost-effectiveness analysis, and other methods, given the nature of the policy options and available evidence?
- In appraising the quantifiable impacts on well-being, have you taken care to avoid 'double counting' outcomes?
- Where monetization of well-being impacts is feasible and appropriate, have you identified appropriate valuation method(s) and evidence?
- Where well-being impacts are not quantified and/or monetized, have you assessed whether these are likely to be decisive and ensured that these are reported alongside the cost-benefit metrics?
- In undertaking your well-being appraisal, have you critically appraised the standard of evidence that was available, performed appropriate quality assurance, sense checks, and sensitivity analysis? Have you presented any related risks and uncertainties transparently and objectively?
- Is your distributional analysis in line with the Green Book, and does this give regard to variable well-being impacts across different groups of society?
- Have you incorporated well-being into the monitoring and evaluation plans, in alignment with the HM Treasury's Magenta Book? [The Magenta Book provides guidance for government decision-makers and analysts on the role of evaluation and the processes and methods for conducting an evaluation.]

- Have you taken steps to ensure that the evidence gathered through your evaluation feeds back into future decisions?

Reproduced from HM Treasury. (2021). *Wellbeing guidance for appraisal: Supplementary Green Book guidance.* Social Impacts Task Force. https://assets.publishing.service.gov.uk/government/uploads/system/uploads/attachment_data/file/1005388/Wellbeing_guidance_for_appraisal_-_supplementary_Green_Book_guidance.pdf. Copyright (2021)

Critics of subjective well-being measurement argue that subjective measures do not consider a person's 'real opportunities' (Binder, 2014). For example, it is possible to underrepresent deprivation with the normative use of subjective well-being measurements as a person may judge their own well-being relative to what they think they can expect (Sanborne, 2022). This can result in someone experiencing profound deprivations to survive by passing as 'happy' and advocates of the capability approach belief that such accounts are invalid (Sanborne, 2022; Sen, 1987). To this end, it has been suggested that subjective well-being should be placed alongside measures of non-subjective outcomes, such as income, health, knowledge and skills, safety, environmental quality, and social connections (OECD, 2013).

Why health economists are well-placed to contribute to the well-being and well-becoming agenda

In the UK, health economists are well-placed to contribute to the well-being and well-becoming agenda for evidence-based policy when we widen our evaluative space beyond health to embrace health and well-being (Edwards, 2022; Edwards & McIntosh, 2019). We have a role to play in guiding UK Research and Innovation (UKRI), the National Institute for Health and Care Research (NIHR), and other funding bodies to call for innovative methodological research using big data, including, for example, household panel data, in econometric analysis, and within trials and natural experiments using longer time horizons to address the issue of health, well-being, and well-becoming (Deidda et al., 2019).

It is interesting to think about if and how recent developments in subjective well-being measurement, life satisfaction measurement, and the methods proposed by the Green Book for social CBA converge with a broad evaluative space coming out of traditional health economics. This can be seen as health economists taking a bottom-up approach to widening the evaluative space across sectors beyond health (e.g. building well-being measures into economic evaluation alongside pragmatic RCTs and into other research designs such as natural experiments), whilst economists interested in subjective well-being measurement and life satisfaction may be thought of as taking a top-down approach using population panel data (e.g. through the questions included in Understanding Society—The UK Household Longitudinal Study; see www.understandingsoci ety.ac.uk). More and more interdisciplinary research between health economists; economists interested in well-being, life satisfaction, and happiness; social care economists (e.g. Weatherly et al., 2020); and other social scientists interested in well-being is needed to develop our understanding of what works in terms of policies to improve well-being within and across generations.

As a normative social science, health economics is positioned well to develop and mature into this collaborative interdisciplinary field on the premise that, 'a fairer country is a healthier one, and that a healthier country is a more prosperous one' (Thomas et al., 2022, p. 5) against the backdrop of an overstretched NHS at a time of a cost of living crisis within the health service as well as wider society.

The COVID-19 pandemic has been the most significant health shock in modern history. The pandemic has cost over 226,000 lives across the UK (UK Government, 2023), and far wider health consequences for those who did not receive treatment for cancer and other health conditions during and after the pandemic. The pandemic has taken a toll through record NHS waiting lists, in exacerbating the underlying causes of poor health (e.g. poverty), and through a massive rise in unmet physical and mental health needs (Thomas et al., 2022). Difficult as it is, at a time when health and social care systems are severely overstretched, there seems to be no long-time alternative to shifting the balance of social consciousness and public spending from treatment to prevention with an emphasis on co-production of health across the life-course. Addressing such a challenge requires a fundamental examination of our economic paradigm, placing health, well-being, and well-becoming at its centre. In other words: 'correcting our failures on population health could help alleviate key economic challenges facing the UK, including low growth, low productivity, labour market losses and wide inequality' (Thomas et al., 2022, p. 5). In essence, in thinking about well-being and well-becoming across the life-course, health economics could have a role and potential position of being more of a redistributive, rather than a maximizing, science in future.

Teaching health economics and social theory to our future medical students, public health practitioners, service commissioners, and policymakers

Health and well-being in society is everybody's business. Students who will become future doctors, public health practitioners, service commissioners, and policymakers need to be taught health economics along with social theory. Whilst there is more attention than there used to be on the social determinants of health, there needs to be an unpacking of our understanding of social adversity (Poole & Robinson, 2023). A lack of diversity impedes such unpacking of understanding of life-course health and well-being opportunity architecture within society.

Challenging the Prevailing Evaluative Paradigm and the Way We Use Evidence in Society

In Chapter 1, we presented the Alan Williams (1987) plumbing diagram of health economics (see Figure 1.1), shading in identifying evidence of where we think health economics has a role to play in well-being and well-becoming through the life-course. It was only on reading the work of Raworth (2017) on doughnut economics, which traced the importance of diagrams and pictures through the history of economic thought that it became evident that Williams' plumbing diagram followed in the footsteps of mainstream economists such as Samuelson in 1947 who is well-known for his economic flow diagram (Samuelson, 1948; Samuelson & Nordhaus, 2009).

On thinking about health economics applied to concepts of well-being and well-becoming, in Figure 8.2 we have condensed some thoughts about the future direction of health economics, particularly within the evaluative space relating to public health and preventative economics. We have constructed this as a triangle with the lower portion reflecting an ongoing need, often ignored, for health economists to keep questioning what they are doing in their day-to-day activities. If we are to avoid remaining within an increasingly technical cul-de-sac of economic evaluation and health technology assessment, then it is necessary to do this. Such microeconomic evaluation of new medicines, devices, and services is a legitimate use of our time, but adheres us ever closer to a medical model of health rather than a wider socioeconomic model of health. Embracing the challenges of this latter model of health and well-being requires a far wider evaluative space, illustrated by the middle section of Figure 8.2. This is where we propose the wider use of methods such as capability well-being, social CBA (including subjective well-being measurement), SROI analysis, and multi-criteria decision analysis (MCDA), which can take a societal or multisectoral perspective involving multiple stakeholders and show distributional changes resulting from the use of resources in different ways in society. The top portion of Figure 8.2 argues for an ever-creative approach to policy support by health economists. This can often involve disaggregated costs and outcomes shifting from the use of cost-effectiveness ratios alone to cost-outcome ratios (e.g. in cost consequence analysis; CCA) leaving policymakers to weigh-up the relative importance of these outcomes within overall strategic policy direction.

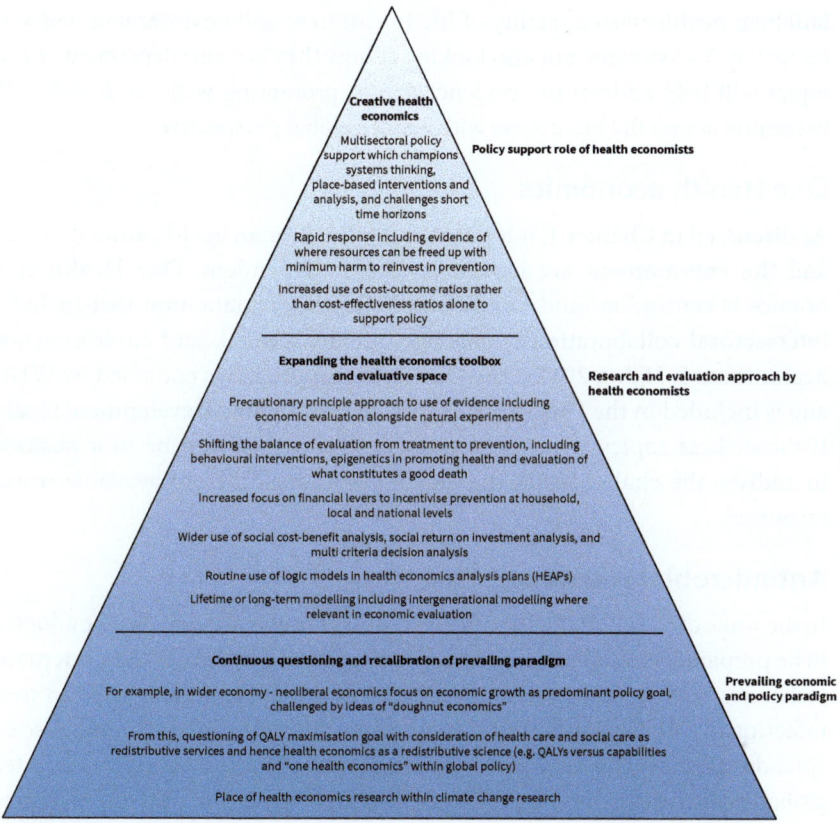

Figure 8.2 From challenging the paradigm to evidence-based policy support: A role for health and well-being economists in future

Diversifying Health Economics as a Way of Addressing the Well-being and Well-becoming Evidence Gap

In July 2023, the 15th International Health Economics Association (IHEA) World Congress took place in South Africa with the theme of 'diversifying health economics'. Diversifying health economics means widening the field, reducing barriers to entry and the inclusion of more topics, people, and regions in the production of cost-effectiveness evidence. Currently, health economics as a discipline is dominated by the Global North, particularly the US and the UK. This means that prospective research interests, standards, viewpoints, and future directions are determined by a minority of the population of the Earth. In this section, we explore some of the themes from the IHEA conference: One Health economics; antimicrobial resistance; indigenous economics and capacity building; health-related quality of life in children; and environment and sustainability, individually but also looking at how they are interdependent. These topics will help address the evidence gap in promoting well-being and well-becoming across the life-course with a more global perspective.

One Health economics

As discussed in Chapter 1, it is paramount that human health, animal health, and the environment are looked at as interdependent. One Health economics is centred around design and policy implementation that includes intersectoral collaboration to manage human, animal, and environmental health (Patz & Hahn, 2012). The One Health approach is endorsed by WHO and is included in the United Nations (UN) Sustainable Development Goals. If these three topics are treated individually, we will not be in a position to address the challenges facing global public health from available scarce resources.

Antimicrobial resistance

In the wake of the COVID-19 pandemic, preventative stances must be adopted to be prepared and reduce the impact of any future pandemics. Antimicrobial resistance takes place when antimicrobials are inappropriately used to treat infections. Consequently, micro-organisms become resistant and disease spreads faster. WHO (2023) has cited antimicrobial resistance as a top ten global health threat and it has been highlighted in the HM Government (2020) National Risk Register in the UK. Antimicrobial resistance has the potential to impact global economies via productivity losses, large health care costs, disruption to trade of crops and livestock, and food system insecurities (WHO, 2023).

Environment and sustainability

At the 2023 IHEA World Congress there was an expressed need for future research in health economics to factor in environmental and sustainability considerations. Martin Hensher, Professorial Research Fellow in Health System Sustainability at the Menzies Institute for Medical Research, Australia, cautioned health economists of an industry research shift ahead, saying, 'Climate change is going to exert an ever greater impact on all of our work as health economists. What you do, what you want to do, what you can no longer do is going to be impacted by climate change.'

At the 2021 UN Framework Convention on Climate Change conference (UNFCCC) in Glasgow, UK, 151 countries committed to significantly cut

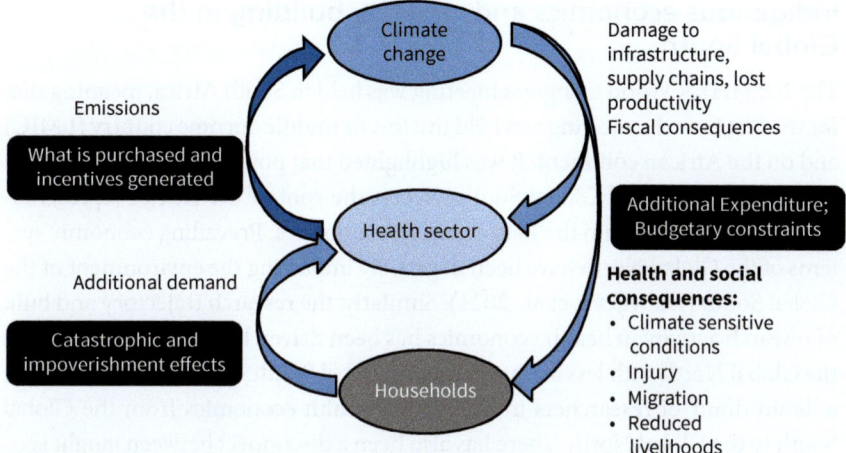

Figure 8.3 Interconnections between climate change and health financing
Reproduced with permission from Borghi, J. (2023, 8–12 July). Is climate change relevant to health financing? [Conference presentation]. 15th IHEA World Congress on Health Economics, Cape Town, South Africa. https://healtheconomics.org/amo-event/2023-congress/ Copyright © 2023 Borghi

their emissions by 2030 in order to limit global temperature rises to 1.5° Celsius and seventy countries committed to develop climate resilient low carbon health systems (Romanello et al., 2021). WHO launched the Alliance for Transformative Action on Climate and Health (ATACH) to address four key areas outlined at the UNFCCC 26th Conference of the Parties (COP26): 1) financing the health commitments on climate resilient and sustainable low carbon health systems; 2) climate resilient health systems; 3) low carbon sustainable health systems; and 4) sustainable supply chains. Currently, we are experiencing extreme levels of heat with record hottest days happening more and more frequently. This can impact societal health, productivity losses at work, and put additional pressure on health and social care services. Extreme heat negatively impacts society's most vulnerable members, which include newborns, infants, and older people. Extreme heat contributes to food system insecurity as a result of droughts, loss in earnings, and increases in food costs (Mehrabi et al., 2022). Climate change will disproportionately affect the Global South more in comparison to the Global North. COP27 focused on the role of the Loss and Damage Fund, which was created to assist the most vulnerable and negatively impacted countries by climate change (Coleman, 2022). Figure 8.3 shows the interconnections between climate change and health financing (Borghi, 2023).

Indigenous economics and capacity building in the Global South

The 2023 IHEA World Congress meeting was held in South Africa, meaning that for the first time the meeting was held in a low or middle-income country (LMIC) and on the African continent. It was highlighted that power imbalances between the Global North and Global South were at the root of the lack of representation and diversity within the field of health economics. Prevailing economic systems of the Global North have been negatively impacting the environment of the Global South (Jakovljevic et al., 2021). Similarly, the research trajectory and bulk of research activity in health economics has been driven by health economists in the Global North with less attention on the Global South. Further, there has been a 'brain drain' of researchers in the field of health economics from the Global South to the Global North. There has also been a disconnect between taught economics and health economics theory and real-world issues specific to the Global South, and disproportionate representation in journals by health economists in the Global North. This can be viewed as 'epistemic injustice'. This epistemic injustice is perpetuated by external funding, externally driven policy implementation, and design, aid dependence, and external technical capacity.

Health-related quality of life in children

The previous sections outline some key issues which will impact future generations if we do not act now. As described in Chapter 3 of this book, a 'good start' to early life is linked with good health and well-being in later life (Clark et al., 2020). Far less attention has been paid to measuring health-related quality of life in children than that of adults. Preference-based measures have been used to determine health-related quality of life in children. Some measures are beginning to be available, for example, the Child Health Utility 9 Dimension (CHU-9D) and the EuroQol five-dimensional questionnaire-youth version (EQ-5D-Y) (Ngwira et al., 2021). A more global perspective means there is a need for age-appropriate preference-based measures relevant to LMICs, as well as those being developed in high income countries (HICs) (Xiong et al., 2023).

Summary

We spend 5 per cent of NHS resources on prevention. There are both efficiency and equity arguments for shifting the balance of resource use from treatment towards prevention, both within the UK NHS and across sectors such as education, housing, transport, and the environment, which all shape our current and future health and well-being. The allocative and technical efficiency arguments relate to the production of health gain across society, and we have evidence that the cost per QALY for public health interventions is one third that of the cost per QALY spent by the NHS. The equity arguments relate to a persistent and worryingly steepening social gradient in lifetime health. Consideration of well-being and well-becoming across the life-course requires health economists to adopt a widening of the evaluative space beyond that which has dominated health technology assessment. For the funders of research, it requires a lengthening of time horizons, and for policymakers it requires a fundamental examination and challenge to the economic paradigm in which our society operates, not least how we view the prevailing goal of economic growth over societal well-being. Climate change is making consideration of future generations a far more tangible requirement than it was fifty years ago.

Concluding Remarks

As soon as a book is published, the evidence in that book is out of date. However, the ideas captured in a book can have longevity and contribute to both the body of knowledge about a topic and help shape research in the future. We entitled this book *The health economics of well-being and well-becoming across the life-course* in order to emphasize the opportunities that exist in investing in early years to promote health and well-being though the life-course and opportunities later in life to intervene in order, in some way, to address factors influencing health and well-being in older age. At present, this feels like an uphill battle given a decade of austerity followed by the COVID-19 pandemic, Brexit, and a cost of living crisis in the UK, as well as the austerity experienced in many other European countries. The UK is forecast to experience five years of lost economic growth, the longest since the Global Financial Crisis of 2008 (National Institute of Economic and Social Research, 2023). By 2040, one in five people (19 per cent) aged twenty years and older are projected to be living with major illness, moving from almost one in six in 2019 (Watt et al., 2023). The public fiscal space for health and social care will continue to be constrained. Prevention of avoidable ill-health, disability, and premature death is the responsibility of all of us. Better health requires co-production and is intrinsically related to well-being and opportunities for well-becoming through the life-course. Health economics as a discipline, as well as continuing to focus on health technology assessment of medicines, surgery, and other health care interventions, is going to need to diversify. As a diversifying discipline, we are well-placed to play a role in supporting evidence-based policy to promote cost-effective, life-course health and well-being opportunity architecture for the population.

Curiosity Questions

- What scope does the field of complexity of economics offer systems level analysis of stocks and flows in the National Health Service and social care system?

- Where is it most likely that resources could be freed up through rational disinvestment for the reinvestment into prevention across the life-course?

- What is the relationship between prevention and well-being across the life-course in terms of policy development with a focus on sustainability goals?

- What do doughnut economics and One Health economics have in common in terms of challenging prevailing paradigms which underpin the methods of economic evaluation that we use in health economics?

- What are the relative merits of future use of legislation and financial levers versus building on positive social norms, nudging, and social networks, to achieve prevention in the pursuit of well-being and well-becoming through the life-course?

- What is the relative potential of precision public health versus a better understanding of human nature and consumption in terms of promoting better health and well-being? And how could they relate to each other in terms of targeted preventative interventions?

- What will the advent of personalized prevention, precision public health, and population pharmacogenomics, including the use of big data and artificial intelligence (AI), mean for the health economics of well-being and well-becoming in future?

- What will health economics look like as a discipline globally by 2040 in terms of the balance between traditional health technology assessments of medicines, surgeries, and other health care interventions; systems level analysis of health and social care services; and a wider focus on prevention and co-production of better health?

References

Almond, D., & Currie, J. (2011). Human capital development before age five. In O. Ashenfelter & D. Card (Eds.), *Handbook of labor economics* (pp. 1315–1486). Elsevier.

Bellis, M. A., Hughes, K., Ford, K., Rodriguez, G. R., Sethi, D., & Passmore, J. (2019). Life course health consequences and associated annual costs of adverse childhood experiences across Europe and North America: A systematic review and meta-analysis. *The Lancet Public Health*, 4(10), e517–e528. https://doi.org/10.1016/S2468-2667(19)30145-8

Ben-Arieh, A., & Frønes, I. (2011). Taxonomy for child well-being indicators: A framework for the analysis of the well-being of children. *Childhood*, 18(4), 460–476. https://doi.org/10.1177/0907568211398159

Bibby, J., & Lovell, N. (2018, March). *What makes us healthy?* The Health Foundation. https://www.health.org.uk/publications/what-makes-us-healthy

Biggeri, M., & Santi, M. (2012). The missing dimensions of children's well-being and well-becoming in education systems: Capabilities and philosophy for children. *Journal of Human Development and Capabilities*, 13(3), 373–395. https://doi.org/10.1080/19452829.2012.694858

Binder, M. (2014). Subjective well-being capabilities: Bridging the gap between the capability approach and subjective well-being research. *Journal of Happiness Studies*, 15(5), 1197–1217. https://doi.org/10.1007/s10902-013-9471-6

Borghi, J. (2023, 8–12 July). *Is climate change relevant to health financing?* [Conference presentation]. 15th IHEA World Congress on Health Economics, Cape Town, South Africa. https://healtheconomics.org/amo-event/2023-congress/

Brazier, J., & Tsuchiya, A. (2015). Improving cross-sector comparisons: Going beyond the health-related QALY. *Applied Health Economics and Health Policy*, 13(6), 557–565. https://doi.org/10.1007/s40258-015-0194-1

Campbell, S. M. (2020). Well-being and the good death. *Ethical Theory and Moral Practice*, 23(3), 607–623. https://doi.org/10.1007/s10677-020-10101-3

Cassidy, C. (2017). Wellbeing, being well or well becoming: Who or what is it for and how might we get there? In M. Thorburn (Ed.), *Wellbeing, education and contemporary schooling* (pp. 13–26). Routledge.

Chowdry, H., & Fitzsimons, P. (2016). *The cost of late intervention: EIF analysis 2016*. Early Intervention Foundation. https://www.eif.org.uk/report/the-cost-of-late-intervention-eif-analysis-2016

Clark, H., Coll-Seck, A. M., Banerjee, A., Peterson, S., Dalglish, S. L., Ameratunga, S., Balabanova, D., Bhan, M. K., Bhutta, Z. A., Borrazzo, J., Claeson, M., Doherty, T., El-Jardali, F., George, A. S., Gichaga, A., Gram, L., Hipgrave, D. B., Kwamie, A., Meng, Q., & Costello, A. (2020). A future for the world's children? A WHO-UNICEF-Lancet Commission. *The Lancet*, 395(10224), 605–658. https://doi.org/10.1016/S0140-6736(19)32540-1

Coleman, C. (2022, 18 November). *COP27: Progress and outcomes*. https://lordslibrary.parliament.uk/cop27-progress-and-outcomes/

Cookson, R., Griffin, S., Norheim, O. F., & Culyer, A. J. (Eds.). (2020). *Distributional cost-effectiveness analysis: Quantifying health equity impacts and trade-offs*. Oxford University Press.

Dahlgren, G., & Whitehead, M. (2006). *European strategies for tackling social inequities in health: Levelling up Part 2*. World Health Organization. https://apps.who.int/iris/bitstream/handle/10665/107791/E89384.pdf

Dalai Lama XIV Bstan-'dzin-rgya-mtsho. (2015). *The wheel of life: Buddhist perspectives on cause and effect*. Wisdom Publications.

Davies, J., Cooper, R. E., Moncrieff, J., Montagu, L., Rae, T., & Parhi, M. (2022). The costs incurred by the NHS in England due to the unnecessary prescribing of dependency-forming medications. *Addictive Behaviors*, **125**, 107143, 1–11. https://doi.org/10.1016/j.addbeh.2021.107143

Deidda, M., Coll-Planas, L., Tully, M. A., Giné-Garriga, M., Kee, F., Roqué i Figuls, M., Blackburn, N. E., Guerra-Balic, M., Rothenbacher, D., Dallmeier, D., & Caserotti, P. (2022). Cost-effectiveness of a programme to address sedentary behaviour in older adults: Results from the SITLESS RCT. *European Journal of Public Health*, **32**(3), 415–421. https://doi.org/10.1093/eurpub/ckac017

Deidda, M., Geue, C., Kreif, N., Dundas, R., & McIntosh, E. (2019). A framework for conducting economic evaluations alongside natural experiments. *Social Science & Medicine*, **220**, 353–361. https://doi.org/10.1016/j.socscimed.2018.11.032

Dodge, R., Daly, A., Huyton, J., & Sanders, L. (2012). The challenge of defining wellbeing. *International Journal of Wellbeing*, **2**(3), 222–235. https://doi.org/10.5502/ijw.v2i3.4

Dolan, P. (2014). *Happiness by design: Finding pleasure and purpose in everyday life*. Penguin Books Limited.

Dolan, P., Layard, R., O'Donnell, G., Delaney, L., Krekel, C., Sanders, J., Blanco-Jimenez, C., Laffan, K., Kavetsos, G., & Kudrna, L. (2021, 1 March). *Shaping the post-Covid World: Moving towards wellbeing over the lifetime as the unit of analysis in policy*. https://www.lse.ac.uk/PBS/assets/documents/SPCW-WELLBEING-FINAL.pdf

Donaldson, C., Bate, A., Mitton, C., Dionne, F., & Ruta, D. (2010). Rational disinvestment. *QJM: An International Journal of Medicine*, **103**(10), 801–807. https://doi.org/10.1093/qjmed/hcq086

Doungsong, K., Hartfiel, N., Gladman, J., Harwood, R., & Edwards, R. T. (2023). RCT-based social return on investment (SROI) of a home exercise programme for people with early dementia comparing in-person and blended delivery before and during the COVID-19 pandemic. *medRxiv*. https://doi.org/10.1101/2023.08.25.23294408

Dowell, S. F., Blazes, D., & Desmond-Hellmann, S. (2016). Four steps to precision public health. *Nature*, **540**(7632), 189–191. https://doi.org/10.1038/540189a

Edwards, R. T. (2001). Paradigms and research programmes: Is it time to move from health care economics to health economics? *Health Economics*, **10**(7), 635–649. https://doi.org/10.1002/hec.610

Edwards, R. T. (2022). Well-being and well-becoming through the life-course in public health economics research and policy: A new infographic. *Frontiers in Public Health*, **10**, 1–8. https://doi.org/10.3389/fpubh.2022.1035260

Edwards, R.T., & McIntosh, E. (Eds.). (2019). *Applied health economics for public health practice and research*. Oxford University Press.

EuroHealthNet. (2023, 21 February). *Invest4Health—New Horizon Europe Project to mobilise novel finance models for health promotion and disease prevention*. https://eurohealthnet.eu/publication/invest4health-new-horizon-europe-project-to-mobilise-novel-finance-models-for-health-promotion-and-disease-prevention/

Falkenberg, T. (2015, 19 November). *Understanding and assessing well-being and well-becoming in Manitoba schools* [Conference opening address]. Faculty of Education, University of Manitoba.

Falkenberg, T. (2019). *Framing human well-being and well-becoming: An integrated systems approach* (Well-being in schools paper series no. 2). Well-being and well-becoming in schools research initiative. http://wellbeinginschools.ca/wp-content/uploads/2019/09/WBIS-Paper-No-2-Falkenberg-2019-2.pdf

Findlay, P., Lindsay, C., McIntyre, S., Roy, G., Stewart, R., & Dutton, E. (2021). *CIPD Good Work Index 2021: UK Working Lives Survey*. Chartered Institute of Personnel Development. https://www.cipd.org/globalassets/media/zzz-misc---to-check/good-work-index-survey-report-2021-1_tcm18-96105.pdf

Frew, E., Afentou, N., Mohtashami Borzadaran, H., Candio, P., & Pokhilenko, I. (2022). Using economics to impact local obesity policy: Introducing the UK Centre for Economics of Obesity (CEO). *Applied Health Economics and Health Policy*, 20(5), 629–635. https://doi.org/10.1007/s40258-022-00738-9

Gokal, K., Amos-Hirst, R., Moakes, C. A., Sanders, J. P., Esliger, D. W., Sherar, L. B., Ives, N., Biddle, S.J.H., Edwardson, C., Yates, T., Frew, E., Greaves, C., Greenfield, S. M., Jolly, K., Skrybant, M., Maddison, R., Mutrie, N., Parretti, H. M., & Daley, A. J. (2022). Views of the public about Snacktivity™: A small changes approach to promoting physical activity and reducing sedentary behaviour. *BMC Public Health*, 22(1), 1–12. https://doi.org/10.1186/s12889-022-13050-x

Heckman, J. J. (2008). The case for investing in disadvantaged young children. *CESifo DICE Report*, 6(2), 3–8. https://www.ifo.de/en/publications/2008/article-journal/case-investing-disadvantaged-young-children

Heggie, R., Boyd, K., Kamaruzaman, H. F. B., & Wu, O. (2023, 21–23 June). *What methods are currently available for incorporating implementation considerations within the economic evaluation of health technologies? A systematic review* [Conference presentation]. Health Economists' Study Group Summer 2023 Meeting, Oxford, United Kingdom. https://hesg.org.uk/meetings/summer-2023-university-of-oxford/

HM Government. (2020). *National risk register. 2020 edition*. https://assets.publishing.serv ice.gov.uk/government/uploads/system/uploads/attachment_data/file/952959/6.6920_CO_CCS_s_National_Risk_Register_2020_11-1-21-FINAL.pdf

HM Treasury. (2021). *Wellbeing guidance for appraisal: Supplementary Green Book guidance*. Social Impacts Task Force. https://assets.publishing.service.gov.uk/government/uplo ads/system/uploads/attachment_data/file/1005388/Wellbeing_guidance_for_apprais al_-_supplementary_Green_Book_guidance.pdf

Hunter, R., Gorely, T., Beattie, M., & Harris, K. (2022). Realist review. *International Review of Sport and Exercise Psychology*, 15(1), 242–265. https://doi.org/10.1080/17509 84X.2021.1969674

Illich, I. (1982). *Medical nemesis: The expropriation of health*. Random House USA.

Jakovljevic, M., Liu, Y., Cerda, A., Simonyan, M., Correia, T., Mariita, R. M., Kumara, A. S., Garcia, L., Krstic, K., Osabohein, R., Toan, T. K., Adhikari, C., Chuc, N. T. K., Khatri, R. B., Chattu, V. K., Wang, L., Wijeratne, T., Kousassi, E., Khan, H. N., & Varjacic, M. (2021). The Global South political economy of health financing and spending landscape—history and presence. *Journal of Medical Economics*, 24(S1), 25–33. https://doi.org/10.1080/13696998.2021.2007691

Kahneman, D., Diener, E., & Schwarz, N. (Eds.). (1999). *Well-being: Foundations of hedonic psychology*. Russell Sage Foundation.

Kane, P. (2007, 26 February). Not wellbeing, but wellbecoming. *The Guardian*. https://www. theguardian.com/commentisfree/2007/feb/26/theresbeensomuchthats

Langford, B. H., Krauss, S. M., & Legters, L. (2021). *Investing in the well-being and well-becoming of America's young people: Recommendations for philanthropy, policy, and practice*. Youth Transition Funders Group. https://static1.squarespace.com/static/648c5

a930f2c617be853e549/t/650205131c36cb514edaa5ea/1694631189397/ytfg-well-being-2021.pdf

Lee, C., Burgess, G., Kuhn, I., Cowan, A., & Lafortune, L. (2020). Community exchange and time currencies: A systematic and in-depth thematic review of impact on public health outcomes. *Public Health*, **180**, 117–128. https://doi.org/10.1016/j.puhe.2019.11.011

Livingston, G., Huntley, J., Sommerlad, A., Ames, D., Ballard, C., Banerjee, S., Brayne, C., Burns, A., Cohen-Mansfield, J., Cooper, C., & Costafreda, S. G. (2020). Dementia prevention, intervention, and care: 2020 report of the Lancet Commission. *The Lancet*, **396**(10248), 413–446. https://doi.org/10.1016/S0140-6736(20)30367-6

Magavern, E. F., Daly, A. K., Gilchrist, A., & Hughes, D. (2021). Pharmacogenomics spotlight commentary: From the United Kingdom to global populations. *British Journal of Clinical Pharmacology*, **87**(12), 4546–4548. https://doi.org/10.1111/bcp.14917

Marmot, M. (2017). Social justice, epidemiology and health inequalities. *European Journal of Epidemiology*, **32**(7), 537–546. https://doi.org/10.1007/s10654-017-0286-3

Marmot, M., Allen, J., Boyce, T., Goldblatt, P., & Morrison, J. (2020). *Health equity in England: The Marmot review 10 years on*. Institute of Health Equity. https://www.health.org.uk/publications/reports/the-marmot-review-10-years-on

Marmot, M., Allen, J., Goldblatt, P., Boyce, T., McNeish, D., Grady, M., & Geddes, I. (2010). *Fair society, healthy lives: The Marmot review. Strategic review of health inequalities in England post-2010*. https://www.instituteofhealthequity.org/resources-reports/fair-society-healthy-lives-the-marmot-review

Martela, F., & Sheldon, K. M. (2019). Clarifying the concept of well-being: Psychological need satisfaction as the common core connecting eudaimonic and subjective well-being. *Review of General Psychology*, **23**(4), 458–474. https://doi.org/10.1177/1089268019880886

Maslow, A. H. (1943). A theory of human motivation. *Psychological Review,* **50**(4), 370–396. https://doi.org/10.1037/h0054346

Maslow, A. H. (2017). *A theory of human motivation*. BN Publishing.

Meagher, K. M., McGowan, M. L., Settersten, R. A., Jr., Fishman, J. R., & Juengst, E. T. (2017). Precisely where are we going? Charting the new terrain of precision prevention. *Annual Review of Genomics and Human Genetics*, **18**, 369–387. https://doi.org/10.1146/annurev-genom-091416-035222

Medvedev, O. N., & Landhuis, C. E. (2018). Exploring constructs of well-being, happiness and quality of life. *PeerJ*, **6**, e4903. https://doi.org/10.7717/peerj.4903

Mehrabi, Z., Delzeit, R., Ignaciuk, A., Levers, C., Braich, G., Bajaj, K., Amo-Aidoo, A., Anderson, W., Balgah, R. A., Benton, T. G., Chari, M. M., Ellis, E. C., Gahi, N. Z., Gaupp, F., Garibaldi, L. A., Gerber, J. S., Godde, C. M., Grass, I., Heimann, T., . . . You, L. (2022). Research priorities for global food security under extreme events. *One Earth*, **5**(7), 756–766. https://doi.org/10.1016/j.oneear.2022.06.008

Mitchell, P. M., Husbands, S., Byford, S., Kinghorn, P., Bailey, C., Peters, T. J., & Coast, J. (2021). Challenges in developing capability measures for children and young people for use in the economic evaluation of health and care interventions. *Health Economics*, **30**(9), 1990–2003. https://doi.org/10.1002/hec.4363

Moore, G. F., Evans, R. E., Hawkins, J., Littlecott, H., Melendez-Torres, G. J., Bonell, C., & Murphy, S. (2019). From complex social interventions to interventions in complex social systems: Future directions and unresolved questions for intervention development and evaluation. *Evaluation*, **25**(1), 23–45. https://doi.org/10.1177/13563 89018803219

Morgan, A., & Ziglio, E. (2007). Revitalising the evidence base for public health: An assets model. *Promotion & Education*, **14**(2 Suppl), 17–22. https://doi.org/10.1177/102538 23070140020701x

Morgan, D., & James, C. (2022). *Investing in health systems to protect society and boost the economy: Priority investments and order-of-magnitude cost estimates* (OECD Health Working Papers No. 144). https://dx.doi.org/10.1787/d0aa9188-en

National Institute for Health and Care Excellence. (2013). *Guide to the methods of technology appraisal 2013* (PMG9). https://www.nice.org.uk/process/pmg9/

National Institute for Health and Care Excellence. (2022). *NICE health technology evaluations: The manual* (PMG36). https://www.nice.org.uk/process/pmg36

National Institute of Economic and Social Research. (2023). *National Institute UK Economic Outlook. Summer 2023* (Series A. No. 11). https://www.niesr.ac.uk/wp-cont ent/uploads/2023/08/JC737-NIESR-Outlook-Summer-2023-UK-v10-AC.pdf

Ngwira, L. G., Khan, K., Maheswaran, H., Sande, L., Nyondo-Mipando, L., Smith, S. C., Petrou, S., & Niessen, L. (2021). A systematic literature review of preference-based health-related quality-of-life measures applied and validated for use in childhood and adolescent populations in sub-Saharan Africa. *Value in Health Regional Issues*, **25**, 37–47. https://doi.org/10.1016/j.vhri.2020.11.009

Nsamenang, A. B. (2010). Fathers, families, and children's well-becoming in Africa. In M. E. Lamb (Ed.), *The role of the father in child development* (5th ed., pp. 388–412). John Wiley & Sons.

Organisation for Economic Co-operation and Development. (2013). *OECD guidelines on measuring subjective well-Being*. OECD Publishing. https://doi.org/10.1787/9789264191 655-en

Patz, J. A., & Hahn, M. B. (2012). Climate change and human health: A One Health approach. In J. S. Mackenzie, M. Jeggo, P. Daszak, & J. A. Richt (Eds.), *One Health: The human-animal-environment interfaces in emerging infectious diseases: Food safety and security, and international and national plans for implementation of one health activities* (pp. 141–171). Springer.

Plsek, P. (2002). Foreword. In K. Sweeney & F. Griffiths (Eds.), *Complexity and healthcare: An introduction* (p. v). Radcliffe Publishing.

Poole, R., & Robinson, C. A. (2023). Breaking out of the citadel: Social theory and psychiatry. *British Journal of Psychiatry Bulletin*, **47**(3), 146–149. https://doi.org/10.1192/bjb.2022.17

Public Health England. (2021). *A brief introduction to realist evaluation*. https://assets.pub lishing.service.gov.uk/government/uploads/system/uploads/attachment_data/file/1004 663/Brief_introduction_to_realist_evaluation.pdf

Raworth, K. (2017). *Doughnut economics: Seven ways to think like a 21st-century economist*. Chelsea Green Publishing.

Romanello, M., McGushin, A., Di Napoli, C., Drummond, P., Hughes, N., Jamart, L., Kennard, H., Lampard, P., Rodriguez, B. S., Arnell, N., Ayeb-Karlsson, S., Belesova, K., Cai, W., Campbell-Lendrum, D., Capstick, S., Chambers, J., Chu, L., Ciampi, L., Dalin, C., . . . Hamilton, I. (2021). The 2021 report of the Lancet Countdown on health and climate change: Code red for a healthy future. *The Lancet*, **398**(10311), 1619–1662. https://doi.org/10.1016/S0140-6736(21)01787-6

Ross, D. A., Hinton, R., Melles-Brewer, M., Engel, D., Zeck, W., Fagan, L., Herat, J., Phaladi, G., Imbago-Jácome, D., Anyona, P., & Sanchez, A. (2020). Adolescent well-being: A definition and conceptual framework. *Journal of Adolescent Health*, **67**(4), 472–476. https://doi.org/10.1016/j.jadohealth.2020.06.042

Ryan, R. M., & Deci, E. L. (2001). On happiness and human potentials: A review of research on hedonic and eudaimonic well-being. *Annual Review of Psychology*, **52**, 141–166. https://doi.org/10.1146/annurev.psych.52.1.141

Ryff, C. D., & Singer, B. (1998). The contours of positive human health. *Psychological Inquiry*, **9**(1), 1–28. https:doi.org/10.1207/s15327965pli0901_1

Samuelson, P. (1948). *Economics*. McGraw-Hill.

Samuelson, P., & Nordhaus, W. D. (2009). *Economics* (19th ed.). McGraw-Hill.

Sanborne, E. (2022). *Why world leaders should prioritize the well-being of their people* [Unpublished doctoral dissertation]. University of Minnesota Twin Cities. https://conservancy.umn.edu/bitstream/handle/11299/226179/Sanborne_prelim.pdf

Sen, A. (1987). *On ethics and economics*. Blackwell.

Sen, A. (2010). Equality of what? In S. M. MacMurrin (Ed.), *The Tanner lectures on human values* (Vol 4, 2nd ed., pp. 195–220). Cambridge University Press.

Skarda, I., Asaria, M., & Cookson, R. (2021). LifeSim: A lifecourse dynamic microsimulation model of the Millennium birth cohort in England. *International Journal of Microsimulation*, **14**(1), 2–42. https://doi.org/10.34196/IJM.00228

Skivington, K., Matthews, L., Simpson, S. A., Craig, P., Baird, J., Blazeby, J. M., Boyd, K. A., Craig, N., French, D. P., McIntosh, E., Petticrew, M., Rycroft-Malone, J., White, M., & Moore, L. (2021). Framework for the development and evaluation of complex interventions: Gap analysis, workshop and consultation-informed update. *Health Technology Assessment*, **25**(57), 1–132. https://doii.org/10.3310/hta25570

Sweeney, K., & Griffiths, F. (Eds.). (2002). *Complexity and healthcare: An introduction*. Radcliffe Publishing.

The Health Foundation. (2020, 2 April). *Four research projects selected to investigate how the health of a population shapes its social and economic outcomes*. https://www.health.org.uk/news-and-comment/news/four-research-projects-selected-to-investigate-how-the-healt

Thomas, C., Jung, C., Patel, P., & Quilter-Pinner, H. (2022). *Health and prosperity: Introducing the IPPR commission on health and prosperity*. Institute for Public Health Research. https://www.ippr.org/files/2022-04/health-and-prosperity-april22.pdf

United Kingdom Government. (2023, 25 May). *Deaths in United Kingdom*. https://coronavirus.data.gov.uk/details/deaths

United Nations Children's Fund. (2007). *Child poverty in perspective: An overview of child wellbeing in rich countries* (Report Card 7). UNICEF Innocenti Research Centre. https://www.unicef-irc.org/publications/pdf/rc7_eng.pdf

Watt, T., Raymond, A., Rachet-Jacquet, L., Head, A., Kypridemos, C., Kelly, E., & Charlesworth. (2023). *Health in 2040: Projected patterns of illness in England*. The Health Foundation REAL Centre. https://www.health.org.uk/publications/health-in-2040

Weatherly, H., Drummond, M., Claxton, K., Cookson, R., Ferguson, B., Godfrey, C., Rice, N., Sculpher, M., & Sowden, A. (2009). Methods for assessing the cost-effectiveness of public health interventions: Key challenges and recommendations. *Health Policy*, 93(2–3), 85–92. https://doi.org/10.1016/j.healthpol.2009.07.012

Weatherly, H., Faria, R., Van den Berg, B., Sculpher, M., O'Neill, P., Nolan, K., Glanville, J., Isojarvi, J., Baragula, R., & Edwards, M. (2020). Economic evaluation methods in social care: A scoping review. In L. Curtis & A. Burns (Eds.), *Unit costs of health and social care report* (pp. 18–26). Canterbury: Personal Social Services Research Unit, University of Kent. https://www.pssru.ac.uk/pub/uc/uc2020/weatherly.pdf

Weiss, C. H. (1977). Research for policy's sake: The enlightenment function of social research. *Policy Analysis*, 3(4), 531–545. https://www.jstor.org/stable/42783234

Welsh Government. (2015). *Well-being of Future Generations (Wales) Act 15*. Acts of the National Assembly for Wales. https://www.legislation.gov.uk/anaw/2015/2/contents

Williams, A. (1987). Health economics: The cheerful face of a dismal science. In A. Williams (Ed.), *Health and economics* (pp. 1–11). Macmillan.

Wong, G., Westhorp, G., Manzano, A., Greenhalgh, J., Jagosh, J., & Greenhalgh, T. (2016). RAMESES II reporting standards for realist evaluations. *BMC Medicine*, 14(1), 1–18. https://doi.org/10.1186/s12916-016-0643-1

World Health Organization. (2005). *Preventing chronic diseases: A vital investment*. https://apps.who.int/iris/bitstream/handle/10665/43328/9241593598_eng.pdf

World Health Organization. (2011). *Health at key stages of life: The life-course approach to public health* (No. WHO/EURO: 2011-4335-44098-62200). WHO Regional Office for Europe. https://apps.who.int/iris/handle/10665/349932

World Health Organization. (2023, 23 June). *WHO outlines 40 research priorities on antimicrobial resistance*. https://www.who.int/news/item/22-06-2023-who-outlines-40-research-priorities-on-antimicrobial-resistance

Xiong, X., Dalziel, K., Huang, L., Mulhern, B., & Carvalho, N. (2023). How do common conditions impact health-related quality of life for children? Providing guidance for validating pediatric preference-based measures. *Health and Quality of Life Outcomes*, 21(1), 8. https://doi.org/10.1186/s12955-023-02091-4

Zhou, Y., & Lauschke, V. M. (2022). Population pharmacogenomics: An update on ethnogeographic differences and opportunities for precision public health. *Human Genetics*, 141(6), 1113–1136. https://doi.org/10.1007/s00439-021-02385-x

Index

For the benefit of digital users, indexed terms that span two pages (e.g., 52–53) may, on occasion, appear on only one of those pages.

Note: Tables, figures, and boxes are indicated by an italic *t*, *f*, and *b* following the page number.